MEDICINE
AND
MODERN WARFARE

CLIO MEDICA

THE WELLCOME SERIES IN THE HISTORY OF MEDICINE

The *Clio Medica* series editors are

V. Nutton, C. J. Lawrence and M. Neve.

Please send all queries regarding the series to Michael Laycock,

The Wellcome Trust Centre for the History of Medicine at UCL,

24 Eversholt Street, London NW1 1AD, UK

MEDICINE
AND
MODERN WARFARE

edited by
Roger Cooter, Mark Harrison and Steve Sturdy

Amsterdam – Atlanta, GA 1999

First published in 1999
by Editions Rodopi B. V., Amsterdam – Atlanta, GA 1999.

© 1999 Cooter, Harrison, Sturdy (eds)
2nd edition, 2004.

Design and Typesetting by Alex Mayor, the Wellcome Trust.
Printed and bound in The Netherlands by Editions Rodopi B. V.,
Amsterdam – Atlanta, GA 1999.

British Library Cataloguing in Publication Data
A catalogue record for this book is available from the British Library
ISBN 90-420-0536-X (Paper)
ISBN 90-420-0546-7 (Bound)

Cooter, Harrison, Sturdy (eds)
Medicine and Modern Warfare –
Amsterdam – Atlanta, GA:
Rodopi. – ill.
(Clio Medica 55 / ISSN 0045-7183;
The Wellcome Series in the History of Medicine)

Front cover:
World War One: an exhibition poster with illustration of the
Royal Army Medical Corps on active service.
Colour halftone after a painting by H. Mackey.

© Editions Rodopi B. V. Amsterdam – Atlanta, GA 1999
Transferred to digital printing 2004
Printed in The Netherlands

Contents

Acknowledgements

With the exception of the papers by Claire Herrick and J.T.H. Connor, the essays collected together in this volume were originally presented at a conference on 'Medicine and the Management of Modern Warfare', held at the Wellcome Institute for the History of Medicine in July 1995. The conference also marked the Silver Jubilee Anniversary of the Society of the Social History of Medicine. The editors wish to thank the Society and those who assisted with the organisation of the conference, particularly Frieda Houser of the Wellcome Institute. We also wish to thank all those who attended the conference for making it such a successful event, as well as the contributors to this volume, for allowing us to publish their work. Lastly, we wish to thank the anonymous referee for his/her comments on the original manuscript of this book.

Contributors

Leo van Bergen is author of a study of the Dutch Red Cross – *De Zwaargewonden Eerst?* – (Erasmus, 1994) and is currently working on a study of the Dutch Military Health Service. He is attached to the University of Nijmegen.

J.T.H. Connor is the author of many articles on the history of medicine in North America. He was formerly a professor at the Hannah Institute for the History of Medicine in Toronto.

Roger Cooter is Professor of Social History and Director of the Wellcome Unit for the History of Medicine at the University of East Anglia, Norwich. He is the author of *The Cultural Meaning of Popular Science* (Cambridge University Press, 1984) and *Surgery and Society in Peace and War* (Macmillan, 1992). He is also editor with Mark Harrison and Steve Sturdy of *War, Medicine and Modernity* (Sutton, 1998) and several books on the history of accidents and health care.

Mark Harrison is Senior Lecturer in History at Sheffield Hallam University. He is the author of *Public Health in British India* (Cambridge University Press, 1994), *Climates and Constitutions* (Oxford University Press, 1999), *Medicine and British Warfare* (Sutton, forthcoming). He is also editor with Roger Cooter and Steve Sturdy of *War, Medicine and Modernity* (Sutton, 1998).

Lesley A. Hall is Senior Archivist at the Wellcome Institute for the History of Medicine, London. She has written extensively on the history of sexuality and medicine and is author of *Hidden Anxieties: Male Sexuality, 1900-1950* (Polity, 1991) and, with Roy Porter, *The Facts of Life: The Creation of Sexual Knowledge in Britain, 1650-1950* (Yale University Press, 1995).

Claire E.J. Herrick completed her Ph.D. on the treatment of wounds and wounded during the First World War in 1996, at the Wellcome Unit for the History of Medicine, University of Manchester. During 1997-8 she was the Caird Senior Fellow at the National Maritime Museum, Greenwich, where she was researching the history of naval medicine between 1914 and 1918.

Hans Pols was, until recently, a graduate student in the Department of the History of Science at Harvard University. He has recently been awarded his Ph.D. on the history of the mental hygiene movement in America.

Cay-Rüdiger Prüll is Research Assistant at the Institute for the History of Medicine in Freiburg. His main areas of research are the social history of medicine, especially the history of pathology and psychiatry. He has published papers on the history of pathology in Germany and has edited a book on *Pathology in the 19th and 20th Centuries* (EAHMH, forthcoming). He is currently working on a study of pathology in Berlin and London, 1900-1945.

Ian Whitehead is Lecturer in History at the University of Derby. He is the author of several articles on the history of medicine in the British Army during the First World War and is currently completing a book on the British medical officer on the Western Front.

Michael Worboys is Professor in the History of Medicine at Sheffield Hallam University and Director of the Cultural Research Institute. He has written extensively on the history of modern medicine, especially upon tropical medicine and infectious diseases. His forthcoming book on germ theories is shortly to be published by Cambridge University Press. He is also editor with Lara Marks of *Minorities, Migrants and Health* (Routledge, 1997).

Steve Sturdy is a lecturer and holds a Wellcome Trust University Award in the History of Medicine, in the Science Studies Unit at the University of Edinburgh. He is the author of numerous articles on the political and social construction of disease and medicine and editor, with Roger Cooter and Mark Harrison, of *War, Medicine and Modernity* (Sutton, 1998).

Medicine and the Management of Modern Warfare: an Introduction

Mark Harrison

Despite a large and often impressive body of work written by serving and retired medical officers,[1] the role of medicine in warfare and the management of armed forces has yet to receive the attention it deserves. It is only quite recently, following the publication of John Keegan's acclaimed book *The Face of Battle* (1976),[2] that military historians have acknowledged the central place of health and medicine in war; both in terms of the experience of combat[3] and the contribution of medicine to military efficiency.[4] With few recent exceptions,[5] medical historians have been equally reticent to tackle military topics, for the subject has been regarded as unfashionable and somewhat remote from the mainstream of social and intellectual history. While the reluctance of medical historians to examine military subjects may simply reflect histriographical fashion, there is, perhaps, a deeper and more fundamental reason for the obscurity of military medical history – the idea that war is something exceptional, something that occurs beyond the realm of ordinary human experience. As Arthur Marwick has noted,[6] there has been (and arguably still is) a tendency to think of war as separate from 'society'; to speak of its impact *on* society, rather than to see war as a particular state *of* society, as Marwick prefers. The tendency to see war as extrinsic to society is equally evident in that literature which does exist on medicine and war. War is credited with having effected revolutions in medical practice and medical science,[7] and even in the improvement of medical provisions.[8] These often exaggerated claims have recently been called into question,[9] but the problem of how to conceptualise the relationship between war and medicine remains.

The essays in this volume illuminate at least some aspects of this relationship. Although its primary focus is on medicine within the armed services, we view both medicine and the military as intrinsically social phenomena. Moreover, we wish to consider the relationship between medicine and the military in terms of the *modernisation* of advanced industrial societies over the past two

1

centuries. While the growing importance of medicine in the armed forces has traditionally been seen as a function of scientific and technological advances (of the emergence of bacteriology, antiseptic surgery and so forth), we see these developments as facets of a more general process, famously described by Max Weber as 'rationalization'. The essence of rationalization for Weber was the mathematization of experience and knowledge: the extension of secular, scientific rationality to every sphere of life – the biological and the social, as well as the material. Although Weber prized the improvements in efficiency that rationalization brought about, he was uneasy about the subjugation of human beings to what he termed a 'means-ends' rationality,[10] (what others have subsequently called 'technological rationality'[11]) which objectified and depersonalised the individual.

Weber saw rationalization as the outcome of pressures generated by industrial capitalism and associated developments in the public sphere, including the changing nature of warfare and military organisation. According to Weber, there had been an interchange of ideas between industry and the military which led to a broad – though often loose – consensus about the desirability of certain forms of discipline and organisation, centred around specialisation, division of labour, and the maximisation of material and human resources. This trend was epitomised by the rise of 'scientific management' and the practises espoused by Frederick Taylor, among others, at the end of the nineteenth century. While specifically Taylorian managerial ideas found few unequivocal supporters – even in America – the general principles of scientific management gained acceptance in most advanced industrial nations during, or shortly after, the First World War.[12] Outside the realms of industry and public administration, the process of rationalization was also apparent in new forms of discipline which were more appropriate to a complex and increasingly urbanised society, where power was more widely diffused. These new forms of discipline were based on dressage, surveillance, and the scientific management of populations, rather than on physical punishment and spectacle.[13]

The armed forces, while clearly, to some degree, separate from civil society (and increasingly so as they professionalised during the nineteenth century[14]), were nevertheless affected by most of the trends described above. Warfare increasingly reflected the emergence of a mass, industrial society, not only in the technology utilised by armed forces but in their very organisation. From around the middle of the nineteenth century, the profession of arms became increasingly specialised and training far more systematic. Modern wars were wars in which 'experts' – scientists, engineers, wireless operators, and others – came to play a crucial role.[15] Armed forces also began to evolve new forms of discipline during the nineteenth century, relying less on summary corporal punishment and more on surveillance and indoctrination. This trend – though it should not be exaggerated in view of the persistence of certain forms of corporal punishment into the twentieth century – has traditionally been seen as a outgrowth liberal, humanitarian reforms in the civilian sphere, which manifested itself also in the formation of such bodies as the Red Cross and new legal constraints upon warfare (the Geneva Convention).[16] While these humanitarian impulses should not be dismissed in Michel Foucault's notorious phrase as 'so much incidental music',[17] the gradual changes that were occurring in military discipline mirrored the new disciplinary regime which Foucault discerned in civil society.

What, then, did medicine contribute to this 'rationalization' of military management? Firstly, and most obviously, it enhanced military efficiency by reducing wastage from disease and by improving the rate of return of casualties to active service.[18] Medical knowledge was also vital in achieving the standardisation of men and materials without which no large armed force could function.[19] As well as the physical examination of prospective recruits, medical men were involved in the calculation of dietary requirements and in deriving limits to physical and mental endurance. Medical officers (MOs) also played an increasing role in the maintenance of discipline and morale. The regimental MO closely monitored the mental and physical health of the men in his unit,[20] and was the principal conduit of propaganda in matters of health and morals. Hygienic rituals, themselves, formed part of the new forms of discipline which began to emerge in the European armed forces during the eighteenth and early nineteenth centuries.[21]

The growing influence of technical experts in the armed forces was both a cause and a consequence of the declining authority of the landed elite, with its culture of the 'gentleman amateur'. Appointments were made increasingly on the basis of merit and technical competence, rather than on seniority and the ability to purchase commissions. These changes were, themselves, linked to the evolution of mass democracy in the public sphere. This democratisation had a significant impact on the development of military medicine in countries such as Great Britain and the United States, where the humanitarian movement was particularly strong.

The extension of the electoral franchise meant that the public could now express its indignation over the poor treatment of soldiers through the ballot box, and public pressure was to prove at least as significant in the development of military medicine as the drive for administrative rationalization. Notions of 'entitlement' which emerged during the twentieth century as part of a new culture of social citizenship also had important implications for military medical provisions. There had always been some measure of medical care for servicemen (often performed by external bodies such as the Church) and this became more systematic after the foundation of standing armies during the seventeenth century. By the nineteenth century, most large European nations provided some form of institutional care for sick, wounded and invalided veterans.[22] However, by the end of the century, servicemen were beginning to demand health care as a right, and to regard it as a kind of 'social wage' earned in the service of their country. They appealed not only to the paternalistic and humanitarian inclinations of certain sections of the community but also to modern concepts of citizenship and social justice.[23]

* * *

The essays collected in this volume amplify different aspects of these processes: the 'medicalization' of warfare and its corollary, the 'militarization' of medicine. By medicalization, we mean the gradual extension of medical authority into new areas such as discipline and administration, together with the growing authority of medical men in the planning and conduct of military campaigns. While recognising that the process of medicalization was partial and often highly contested, the term nevertheless encompasses a complex of interconnected changes that occurred in the armed forces of most industrialised nations from the middle of the nineteenth century. The concept of 'militarization' is no less problematic, not least because it is sometimes held to apply only to certain states (most notably Prussia, and later Imperial Germany)[24] in which the military exercised an overwhelming political influence. However, if we accept Alfred Vagts' argument that militarism is a cultural as much as a political phenomenon (where military values are prized in civil society), then the term can be more widely applied.[25] Indeed, a number of historians have sought evidence of a culture of militarism in Great Britain, which has traditionally been regarded as a liberal nation and the antithesis of militaristic Prussia. Anne Summers, among others, has argued that a peculiar form of militarism was

4

much in vogue in Britain prior to the First World War, evident in mass support for 'militaristic' organisations such as the Boy Scouts and Rifle Brigades, not to mention those dedicated to the introduction of conscription and military and naval reform.[26] The military trappings of such organisations as the Boy Scouts have probably been exaggerated, nevertheless there is a consensus emerging among historians that Britain – along with other major powers – was more militaristic in the decade or so before the Great War than before or since.[27] Britain's may have been a peculiar form of militarism – 'Liberal Militarism', to borrow David Edgerton's phrase – but it was militarism nonetheless.[28]

It is not surprising, therefore, that the medical profession in Britain, as well as Germany and other more patently militaristic nations, should have adopted the values and organisational forms of the military. This was, perhaps, most evident in the case of nursing, the professionalisation of which was closely bound up with military-medical reform, and which carried military-style uniforms into civilian practice.[29] But doctors were equally – though, perhaps, less obviously – affected by the militarization of society before the Great War. Military associations helped to overcome the stigma of domesticity (femininity, even) attached to certain aspects of medical practice.[30] Moreover, it should be remembered that the authority of the profession as a whole was still precarious in the middle of the nineteenth century and that involvement with what many regarded as the most senior profession could do no harm to the status of medical men (and increasingly of women). In many continental countries such as France and Germany, where conscription was in force, doctors were automatically brought into the armed forces, meaning that the connection between the professions of arms and medicine was very close. Accordingly, doctors enjoyed a high reputation in the armed forces and in society more generally. In countries such as Britain, however, the association was more tenuous. Those doctors who volunteered for military service were often the dregs of their profession, unable to find lucrative employment in civilian life.[31] Consequently, they were regarded by their combatant colleagues as professional and social inferiors, and, until the very end of the nineteenth century, were denied combatant rank and its associated privileges. The low status of the medical services in nations without conscription also meant that they tended to be poorly funded and singled out for the deepest cuts at times of retrenchment.

But the very weakness of the medical services in such countries meant that the armed forces had to rely increasingly on civilian doctors to make good deficiencies in wartime. Notwithstanding the poor reputation that the armed forces had for the treatment of medical men, doctors and nurses volunteered in large numbers to serve their countries. Sometimes they served in the armed forces on temporary commissions, and sometimes in supposedly neutral organisation such as the Red Cross, which were often little more than appendages of the military medical services.[32] Active involvement in matters of national importance improved the professional status of nurses and doctors. While this was true of these professions generally, many individuals rose to national prominence as a result of their service in wartime and continuing associations with the military. War (and even military requirements in peacetime) also provided the conditions under which medical specialisation could develop: bacteriology, psychiatry, orthopaedics, all benefited from the military's preoccupation with manpower efficiency.[33] However, the link between professional advancement and military service is a complex one and it is by no means true that war is always 'good for medicine'.[34] The exigencies of war led some areas of medicine to be privileged at the expense of others and gains made in wartime were not always consolidated in the very different conditions of peace. Nor do specialisms advance simply because there is an evident demand for them in wartime: demand arises from a series of negotiations between specialists aiming to promote their interests and officials concerned with maximising the effectiveness of manpower. The latter may be faced with many conflicting suggestions from among medical practitioners as to how best to address their needs.

Whatever the precise relationship between the armed forces and the medical profession – and this depended very much on the presence or absence of conscription – the increasingly close relationship between the two led to the adoption of a military ethos in medicine, which survives in attenuated form until the present day. By way of qualification, it is important to emphasise that the majority of doctors who entered military service in the course of the last century did so because they were conscripted into the armed forces, or because they made a professional judgement that this was the best way to advance their career. They were not necessarily militaristic in the sense that they valued the military way of life in itself. However, the prevailing mood of militarism at the end of the nineteenth century, and the growing participation of doctors in military work, left its mark on the very language with which they have chosen to describe the achievements of their profession. Titles such as *Victory with Vaccines*, *The Battle against Bacteria*, and

Crusading Doctor, may reveal far more about the profession of medicine than their authors ever intended.[35]

* * *

Medicine and Modern Warfare begins with Connor's study of the US Army medical service during the Spanish-American War of 1898. One of the main themes running throughout Connor's paper is the struggle of US Army doctors for professional recognition. While he places this in the context of the broader professionalization of medicine during the Progressive era, it is clear from Connor's account that the military medical service was seen as inferior to the civilian profession (as it was in Britain). Connor argues that US Army doctors were engaged in a campaign on two fronts: in the Cuban theatre itself, where they faced poor sanitary conditions and high wastage from diseases such as yellow fever; and at home, where they fought vigorously for a rank in the army consistent with their civilian status.

As far as the first of these campaigns is concerned, the Spanish-American War revealed the limitations of the new technologically-based optimism which ran through American medicine at the end of the nineteenth century. The problems encountered by military doctors were incapable of solution by a quick technological fix. Investigations revealed that many of the problems concerned were due not so much to the inadequacies of individual physicians but to the low status accorded to medicine in the US Army; to the fact that few combatant officers and men had even the most rudimentary understanding of hygiene; to the fact the service was underfunded; and to the fact that medical officers lacked the rank and authority of other officers of corresponding age and experience. These deficiencies were virtually identical to those revealed in the British Army's medical service by the South African War which began the following year. And, as in Britain, the audit of war led to a substantial reorganisation of the medical services, although military doctors continued to complain about their lowly status until at least the First World War. Connor also makes the intriguing suggestion that the campaigns for professional recognition launched by the American Medical Association during and after the war may account for its more effective 'mobilization' after 1899; a suggestion which takes us back once again to the theme of medicine's militarization at the end of the nineteenth century. After the conclusion of the Spanish-American War, the Association's journal developed into an aggressive lobbying organisation on behalf of American doctors, their professional demands being couched in the rhetoric of efficiency and rational use of resources.

Some of these themes are echoed in van Bergen's chapter on the Dutch Military Health Service. The Netherlands did not have a system of conscription and, as in Britain and the United States, the medical services did not attract a high standard of recruit. The decision to enter the MHS was essentially an economic one: although poorly paid, the MHS offered a stable income to recruits who often came from lower class homes. Yet conditions were so poor that the service was often left with a shortfall of recruits. This was due, to some extent, to the increasing professionalization of Dutch military medicine in the late nineteenth century, which raised qualifications for entry into the service. But it was also due to the fact that the MHS was singled out for the deepest cuts whenever the armed forces were subject to retrenchment. Since Holland was a declining military power, these cuts were frequent and often devastating. When mobilisation of the Dutch army occurred during the First World War, the MHS was clearly unable to offer the level of medical support which the army required, even though the Netherlands never became involved in the conflict. Senior military doctors, however, blamed the problems encountered by the medical services on 'malingerers' who occupied hospital beds for no good reason. Indeed, malingering was something of an obsession in the Dutch MHS, as it was in its counterparts in other nations. Medical officers felt they had something to prove to their combatant colleagues, some of whom tended to view the medical services with suspicion. They wanted to show that they were not being soft on the men under their charge but, in so doing, often seemed far more concerned about malingering than combatants.

While doctors in volunteer forces such as the Dutch and British armies had to fight hard for professional recognition, the armed forces did provide almost unrivalled opportunities for medical men interested in research. This is the main theme of Worboys's chapter on the career of Almroth Wright, a civilian who held the post of Professor of Pathology at the British Army's Medical College at Netley from 1890 to 1902. Almroth Wright was one of the most famous (some would say infamous) medical scientists of his generation; the inspiration for the character of Sir Colenso Rigeon in George Bernard Shaw's play *The Doctor's Dilemma* – an outspoken opponent of women's suffrage and a champion of vaccine therapy in the face of increasing scepticism from clinicians. However, Wright's reputation rested, above all, on his work on the anti-typhoid vaccine during the 1890s; work conducted during his tenure at the Army Medical College.

That a pioneering 'research school' could flourish at Netley surprised many of Britain's leading medical scientists. English medical schools were generally unpromising environments for science-based research and the army was not known for its sympathy with medical aspirations. Further, Netley was geographically and professionally isolated from the main centres of medical research in Britain, being located on the south coast near Southampton. Contemporaries and historians have been convinced that the counterweight to these unfavourable circumstances was Wright's own genius and fiery personality but Worboys questions this account and suggests that the army was not so antithetical to research as is sometimes claimed. He argues that the changing culture of the British Army was actually supportive of medical research and innovation. He notes that the antityphoid vaccine, whilst resisted tooth and nail by certain of Wright's enemies, was tested and recommended as a standard procedure in the army only a decade or so after it was first developed by Wright in 1896. Such innovations were congruent with the wider change in the role of medicine in modern armed forces, and especially the drive to improve manpower economy. For those, like Wright, who wanted to pursue a career in medical research, the armed forces also provided a wide range of problems to be solved and a captive population of fit young men on which to test new vaccines and the like. Such measures were at the cutting edge of preventive medicine, being specific measures targeted on individuals rather than general environmental management.[36] Carrying immunity to typhoid fever, the inoculated soldier was immunologically superior and more standardised than his predecessor; advantages which would be reflected in effective control of typhoid in most armed forces during the First World War.

Almroth Wright made many enemies inside the British Army on account of his impatience with military 'red tape' and the fact that he – a civilian – had been appointed to a position sought after by ambitious members of the Army Medical Service. However, these very qualities endeared him to some prominent military figures – not least, Britain's best-known general, Lord Roberts – who regarded Wright as a guiding light of military medical reform. During the South African War there had been an uproar over the British Army's neglect of elementary hygiene, which had led to no less than 60,000 casualties among its ranks from typhoid. Care of the sick and wounded was also found to be gravely deficient. As with the Spanish-American War, the events of 1899-1902 placed military medical reform on the political agenda but, in the period immediately after the conflict, the momentum behind reform began to flag. But reformers who despaired at deep retrenchment of the military budget soon found a new focus for their efforts – the Russo-Japanese War of 1904-5.[37]

Herrick's chapter considers the war in the light of this campaign for reform, examining the ways in which the war was reported to the public and the military in Britain. Herrick argues that the war was represented by doctors in such a way as to present 'scientific medicine' as the key to military efficiency. Reporting of the war was characterised by immense admiration for the Japanese, and their capacity for adopting and improving upon techniques learnt in the West. The Japanese and their martial qualities stood in stark contrast to a 'degenerate' Britain, in which the military were accorded second-class status. Those who highlighted Japanese achievements in the field of medicine sought to persuade the War Office to allot more funds to the medical services and to encourage combatant officers, in particular, to take seriously the neglected matter of sanitation. Many British officers were, indeed, convinced by the example of the Russo-Japanese War that hygienic discipline could significantly improve military efficiency, as it was shown to have given the Japanese a significant edge over the Russians. Indeed, the Russo-Japanese War was the first conflict in which the number of fatal casualties from disease was less than those from wounds inflicted in battle; in the Japanese forces at least. Japan continued to provide an example to medical reformers until well into the First World War, and it is clear that the climate of opinion created by reports of Japanese medical successes enabled medical reformers to secure a number of important gains in the period after 1905 (although these owed as much to the new Liberal government and a receptive secretary of state for war in the person of R.B. Haldane). Among these reforms was the creation of a medical wing for the new Territorial Force, which formalised existing arrangements for voluntary aid in time of war (the Japanese had made good use of reserve and volunteer forces), and instruction for combatants in the elements of hygiene.

Medical officers, of course, continued to advise on hygiene, but it was now the responsibility of commanding officers to ensure that all reasonable precautions were taken to prevent disease. The importance attached to sanitation was therefore far higher when the British Army entered the First World War than in any previous conflict. However, the rapid expansion of the Army led to the introduction of many officers and men without sanitary training or experience, leading to a number of scandals early in the war when disease broke out amongst British troops. Troops of all nationalities serving on the Western Front were often afflicted by epidemics of typhoid (until inoculation was extended to virtually all soldiers in 1915), dysentery, measles, and respiratory diseases; not to mention the devastation caused by influenza in 1918. But in Europe, at least, disease never threatened to undermine military operations and deaths from disease were lower than those from wounds inflicted in battle. It was only away from the Western Front – in Gallipoli, Macedonia, Mesopotamia, East Africa and eastern Europe – that disease remained a significant problem. In these theatres, such diseases as malaria, typhoid and typhus were endemic among the local population; further, when faced with mobile operations sometimes extending over thousands of miles, commanding officers often overlooked elementary hygienic precautions.

Yet good sanitation was not simply a matter of educating combatant officers and men, it was also necessary to instruct civilian doctors who had volunteered, or had been conscripted into, military service. As Whitehead points out in his study of the British medical officer on the Western Front, these new recruits had to undergo additional training to make them aware of differences between military and civilian medicine, and to familiarise them with military procedure. Many new recruits found that Royal Army Medical Corps orderlies were far better versed in sanitation than themselves; they also had much to learn about surgical practice under wartime conditions, although both Regulars and those on temporary commissions had to abandon much of what had been learned in South Africa. Conservative, antiseptic surgery may have worked well in the confines of a modern hospital, or the relatively sterile environment of the veldt, but it was inappropriate in the richly-manured soils of France and Flanders.[38] Military service also imposed a new set of priorities on doctors: their primary responsibility was now to the state rather than the individual patient; discipline and surveillance were as important as compassion for the sick and wounded. Nowhere was this more evident than in the view – deliberately cultivated by the medical authorities – that everyone who reported sick was a 'scrimshanker'. The military doctor had also to wrestle with some peculiarly difficult ethical dilemmas, such as overcoming hatred towards enemy patients and their involvement in corporal punishment or courts martial.

Some doctors had, of course, been involved in similar types of work in civilian life. Some had been employed by the state as Medical Officers of Health and Poor Law Medical Officers, and hence had a rather different outlook from those who treated private patients. Some had also been employed by such organisations as friendly societies, and their work would have involved evaluation of whether a patient was 'genuine' or not. Nevertheless, most new recruits to the medical services required some form of specialist training and this was reorganised significantly in 1917, when a new centre was created at Blackpool to provide instruction for medical officers in various medical and non-medical skills necessary for military service. However, the impossibility of providing adequate preparation for every doctor prior to embarkation led to the establishment of training centres overseas. Whether or not the attitudes learnt in the army had any significant and lasting effect on medical practice in peacetime is another subject which awaits further research.

The degree to which medicine became militarized is, however, considered in Rudiger Prüll's chapter on pathology in Germany and Britain during the First World War. Central to Prüll's account is the development of a distinctively German 'war pathology', a sub-discipline founded as a result of interaction between the army medical corps and the civilian pathologist Ludwig Aschoff, head of the University of Freiburg's institute of pathology. *Kriegspathologie* was very different from pathology in wartime Britain. The latter was mostly clinical and laboratory-based – involving few autopsies and offering pragmatic assistance to other branches of the medical service. Unlike German pathologists, their British counterparts did not develop a distinctive identity or agenda of their own. German war pathology, by contrast, drew away from bacteriology and support for clinical medicine. It was static and morphological in complexion, and was based principally on post-mortem examinations. Its aim was to discern the constitutional 'types' thought particularly liable to disease, reflecting contemporary preoccupations with race and degeneration. German pathology was also distinctively militaristic in that it made more extensive use of a military vocabulary of defence and attack.

Prüll suggests that *Kriegspathologie* mirrored Germany's peculiarly conservative and militaristic culture. British pathology, by contrast – with its emphasis on physiological processes and its absence of concern with race and degeneration – was a reflection of Britain's more liberal atmosphere. Although we should be wary of underestimating the extent to which Britain had become militarised in the years before the Great War, Prüll makes a persuasive case for the comparative absence of such concerns in British pathology, at least. The fact that so much of the impetus behind the development of German war pathology came from prominent civilians such as Aschoff, also shows that such views were widely diffused throughout the German medical profession and were, in no sense, the preserve of the military. German medicine, it appears, was more militarized than its British counterpart.

It is important to recollect that the medical and civilian branches of the medical profession had developed differently in Britain and Germany. In the former, the civilian medical profession had only just begun to forge links with the military authorities (the South African War of 1899-1902 being a crucial watershed in this respect) but in Germany, where conscription had long been in force, even the very best medical graduates entered military service, and retained close links after their period of service had come to an end. This may help to explain why German doctors were more ready to take on board the values and the vocabulary of military life, although more research clearly needs to be done on these differences in national styles before any definitive statement can be made.

The final chapter dealing with the First World War is Harrison's study of medicine and morale in the Indian Expeditionary Force in France and England during 1914-15. The main theme of Harrison's chapter is medicine's role in maintaining the bonds which tied the Indian soldier (or sepoy) to the Raj; in sustaining what Harrison calls the 'moral nexus' of the Indian Army. He argues that Indian soldiers came to see health care as part of an implicit bargain between themselves and the imperial state. Although medical provisions for Indian troops had been minimal prior to the war, unfavourable comparisons made between the standard of care available to sepoys and that of French colonial troops (not to mention British soldiers) led to the establishment of new hospitals for Indians in France and in southern England. These provisions were ultimately, in many instances, far more generous than those made for British troops, reflecting the British and Indian governments' fear of political agitation among Indian troops. But while every attention was paid to the requirements of caste and religion – from special diets to the observance of religious rituals – medical care was sometimes administered in ways which were seen as degrading. Hospitals in France and England were subjected to strict discipline and were policed surreptitiously by the Government of India's secret service. Visits by Indian dignitaries and others likely to cause trouble for the authorities were strictly controlled. Military discipline was, of course, a feature of hospital life for all soldiers regardless of nationality; although its severity did tend to depend on rank (officers being subjected to far fewer restrictions). But Indian soldiers were generally unused to hospitals, many being cared for in India in their own lines, or in smaller regimental institutions. As far as many sepoys were concerned, having to defer to female nurses was demeaning; moreover, restrictions placed upon the liberty of both patients and staff were such that they undermined the sepoys' sense of honour, or *izzat*. This was especially true of the Kitchener Indian Hospital in Brighton, where the imposition of a cordon around the hospital – preventing both patients and Indian staff from visiting the town – caused considerable resentment (the enthusiasm shown by some local women for the Indians having diminished the *izzat* of the Raj).

It is unsurprising, therefore, that hospitals in England and France were among the main foci of dissent and political activity in the Indian Army during the First World War. There were numerous contraventions of hospital discipline – some very serious, including the attempted murder of hospital staff – and letters written by Indian soldiers to their comrades or families reveal that medical provisions were among the principal causes of disaffection. These letters – of which extracts were translated and collected by the Censor of Indian Mails – provide a unique insight into the feelings of the Indian soldier and into Indian attitudes towards Western medicine more generally.

In comparison with the First World War, which has received far more attention from historians of medicine than any other (principally on account of the recent interest in 'shell shock'),[39] the literature on the Second World War is scant in the extreme. Very little, in fact, has been written on the medical aspects of the war since the publication of the official histories in the 1950s and 60s.[40] This is a great pity, as the war provides some classic illustrations of medicine's contribution to military efficiency, the campaigns in the Western Desert and Burma showing that a significant tactical advantage was conferred upon forces which instituted strict hygienic discipline. Other features of the war also invite further attention: the reorganisation of medical services on account of mechanisation and air support; mass blood transfusion; new drugs and therapies (such as mepacrine and penicillin); and the development and use of insecticides such as DDT.[41] However, it is already clear that official histories of medicine during the Second World War were coloured, in the immediate post-war period, by the heroic and triumphalist rhetoric of doctors determined to consolidate their new-found influence in government and military circles. While few would deny the important contribution which medicine made to military victory, it is clear that success in preventing and treating casualties depended crucially on the attitudes of combatant officers. Medical innovation would have counted for little if commanding officers had been as unsympathetic to medical demands as they had been in many previous conflicts. Arguably, the most significant thing about the medical history of the Second World War was not the development and use of new medical technologies, but the transformation which occurred in military-medical relations: the shared conviction that medicine was a vital technical and administrative resource.

One aspect of medical work in wartime which has proved attractive to historians is the abuse of medical power and knowledge. The overriding emphasis here has been on the willing involvement of doctors in human experimentation in Nazi concentration camps[42] and in Japanese biological warfare establishments.[43] Similar concerns underlie recent work on the aftermath of the atomic bombing of Hiroshima and Nagasaki. As Susan Lindee has argued in her excellent study of the American-dominated Atomic Bomb Casualty Commission, the main intentions of those involved in monitoring the long-term effects of exposure to radiation were military rather than humanitarian. Their values were those of the Cold War; their aim to translate the suffering of Japanese survivors of the bombings into data of vital importance those working with radiation.[44]

Another area of military medicine during the Second World War which has begun to receive attention is psychiatry, although there remains tremendous scope for further work. Indeed, the sources for a study of psychiatry during the Second World War are richer and more varied than for 1914-18, and contain much fascinating material on subjects such as group therapy and patient-feedback.[45] This archive is used to good effect by Pols in his chapter on American psychiatry during and after the Second World War. Pols stresses the marked shift in attitudes towards psychiatric casualties of the war that occurred after the victory over Japan in 1945 and the beginning of the Cold War. This made it difficult for wounded servicemen to express and work through their traumatic experiences. While the war was in progress, however, servicemen suffering from anxiety neuroses and other mental disorders associated with combat were treated by military psychiatrists who were usually sympathetic and knowledgeable about conditions at the front. Thus, the basic assumption underlying military psychiatry was that anxiety was a normal reaction to the stresses of combat, rather than the manifestation of some innate predisposition to mental illness.

After the war had ended, psycho-analytically oriented psychiatrists – many of whom had no experience of combat – came to see the problem differently. They related the mental illness of ex-servicemen not to the trauma they had experienced in battle, but to the ways in which these men had been socialised in pre-war America. The blame for the high number of psychiatric casualties (often comprising as much as 30 per cent of battle casualties) was laid at the doorstep of over-protective mothers, who had supposedly smothered the masculinity of the American male. Henceforth, the ex-serviceman was denied the opportunity to express his individual suffering, the anxiety of combat having been displaced by anxieties about the nation's masculinity. While this denied a whole generation of men the opportunity to articulate their experiences of war, psychiatrists themselves had gained by having apparently uncovered a problem which threatened to undermine the American way of life, and the nation's very survival as a vigorous military power.

The last chapters in this volume examine aspects of the history of war and sexually transmitted diseases in Britain. The first of these is Hall's analytical overview of the period 1850-1950, the bulk of which concentrates on the Second World War and Mass Observation's survey of attitudes towards venereal disease. She begins by noting that public anxiety over what were then termed 'venereal diseases' manifested itself especially in times of war, and goes on to suggest that such anxieties had much to do with the perception that these diseases were generated at the unstable interface between military and civilian spheres.[46] These diseases may have possessed a liminal quality, for they were seen to arise in a space between clearly-defined categories, where conventional distinctions broke down. War brought the military into the public domain far more than in times of peace, and this was especially true of wars from the mid-nineteenth century, which involved armies swollen with volunteers and conscripts. Whereas the control of venereal diseases had previously been regarded as a purely military problem, they were increasingly seen as more general problem of the population at large. Thus, Hall suggests that the Contagious Diseases Acts of the 1860s[47] may be seen as an attempt to create a clearly-defined cadre of women to supply the sexual needs of soldiers, thereby establishing a *cordon sanitaire* which protected society at large. The CD Acts, although vigorously and, ultimately, successfully opposed in Britain, heralded the emergence of venereal diseases as a matter of public concern, and these concerns increased during the two world wars as distinctions between the army and the civilian population broke down. Anxieties over the prevention of VD focused not simply on the armed forces but on the potentially harmful effects of these diseases in the population as a whole; a population which was mobilised for total war. The life of the civilian was now as vital to warfare as the life of the soldier. However, as Hall's study of the Mass Observation archive makes clear, the public had radically divergent views on which sections of society were the chief disseminators of VD. Some blamed servicemen (especially foreigners), who had traditionally been seen as morally and medically suspect; others blamed women, not just prostitutes but 'cheap loose-living girls' who threw themselves at any man in a uniform. Remedies varied from segregation and various forms of compulsion and punishment, to free and informed discussion. The measures actually taken in Britain during the war to prevent VD were an amalgam of both, although far more emphasis than hitherto was placed on education, reflecting the view that education was essential to active citizenship. Yet while the exact nature of preventative measures and of anxieties over VD changed considerably over the century examined by Hall, one enduring feature was the link between war, soldiers and VD as disruptions of the natural order.

Harrison's study of 'Sex and the Citizen Soldier' develops some of these themes, particularly Hall's notion of war as a social crisis. While accepting the traditional view that the Second World War brought a liberalisation of attitudes towards sex and the discussion of STDs, Harrison argues that influential sections of British society – concerned with the breakdown of traditional moral constraints upon sexual behaviour – sought to reassert control over the bodies of the British people in the name of health, democracy and good citizenship. These attempts at control centred, once again, on venereal disease, and particularly on the armed forces and prostitutes, which were traditionally seen as the main sources of venereal infection. Since traditional moral rhetoric had lost much of its force, the contraction and transmission of VD was portrayed not so much as an offence against God but as an offence against the State. The secularisation of VD control during the Second World was the culmination of a trend evident since the First World War,[48] but the rhetoric of VD control also embodied new ideas of citizenship, which had become increasingly important since the extension of the electoral franchise to all men and women of at least 21 years of age in 1918 and 1928. During the war these notions of citizenship – which stressed the reciprocal duties and rights of government and the state – took on an extra dimension as a result of the conflict against the Axis powers. The typical British male was portrayed as free and self-directed, but his freedom was bounded by a sense of responsibility, moderation and 'good form'. These qualities supposedly distinguished him from members of the Axis forces, who were represented variously as cruel, promiscuous and ill-disciplined. But this new image of the British serviceman was tarnished as both his self-discipline and capacity for education in matters of health were called into question by escalating rates of VD in many foreign theatres.

The failure of British servicemen to heed hygienic advice led to a change of policy in the British and other Allied forces after 1942. Army brothels were closed down and civilian ones were placed out of bounds. Compulsion rather than education was the order of the day, even though such bans were difficult to enforce in practice. However, unlike previous conflicts, it was not so much the military effects of VD that concerned the Allied military authorities. New sulpha drugs and penicillin had dramatically reduced the time taken to treat soldiers suffering from gonorrhoea and syphilis but the political and disciplinary implications of high rates of venereal infection blackened the reputation of the British overseas. Such considerations were vitally important in view of the often awkward relation that existed between the Allied forces and civilian administrations in occupied countries, and also in terms of the blow which VD and rampant promiscuity dealt to images of Britishness, as expressed in propaganda at home.

It is hoped that the essays collected in this volume will encourage others to look seriously at the medical aspects of war. The military medical archive in most countries has only begun to be tapped and it capable of sustaining a wide variety of historical projects. This is especially true of the period before and after the First World War, although much still remains to be said about health and medicine in 1914-18. This is especially true of naval medicine which, as with aviation medicine, has been generally neglected. The essays in this volume also suggest new questions and problematics. There is considerable scope for research into medicine and disciplinary regimes within the armed forces and, more especially, on the place of health and medicine in the 'morale economy' of service life. Other possible lines of inquiry flagged here include the 'militarization' of medicine; the role of the armed forces in medical professionalisation; and the armed forces as sites of medical innovation. However, perhaps the greatest need is for further studies of medicine's contribution to the emergence of modern warfare; a subject which has been framed almost exclusively in terms of weaponry, strategy and tactics. Our aim has been to demonstrate – or, at the very least, to suggest – that medicine's role was central to the emergence of mass, industrialised warfare from the middle of the nineteenth century. Without the administrative and technical support which medicine provided – not to mention its role in the maintenance of discipline and morale – it is hard to conceive how the 'total' wars of the twentieth century could have been fought.

Notes

1   National studies include: H. Fischer, *Der deutsche Sanitätsdienst 1921-1945: Organisation,Dokumente, und persönl Erfahrungen* (Osnabruck: Biblio Verlag, 1984); R.C. Engleman & R.J.T. Joy, *Two Hundred Years of Military Medicine* (Fort Detrick, Maryland, 1975); Sir Neil Cantlie, *A History of the Army Medical Department*, 2 vols. (Edinburgh: Churchill Livingstone, 1974); J. Rieux & J. Hassenforder, *Centenaire de l'École d'Application du Service de Santé et du Val-de-Grâce* (Paris: Charles Lavarzelle, 1951); A. Casarini, *La Medicina Militaire nella Storia* (Rome: Ministero della Geurra, 1929).

2   John Keegan, *The Face of Battle: A Study of Agincourt, Waterloo and the Somme* (London: Jonathan Cape, 1976).

3   See, for example: John Ellis, *The Sharp End of War: The Fighting Man in World War II* (London: David and Charles, 1980); I.W.F. Beckett & Keith Simpson (eds), *A Nation in Arms: A Social Study of the British Army in the First World War* (Manchester: Manchester University Press, 1988); Hugh Cecil & Peter Liddle (eds), *Facing Armageddon: The First World War Experienced* (London: Leo Cooper, 1995).

4   See, for example: Richard A. Gabriel & Karen S. Metz, *A History of Military Medicine*, 2 vols. (New York, Wesport Connecticut, London: Greenwood Press, 1992); Michael B. Tyquin, *Gallipoli: The Medical War. The Australian Army Medical Services in the Dardanelles Campaign of 1915* (Kensington, New South Wales, 1993); Brendan O'Keefe & F.B. Smith, *Medicine at War: Medical Aspects of Australia's Involvement in South East Asian Conflicts 1950-1972* (St. Leonards, New South Wales: Allen & Unwin, 1994).

5   See, for example: Wolfgang U. Eckart & Christoph Gradmann (eds), *Die Medizin und der Erste Weltkrieg* (Pfaffenweiler: Centaurus, 1996); Harold D. Langley, *A History of Medicine in the Early U.S. Navy* (Baltimore & London: Johns Hopkins, 1995); John S. Haller, Jr., *Farmcarts to Fords: A History of the Military Ambulance, 1790-1925* (Carbondale & Edwardsville: Southern Illinois University Press, 1992); John Shepherd, *The Crimean Doctors: A History of the British Medical Services in the Crimean War*, 2 vols. (Liverpool: Liverpool University Press, 1991). For a more comprehensive survey

of existing literature on war and medicine see: Roger Cooter, 'War and Modern Medicine', in W.F. Bynum & Roy Porter (eds), *Companion Encyclopedia of the History of Medicine* (London: Routledge, 1994), 1536-73; Mark Harrison, 'Medicine and the Management of Modern Warfare', *History of Science*, xxxiv (1996), 379-410.

6   Arthur Marwick, 'Preface', *The Deluge* (London: Macmillan; second edition, 1991).

7   For example: Guy Hartcup, *The War of Invention: Scientific Developments, 1914-18* (London: Brassey's Defence Publishers, 1988); T. Reimer, *Die Entwicklung der Flugmedizin in Deutschland* (Cologne: F. Hansen, 1979); F.H.K. Green & Sir Gordon Covell (eds), *Medical Research: Medical History of the Second World War* (London: HMSO, 1953); Z. Cope (ed.), *History of the Second World War United Kingdom Medical Services. Surgery* (London: HMSO, 1953).

8   For example: Jay Winter, *The Great War and the British People* (Basingstoke: Macmillan, 1987); Deborah Dwork, *War is good for Babies and other young Children: A History of the Infant and Child Welfare Movement in England 1898-1918* (London: Tavistock, 1987); Brian Abel-Smith, *The Hospitals, 1800-1948* (Cambridge, Mass.: Harvard University Press, 1964); A.S. MacNalty, *The Civilian Health and Medical Services*, Vol. 1 (London: HMSO, 1953); Richard Titmuss, *Problems of Social Policy* (London: HMSO, 1950).

9   Charles Webster has questioned the existence of a 'consensus' over health-care provisions during and immediately after the Second World War, in his *The Health Services since the War, I: Problems of Health Care. The National Health Service before 1957* (London: HMSO, 1988). Other historians downplay the effects of war to an even greater degree, seeing the extension of health care provisions as the outcome of more general modernising forces in advanced industrial societies. See Daniel M. Fox, *Health Policies, Health Politics: The British and American Experience, 1911-1965* (Princeton: Princeton University Press, 1986); *idem*, 'The National Health service and the Second World War: the elaboration of Consensus', in H.L. Smith (ed.), *War and Social Change: British Society in the Second World War* (Manchester: Manchester University Press, 1986), 32-57. Linda Bryder has challenged Jay Winter's argument [*op. cit.* (note 8)] that the health of the British people improved during the First World War in her article 'The First World War: Healthy of Hungry?', *History Workshop* Journal, xxiv (1987), 141-57. Her critique is developed further in Roger Cooter's essay 'Medicine and the Goodness of War', *Canadian Bulletin of Medical History*, xii

(1990), 147-59.

10 Max Weber, 'The Technical Advantages of Bureaucratic
    Organisations', in *From Max Weber: Essays in Sociology*, ed. & trans.
    H. Gerth & C.W. Mills (New York, 1972), especially 49-51.

11 Herbert Marcuse, 'Some Social Implications of Modern Technology',
    Studies in the Philosophy of Modern Science, vi (1941), 414-39.

12 On scientific management see: Mike Hales, 'Management Science
    and the "Second Industrial Revolution"', in L. Levidoff (ed.), *Radical
    Science* Essays (London: Free Association Books, 1986), 62-87; C.
    Littler, *The Development of the Labour Process in Capitalist Societies: A
    Comparative Study of the Transformation of Work Organisation in
    Britain, Japan and the U.S.A.* (London: Heinemann, 1982); C.S.
    Maier, 'Between Taylorism and Technocracy: European Ideologies
    and the Vision of Industrial Productivity in the 1920s', *Journal of
    Contemporary History*, v (1970), 27-61; S. Haber, *Efficiency and
    Uplift: Scientific Management in the Progressive Era, 1890*-1920
    (Chicago: Chicago University Press, 1964); H. Thistleton-Monk,
    *Efficiency Ideals: A Short Study of the Principles of 'Scientific
    Management'* (London: T. Werner Laurie, 1919). An example of the
    application of specifically Taylorite principles in the surgery of the
    First World War can be found in the work of Dr Pedro Chuto; see
    Roger Cooter, *Surgery and Society in Peace and War: Orthopaedics and
    the Organisation of Modern Medicine, 1880-1948* (London:
    MacMillan, 1993), p.122.

13 See Michel Foucault, 'The Politics of health in the Eighteenth
    Century', in C. Gordon (ed.), *Power/Knowledge: Selected Interviews
    and other Writings by Michel Foucault* (Worcester: Harvester Press,
    1988), 166-82; *idem, Discipline and Punish: The Birth of the Prison*,
    trans. A. Sheridan (Harmondsworth: Penguin, 1977); S. Cohen &
    A. Scull (eds), *Social Control and the State* (Oxford: Oxford
    University Press, 1985); D. Melossi & M. Pavarini, *The Prison and
    the Factory* (London: Macmillan, 1981); Michael Ignatieff, *A Just
    Measure of Pain: The Penitentiary and the Industrial Revolution, 1750-
    1850* (London: Macmillan, 1978); E.P. Thompson, 'Time, Work-
    Discipline, and Industrial Capitalism', *Past and Present*, 38 (1967),
    56-97.

14 On the increasing separation of the army from civil society see Myna
    Trustram, *Women of the Regiment: Marriage and the Victorian Army*
    (Cambridge University Press, 1984).

15 On modern warfare see: Paul Crook, *Darwinism, War and History*
    (Cambridge: Cambridge University Press, 1994); Daniel Pick, *War
    Machine: The Rationalisation of Slaughter in the Modern* Age (New

Haven & London: Yale University Press, 1993); Edward Hagerman, *The American Civil War and the Origins of Modern Warfare: Ideas, Organization, and Field Command* (Bloomington & Indianapolis: University of Indiana Press, 1992); Tim Travers, *The Killing Ground: The British Army, the Western Front and the Emergence of Modern Warfare* (London: Macmillan, 1987), *idem, How the War was Won: Command and Technology in the British Army on the Western Front 1917-1918* (London & New York: Routledge, 1992).

16   Geoffrey Best, *Humanity in Warfare: The Modern History of the International Law of Armed Conflicts* (London: Weidenfeld & Nicolson, 1980).

17   Quoted in A. Scull, 'Humanitarianism or Social Control? Some Observations on the Historiography of Anglo-American Psychiatry', in Cohen & Scull (eds), *op. cit.* (note 13), 133.

18   See Philip D. Curtin, *Death By Migration: Europe's Encounter with the Tropical World in the Nineteenth Century* (Cambridge: Cambridge University Press, 1989); *idem, Disease and Empire: The Health of European Troops in the Conquest of Africa* (Cambridge: Cambridge University Press, 1998). On medicine and efficiency more generally, see: Joel D. Howell, *Technology in the Hospital: Transforming Patient Care in the Early Twentieth Century* (Baltimore & London: Johns Hopkins Press, 1995); Steve Sturdy, 'The Political Economy of Scientific Medicine: Science, Education and the Transformation of Medical Practice in Sheffield, 1890-1922', *Medical History*, xxxvi (1992), 125-59; Susan Reverby, 'Stealing the Golden Eggs: Ernest Amory Codman and the Science and Management of Medicine', *Bulletin of the History of Medicine*, lv (1981), 156-71; C.E. Rosenberg, 'Inward Vision and Outward Glance: The Shaping of the American Hospital, 1880-1914', *Bulletin of the History of Medicine*, liii (1976), 346-91; George Rosen, 'The Efficiency Criterion in Medical Care, 1900-1920: An early Approach to an evaluation of Health Service', *Bulletin of the History of Medicine*, l (1976), 28-44.

19   See A.R. Skelley, *The Victorian Army at Home: The Recruitment and Terms and Conditions of the British Regular, 1859-1899* (London: Croom Helm, 1977).

20   One of the most important aspects of the medical officer's work was detecting men thought to be malingering; that is, those who reported sick without good cause. See Ian Whitehead, 'Not a Doctor's Work? The Role of the British Medical Officer in the Field', in Cecil & Liddle (eds), *op. cit.* (note 3), 451-65; Joanna Bourke, *Dismembering the Male: Men's Bodies and the Great War* (London: Reaktion Books, 1996), chapter 2; Roger Cooter, 'Disciplining

Doctors: Malingering and Modernity in World War One', in
R. Cooter, M. Harrison & S. Sturdy (eds), *War, Medicine and
Modernity, 1860-1945* (Stroud: Sutton, 1998), 125-148.

21 See Christopher Lawrence, 'Disciplining Disease: Scurvy, the Navy
and Imperial Expansion' in D. Miller & P. Reill (eds), *Visions of
Empire* (Cambridge: Cambridge University Press, 1994), 80-106.

22 See Colin Jones, 'The Welfare of the French Foot-Soldier from
Richleau to Napoleon', in his *The Charitable Imperative: Hospitals
and Nursing in Ancien Regime and Revolutionary France* (London:
Routledge, 1989); Joachim Moerchel, *Das Österreichische
Militärsanitätswesen im Zeitalter des aufgeklärten Absolutismus*
(Frankfurt: Peter Lang, 1984); Isser Woloch, *The French Veteran from
the Revolution to the Restoration* (Chapel Hill: University of Carolina
Press, 1979); Peter Mathias, 'Swords into Ploughshares: The Armed
Forces, Medicine and Public Health in the late Eighteenth Century',
in J. Winter (ed.), *War and Economic Development: Essays in Memory
of David Joslin* (Cambridge: Cambridge University Press, 1975); H.
Müller-Dietz, *Der russische Militärtz im 18 Jahrhundert* (Berlin:
Osteuropa Institut, 1970); Friedrich Ring, *Zur Geschichte der
Militärmedizin in Deutschland* (Berlin: Deutscher Verlag, 1962).

23 See: Bourke, *op. cit.* (note 20); Seth Koven, 'Remembering and
Dismemberment: crippled Children, wounded Soldiers, and the
Great War in Britain', *American Historical* Review, xciv (1994),
1167-1202; R.W. Whalen, *Bitter Wounds: German Victims of the
Great War, 1914-1939* (Ithaca & London: Cornell University Press,
1984); Antoine Prost, *Les Anciens Combatants et la Societé Francaise,
1914-1939* (Paris: Presses de la Foundation Nationale des Sciences
Politiques, 1977).

24 On militarism in Germany see: F. Fischer, *Germany's War Aims in the
First World War* (London: Chatto & Windus, 1977), 3-49; Gerhard
Ritter, *The Sword and the Sceptre: The Problem of Militarism in
Germany*, trans. C. Gables (Florida, 1970); K. Demeter, *The German
Officer Corps in Society and State 1650-1945*, trans. A. Martin
(London: Weidenfeld & Nicolson, 1965); G.A. Craig, *The Politics of
the Prussian Army 1640-1945* (Oxford University Press, 1964).

25 Alfred Vagts, *A History of Militarism* (London: Hollis & Carter, 1959).

26 See: I.F.W. Beckett, *The Amateur Military Tradition* (Manchester
University Press, 1991); R.J.Q. Adams & P. Poirier, *The Conscription
Controversy in Britain 1900-18* (London: Macmillan, 1987); J.
Springhall, 'Building Character in the British Boy: the attempt to
extend Christian manliness to working-class Adolescents, 1880 to
1914', in J.A. Mangan & J. Walvin (eds), *Manliness and Morality:*

Middle-Class Masculinity in Britain and American, 1880-1940
(Manchester: Manchester University Press, 1987), 52-74; J.M.
MacKenzie (ed.), *Propaganda and Empire: The Manipulation of
British Public Opinion 1880-1960* (Manchester: Manchester
University Press, 1985); *idem* (ed.), *Imperialism and Popular Culture*
(Manchester: Manchester University Press, 1986); Anne Summers,
'Militarism in Britain before the Great War', *History Workshop
Journal,* ii (1976), 104-23; Hugh Cunningham, *The Volunteer Force*
(London: Macmillan, 1972); Olive Anderson, 'The growth of
Christian militarism in mid-Victorian Britain', *English Historical
Review,* lxxxvi (1971), 46-72. These accounts should be read
alongside R. Price, *An Imperial War and the British Working Class*
(London: Routledge, 1972), which downplays the enthusiasm for
the Boer War among the British working class.

27   Edward Spiers, 'The late Victorian Army 1888-1914', in
D. Chandler & I. Beckett (eds), *The Oxford Illustrated History of the
British Army* (Oxford: Oxford University Press, 1994), 189-214.

28   David Edgerton, 'Liberal Militarism and the British State', *New Left
Review*, 185 (1991), 138-69.

29   Anne Summers, *Angels and Citizens: British Women as Military Nurses
1854-1914* (London: Routledge, 1988); Penny Starns, 'Fighting
Militarism? British Nursing During the Second World War', in
Cooter *et al.* (eds), *op. cit.* (note 20).

30   See M. Pelling, 'Compromised by Gender: The Role of the Male
Medical Practitioner in Early Modern England', in M. Pelling & H.
Marland (eds), *The Task of Healing: Medicine, Religion and Gender in
England and the Netherlands 1450-1800* (Rotterdam: Erasmus,
1996), 101-33.

31   See Nelson D. Lankford, 'The Victorian Medical Profession and
Military Practice: Army Doctors and National Origins', *Bulletin of
the History of Medicine*, 54 (1980), 511-28; *idem, Status,
Professionalism and Bureaucracy: The Surgeon in the British Army,
1860-1914* (Ph.D. thesis, Indiana University, 1976).

32   See: Eileen Crofton, *The Women of Royaumont: A Scottish Hospital on
the Western Front* (East Linton: Tuckwell press, 1997); John F.
Hutchinson, *Champions of Charity: War and the Rise of the Red Cross*
(Oxford: Westview Press, 1996); Leo van Bergen, *De Zwaargewonden
Eerst? Het Nederlandsche Roode Kruis en het Vraagstuk van Oorlog en
verde 1867-1945* (Rotterdam: Erasmus, 1994); Leah Leneman, *In the
Service of life: The Story of Dr Elsie Inglis and the Scottish Women's
Hospitals* (Edinburgh: Mercat Press, 1994).

33   On war and medical specialisation see: Cooter, *op. cit.* (note 12);

Steve Sturdy, 'From the Trenches to the Hospitals at Home: Physiologists, Clinicians and Oxygen Therapy, 1914-30', in J.V. Pickstone (ed.), *Medical Innovation in Historical Perspective* (London: Macmillan, 1992), 104-23; Joel D. Howell, 'Soldier's Heart: the redefinition of Heart Disease and Speciality formation in early twentieth-century Great Britain', *Medical History*, suppl. v (1985), 34-52; Martin Stone, 'Shellshock and the Psychiatrists', in W.F. Bynum *et al.* (eds), *The Anatomy of Madness*, vol.2 (London: Routledge, 1985), 242-271.

34 See Cooter *op. cit.* (note 9).

35 Michael A. Shadid, *Crusading Doctor: My Fight for Cooperative Medicine* (Oklahoma, 1992); H.J. Parish, *Victory with Vaccines: The Story of Immunization* (London, 1968); P.E. Baldry, *The Battle against Bacteria: A History of the Development of Anti-Bacterial Drugs, for the General Reader* (Cambridge, 1965).

36 See David Armstrong, *The Political Anatomy of the Body: Medical Knowledge in Britain in the Twentieth Century* (Cambridge: Cambridge University Press, 1993).

37 See Mark Harrison, *Medicine and British Warfare: The Army Medical Services and the Management of Modern Warfare, 1899-1945* (forthcoming).

38 C.E.J. Herrick, *Of War and Wounds: The Propaganda, Politics and Experience of Medicine in World War I* (unpublished Ph.D. thesis, University of Manchester, 1996).

39 On 'shell shock' see: Paul Lerner, *Hysterical Men: War, Neurosis and German Mental Medicine, 1914-1921* (Unpublished Ph.D. thesis, Columbia University, 1996); Mark Oliver Roudebush, *A Battle of Nerves: Hysteria and its Treatment in France During World War I* (Unpublished Ph.D. thesis, University of California at Berkeley, 1995); Ben Shephard, '"The Early Treatment of Mental Disorders": R.G. Rows and Maghull 1914-1916', in G. Berrios & H. Freeman (eds), *150 Years of British Psychiatry, Volume 2: The Aftermath* (London: Gaskell, 1996), 434-64; Keith Simpson, 'Dr James Dunn and Shell-Shock', in Liddle & Cecil (eds), *op. cit.* (note 3), 502-22; Harold Merksey, 'Shell-shock', in G. Berrios & H. Freeman (eds), *150 Years of British Psychiatry, 1841-1991* (London: Gaskell, 1991), 245-67; Ted Bogacz, 'War Neuroses and Social Cultural Change in England, 1914-22: the Work of the War Office Committee of Enquiry into "Shell-Shock"', *Journal of Contemporary History*, xxiv (1989), 237-56; Stone, *op. cit.* (note 33); P.J. Lynch, *The Exploitation of Courage: Psychiatric Care in the British Army, 1914-1918* (Unpublished M.Phil. thesis, University of London, 1977). For a

fuller bibliography see Paul Lerner & Mark S. Micale, 'Trauma, Psychiatry and History: An Introduction', in Lerner & Micale (eds), *Traumatic Pasts: Studies in History, Psychiatry and Trauma in the Modern Age* (Cambridge University Press, forthcoming).

40 With the exception of: Mark Harrison, 'Medicine', in I.C.B. Dear & M.R.D. Foot (eds), *The Oxford Companion to the Second World War* (Oxford: Oxford University Press, 1995), 723-31; E. Guth (ed.), *Vorträge zur Militärgeschichte, Band II: Sanitätswesen im Zweiten Weltkrieg* (Bonn: E.S. Mittler & Sohn, 1990); J. Bringmann, *Problemkries Schussbruch bei der deutschen Wehrmacht im Zweiten Weltkrieg* (Dusseldorf: Droste Verlag, 1981); R. Valentin, *Die Krankenbatallione Sonderformation der deutschen Wehrmacht im Zweiten Weltkrieg* (Dusseldorf: Droste, 1981).

41 For a recent study of penicillin production during the Second World War, see Peter Neushul, 'Science, Government and the Mass Production of Penicillin', *Journal of the History of Medicine and Allied Sciences*, xxxviii (1993), 371-95. On the use of mepacrine during the war see Mark Harrison, 'Medicine and the Culture of Command: The Case of Malaria Control in the British Army during the Two World Wars', *Medical History*, xl (1996), 437-452.

42 Paul Weindling, *Health, Race and German Politics between National Unification and Nazism 1870-1945* (Cambridge: Cambridge University Press, 1989); Benno Müller-Hill, trans. G.R. Fraser, *Murderous Science: Extermination by Scientific Selection of Jews, Gypsies and Others: Germany 1933-1945* (Oxford: Oxford University Press, 1988).

43 See Sheldon H. Harris, *Factories of Death: Japanese Biological Warfare 1932-45 and the American Cover Up* (London & New York: Routledge, 1994).

44 M. Susan Lindee, *Suffering Made Real: American Science and the Survivors at Hiroshima* (Chicago and London: Chicago University Press, 1994).

45 With the exception of: Anne-Marie Condé, '"The Ordeal of Adjustment": Australian Psychiatric Casualties of the Second World War', *War and Society*, (1997); Terry Copp & Bill McAndrew, *Battle Exhaustion: Soldiers and Psychiatrists in the Canadian Army, 1939-1945* (Montreal: McGill-Queen's University Press, 1990); R.H. Ahrenfeldt, *Psychiatry in the British Army in the Second World War* (London: Routledge & Kegan Paul, 1958).

46 This was also true of other diseases such as cholera and plague, particularly in colonial contexts where military/civilian anxieties overlay racial ones. See, for example, Mark Harrison, *Public Health*

in British India: Anglo-Indian Preventive Medicine 1859-1914 (Cambridge: Cambridge University Press, 1994); David Arnold, *Colonizing the Body: State Medicine and Epidemic Disease in Nineteenth Century India* (Berkeley: University of California Press, 1993).

47 On the CD Acts and related issues see: Douglas M. Peers, 'Soldiers, Surgeons and the Campaigns to Combat Sexually Transmitted Diseases in Colonial India, 1805-1860', *Medical History*, 42 (1998), 137-160; Philippa Levine, 'Venereal Disease, Prostitution, and the Politics of Empire: the Case of British India', *Journal of the History of Sexuality*, iv (1994), 579-602; Richard Davenport-Hines, *Sex, Death and Punishment: Attitudes to Sex and Sexuality in Britain since the Renaissance* (London: Collins, 1990); Frank Mort, *Dangerous Sexualities: Medico-Moral Politics in England since* 1830 (London: Routledge & Kegan Paul, 1987); Judith R. Walkowitz, *Prostitution and Victorian Society: Women Class and the State* (Cambridge: Cambridge University Press, 1980); Kenneth Ballhatchet, *Race, Sex and Class under the Raj: Imperial Attitudes and their Critics* (London, 1980); Edward J. Bristow, *Vice and Vigilance: Purity Movements in Britain since 1700* (Dublin: Gill & Macmillan, 1979); F.B. Smith, 'Ethics and Disease in the Late-Nineteenth Century: The Contagious Diseases Acts', *Historical Studies*, xv (1971), 118-35.

48 See Lutz Sauerteig, 'Militär, Medizin und Moral: Sexualität im Ersten Weltkrieg', in Eckart & Gradmann (eds), *Die Medizin und der Erste Weltkrieg*, 197-226; Mark Harrison, 'The British Army and the Problem of Venereal Disease in France and Egypt during the First World War', *Medical History*, xxxix (1995), 133-158; Bridget A. Towers, 'Health Education Policy 1916-1926: Venereal Disease and the Prophylaxis Dilemma', *Medical History*, xxiv (1980), 70-87; Suzann Buckley, 'The Failure to resolve the Problem of Venereal Disease among the British Troops during World War I', in B. Bond & I. Roy (eds), *War and Society: A Yearbook of Military History*, Vol.2 (London: Croom Helm, 1977); Edward H. Beardsley, 'Allied against Sin: American and British Responses to Venereal Disease in World War I', *Medical History*, xx (1976), 189-202.

1

'Before the World in Concealed Disgrace': Physicians, Professionalization and the 1898 Cuban Campaign of the Spanish American War

J. T. H. Connor

The Cuban campaign of 1898 and the ensuing 'splendid little war' between the United States and Spain was the first major American military operation since the Civil War; it also marked the first time that American troops engaged in formal warfare on foreign soil. Furthermore, it whetted the American appetite for imperialistic activities, now familiar to us through the rhetoric of 'surgical strikes' and 'military incursions' used to describe combat in tropical and desert regions. Tangentially, the Cuban campaign also introduced the United States to the field of tropical medicine, already occupied by other industrialized and 'advanced' nations of the time.

America's physicians quickly became involved in the conflict, but they were to become engaged in a battle on two fronts: first, in the Cuban theatre of operations where they faced new battle injuries caused by modern weapons, appalling sanitary conditions, lack of medical supplies, and epidemic disease such as yellow fever; and second, on the home front in army/political bureaucracy where military medical personnel sought higher rank consistent with their status in civilian life – an extension of the ever-strengthening struggle for the professionalization of American medicine during the Progressive Era.

This discussion analyzes this campaign and its aftermath to show how medical personnel coped with the exigencies of 'modern' warfare through the employment of 'modern' medicine on the battlefield. And, more importantly, it argues that any technologically-based optimism that American doctors displayed was quickly dispelled by widespread criticism in both the professional and lay press – an early example of the powerful effect of the 'media' on both medicine and warfare – which drew attention to physicians' apparent ill-preparedness and incompetence. This tension between potential performance and battlefield reality, however, gave extra stimulus for the professionalizing of American medicine in the Progressive Era, for the relative impotence of military doctors as contrasted with the increasing power of practitioners in civilian life embarrassed American doctors and prompted them to lobby for additional powers within the United States Army. While their public rhetoric of pre-war fear and post-war failure was problematic for American doctors, they nonetheless were able to employ it to their eventual advantage to help forge a consensus in their drive for professional organization at the turn of the century. These actions further strengthened the American medical profession by raising the profile of doctors in yet another facet of American society.

The Context of the Cuban Campaign

A particularly brief conflict, the war between the United States and Spain officially existed for only about eight months; the Cuban campaign itself was even shorter, lasting from late June until mid-July 1898. Briefly, from 1896 tensions between the Cuban people and their Spanish overlords increased to the point of open revolt. Concomitant with this unrest was one particular incident: on 15 February 1898 the United States battleship *Maine* was blown up in Havana harbour, with the loss of 260 American sailors. This event, and the belief that the Spanish were inhumane oppressors, stirred American popular feeling such that diplomatic relationships between the U.S. and Spain became strained. When diplomacy finally failed, President McKinley sent a war message to Congress on 11 April; by the end of April, Congress declared that a state of war had existed between the United States and Spain since 21 April 1898.

America was particularly ill-prepared to enter into a war because her regular army consisted of only 26,000 men who were poorly trained, ill-equipped and scattered throughout the states in small groups. To augment this force, McKinley called for 200,000 volunteers, who were to congregate at mustering-in camps in the southern states. By mid-June, the first contingent of men sailed from Tampa, Florida and reached Santiago de Cuba within a week; thus by 22 June conflict officially began. Other troops followed to other Cuban battle zones and engaged Spanish troops (the total complement of men numbered around 59,000 Regulars and 216,000 volunteers). On 17 July the Spanish Commander surrendered in Santiago, and by late July and early August American troops were returning to their homeland. There the mustering-out of disease-stricken men took place; the Cuban campaign had ended.

Earlier scholars of this war have tended to concentrate on the causes and consequences of the conflict rather than on its conduct. Two major themes dominate their works: American imperialism; and the United States as liberator of Cuba's inhabitants, who were perceived as oppressed and cruelly treated by their Spanish overlords.[1] (These studies are also sprinkled liberally with stories about the heroic exploits of such soldiers as Theodore Roosevelt.) Other historians have studied the relationship between the popular press, public opinion, and the course of the war, focusing in particular on the role of newspaper magnates (for example, William Randolph Hearst) who encouraged their papers to publish sensationalist accounts of the Cuban situation.[2] More recent studies of the Spanish-American war have either sought improved descriptions and explanation of an event generally recognized as 'one of the most important turning points in the national experience',[3] or have singled out specific components of the conflict for analysis. One issue, not surprisingly, is military history. Graham Cosmas fully documents the successes, failures and problems of the American army during the war.[4] Other analyses have centred on the issue of military reform around the turn of the century.[5] And another is medical history. Although an historical study of the role of medicine in warfare is justifiable in itself, the war of 1898 assumes some importance in light of its mortality statistics: for the duration of the entire war approximately 4,000 men died, of whom only about 300 were killed in combat; the remaining 3,700 died of some form of fever (particularly typhoid, malaria, and yellow fever).[6] During the actual Cuban campaign, 1,014 men died: 243 in combat, and 771 of fevers.[7] In other words, 93 per cent of soldiers' deaths in the whole war, and 76 per cent of those in the Cuban campaign were not combat-related, but were, technically speaking, of a 'medical nature'.

Several studies have thus dealt with disease, public health and warfare, especially their relationship in army-camp life.[8] The 'embalmed beef' scandal has also received attention from Edward Keuchel, who described how army politics and rivalries, combined with the general drive of the 'pure food movement', had more to do with the furore surrounding charges that army beef had been adulterated, than did the presence of any untoward preservative in army rations.[9] The most successful treatment of medical issues, however, is Cosmas' *An Army for Empire*.[10] Using especially the multi-volume report of the War Investigating Commission (otherwise known as the Dodge Commission after its chairman General Grenville M. Dodge), which sought to assuage the public outcry of army incompetence and negligence during the war, Cosmas concluded first, that there had been a 'near collapse' of the army medical service, attributable in great part to Surgeon-General Dr. George M. Sternberg, a 'research scientist not an organizer'.[11] Second, problems associated with returning sick troops had been exacerbated owing to a 'mixture of scientific ignorance, misunderstanding between the field commander and his superiors in Washington, and poor distribution of responsibility'. Battle weary, disease-ridden soldiers returned to camps that were either not fully built or lacking essential medical equipment and supplies. Finally, Cosmas notes that specific problems were compounded by the 'complex, fluctuating political and military circumstances of the conflict, the deficiencies of an as yet primitive medical science, and a generation of public and congressional neglect of the Army were the principal causes of the war's waste and disorder'.[12]

Cosmas' conclusions are wholly reasonable, for administrative and communication problems abounded during this campaign, thereby adding to the usual confusion that is part of warfare. But they also invite other questions: Were American doctors prepared for a war, especially in a tropical region; and if so, what was the nature of their preparation? How did military medical men conduct themselves during and after the period of conflict? Did the physicians and surgeons involved in the war effort realize the predicament they were in vis-à-vis fever deaths outweighing combat deaths? Did members of the medical profession offer any explanation, or assume any responsibility for the unfortunate outcome of the Cuban campaign with respect to medical activities? Finally, Cosmas' judgements such as 'scientific ignorance' and 'primitive medical science' prompt reflection on the state of medical knowledge at this time. While his portrayal may appropriately describe medical activity during the American Civil War,[13] it seems problematic for the late 1890s, when such clinical developments as aseptic surgery and x-rays, for example, had become fully integrated into medical practice, thus greatly augmenting the physician's armamentarium. Given Cosmas' interpretation, then, it seems reasonable to ask whether American physicians availed themselves of these innovations.

Yet another issue involves the professional status of American physicians and its relationship to the Cuban campaign and its aftermath. From 1897 to 1898, Surgeon-General Sternberg was also President of the American Medical Association, an organization that was striving to become the lobby group par excellence of the medical profession in the United States. During the last decades of the nineteenth century, too, American doctors increasingly gained autonomy over their occupation with the re-institution of licensing regulations, the beginnings of medical educational reform, and the re-orientation of the general hospital from lay-charity institution to temple of bio-medical science.[14] Hence, it is appropriate to ask whether or not the criticism aimed at physicians in the aftermath of the Cuban campaign (as well as their response to it) was grounded in the changing professional medical climate of the late 1890s. In particular, how did American doctors reconcile their increasing civilian power with the apparent relative disdain displayed towards them in military life?

Major American medical journals reveal much about the attitudes, opinions, and concerns of American physicians about the Spanish-American conflict. Emanating from the medical centres of Boston, New York, Chicago and Philadelphia[15] these journals, while they may underrepresent the views of all regions of the United States, nevertheless, provide insights into issues related to medical professionalization.

The Cuban Campaign Conflict

The new philosophy, tactics and technology of 1890s warfare presented difficulties that American physicians were quick to appreciate. One thoughtful doctor articulated the changing nature of war, with fighting becoming a business in which victory was decided by the side which could 'kill the most men possible in the briefest space of time'.[16] Similarly, the editor of the *Philadelphia Medical Journal* considered war the 'brutes' method of settling disputes." He lamented how 'Hundreds of millions of dollars are eagerly voted to destroy property, create disease, mangle and kill human beings, and if one-hundredth or one-thousandth of this amount were asked of our jingo political bosses for preventing disease and death, the request would be laughed at. How far are we from rationality, religion, or true civilization!'[17]

And the *Journal of the American Medical Association* one month before the declaration of war specifically identified two medical-military problems: lack of time to prepare properly for conflict, and the probable high incidence of disease among invading troops. Two other potential outcomes of modern technology and warfare about which American practitioners had little knowledge and no experience also loomed large. New types of injuries could arise from splinters of steel or flying bolts and rivets from iron-hulled ships; such injuries would differ from those sustained by sailors on earlier wooden-hulled ships. They could also come from the newly introduced small-calibre, steel-coated bullet which, it was believed, was more likely to wound its victim than kill him – thus creating the added problem of an increased number of battlefield casualties.[18]

The *Boston Medical and Surgical Journal* echoed these concerns in several editorials. It seemed inevitable that the 'proportion of severe and fatal injuries would be greater than before, and that minor casualties will be fewer. The crushing and shattering of the head and trunk by flying pieces of shell, or steel torn from the decks or machinery by the missiles striking a modern war ship, result in no trifling injuries...'[9] And, owing to the design and construction of the modern battleship which consisted of 'closed water-tight compartments, narrow and tortuous passages', there was likely to be no safe place for the treatment of wounded personnel; indeed, while such a vessel might 'add to the security of the living, they add also to the danger of the wounded in battle'.[20] Related to this line of thought was the prospect of battle-related neurosis. How would men react in war conditions after being subjected to constant bombardment 'cooped up in extremely small spaces' such as those in torpedo boats and torpedo-destroyers? What treatments might be applied to care for those suffering 'nervous shock'? And, what were the consequences of such trauma for military personnel claiming a disability pension?[21]

Another threat came from disease, especially yellow fever, but this was mitigated by faith that Surgeon-General Sternberg, being as knowledgeable as anyone in the United States about disease, could adequately deal with it. Conventional wisdom held that if proper sanitary regulations were observed along with the prompt isolation of infected troops, then subsequent outbreaks of disease would be controllable.[22] Notwithstanding this general faith, occasionally physicians did express their dissent on this matter.[23]

So strong was this belief that an editorial complained that newspapers discussed yellow fever 'so freely that every volunteer considering his risks thinks less of Spanish bullets than of this dangerous pestilence'. Moreover, 'the danger to our troops has been unnecessarily "exploited" and exaggerated. It should be remembered that the discipline and sanitary administration of a military camp afford the very means of preventing the occurrence of the disease or stamping out its infection if it should be introduced.'[24]

But while physicians pondered and philosophized in these medical journals, the politicians acted. During the last week of April, President McKinley called for 125,000 volunteers, and a month later he called for an additional 75,000; his announcements, of course, affected the medical profession as well. Doctors volunteering for military service had a double duty because even before they might be involved in combat, they were charged with the responsibility of selecting healthy individuals from the enthusiastic bands of young men who flocked to recruiting centres. However, before physicians could select soldiers, they in turn had to be selected by passing 'a satisfactory examination as to character and professional ability before a board of army or civilian surgeons, or both, designated by the Surgeon-General of the Army'.[25] This examination was in two parts:[26] a 'physical'; and a written examination on such subjects as anatomy and surgery, practice of medicine, and materia medica. Supplementing these routine medical areas were the two more specialized topics of hygiene and military surgery. On the question of hygiene, the applicant had to demonstrate his knowledge of camp sanitation, treatment of sunstroke, and ways of determining the salubrity of a water supply. Respecting military surgery, one question in particular stands out: what is the 'effect produced by modern small jacketed bullet [sic], compared with the old large calibre missile?' Such questions, no matter how superficial they might have been, indicate that thought was given to the selection of future army surgeons and the medical problems they were likely to encounter in the Cuban campaign.

New army surgeons who needed to augment their knowledge of such specialized topics could do so easily. Increasingly, journals published timely articles such as 'Special Sanitary Instructions for the Guidance of Troops Serving in Tropical Countries'.[27] Information on yellow fever, unsanitary conditions and the genesis of disease, and appropriate therapeutics abounded in America's key medical journals.[28] Generally, these articles reflected the conventional wisdom of disease etiology by noting that malaria and yellow fever could be transmitted by person-to-person contact or by contaminated water.

With respect to the injurious effect of modern weaponry, Dr. Frank Lydston discussed the 'Probable Influence of the Modern Small Arms Projectile on Military Surgery',[29] offering facts and figures about different calibres, muzzle velocities of bullets, and the different characteristics of bullet wounds. However, Lydston's advice was at best conjectural, for as he himself concluded, it remained 'to be shown precisely what effects will be produced by the new projectile upon the living human body, in actual practice. Shooting at cadavers, bags of sand, and steel armour plates proves but little as regards the power of the modern projectile when brought to bear upon living armed enemies. ...' Another consequence of the newly introduced powerful, small arms and ammunition, was their superior range as compared with their older counterparts. This state of affairs, especially its potential effect on army ambulance personnel, caused several physicians great concern. Dr. Edmund Andrews explained how 'old fashioned muskets' had a short firing range, thus the 'danger belt behind the fighting line was so narrow that the ambulances could be driven up pretty close, enabling the litter-bearers easily to bring the wounded to them'. Now, with the German-made Mauser rifles and powerful shells used by the Spanish troops, the 'danger belt' had been widened, which exposed ambulance crews and litter bearers to enemy fire at almost any time. To assist the litter-bearer overcome this new problem, Andrews advocated the use of a wheeled stretcher based on the design of the rickshaw.[30] There is no evidence that Andrews' suggestion was adopted by the American army for use in the Cuban campaign; indeed, owing to the terrain of Cuba such a wheeled appliance would probably have been of little use, but Andrews' idea illustrates that physicians were indeed contemplating the complexities of modern warfare in general, and the Spanish-American war in particular.[31] Another proposal to assist in treating troops in the battle zone was a mobile operating room. This collapsible, wheeled device would have permitted surgeons to set up an operating facility wherever and whenever it was needed; in effect, this suggestion was a forerunner to the Mobile Army Surgical Hospital (MASH) unit of the twentieth century.[32] Considered collectively, these discussions illustrate the American doctor's ingenuity and concern for his potential military patients; but more importantly, they demonstrate the faith of the American medical profession in technology and the scientific knowledge of the period. To a great extent, their faith was buoyed by medical experience in civilian life. After all, should the American physician of the early 1890s cast his mind back to a generation earlier then great strides would appear to have been made in medical practice. Unfortunately, this faith would only serve to underscore these physicians' disappointment when they became part of the military realm.

In addition to considering potential problems posed by combat in a tropical region, army medical practitioners had to contend with many medical problems even before the troops embarked for Cuba. The regular U.S. Army, which was scattered throughout the states, was supplemented by volunteers, all of whom were to congregate in designated geographic areas for basic training and acquisition of equipment; one such place was Chickamauga Park, Georgia. At this location thousands of men (one camp alone had 50,000) encamped for several weeks with the result that many diseases spread among them. Lieutenant-Colonel Nicholas Senn, Chief Surgeon of the Sixth Army Corps, reported that as of 3 June 1898 the most common ailment was diarrhoea, but there had also been outbreaks of measles, pneumonia and typhoid fever, as well as a number of deaths from cerebro-spinal meningitis. Nevertheless, Senn pronounced the general health of the troops to be excellent.[33] Still, the logistics and associated medical problems of such large numbers posed numerous difficulties, many of which were considered to be the responsibility or concern of the army surgeon. Matters pertaining to diet and rations, footwear and clothing, vaccination, venereal disease, the identification and maintenance of potable water supplies, the disposal of human and other waste, the procurement of medical and surgical supplies, the establishment of ambulance and hospital units, and so on, all had to be addressed by army medical personnel. Problems were compounded when medical personnel themselves contracted debilitating diseases such as typhoid fever: what was sometimes a strained situation then often became wholly untenable.[34]

Three other personnel-related mobilization issues surfaced which reflected broader trends in civilian life. First, was the question of the eligibility of sectarian physicians for military medical service. Although much of the strident antagonism between "regular" physicians and their sectarian counterparts had subsided by the late 1890s, tensions continued to exist between them. More important, however, were the desires of patients to be treated by the physician of their choice; as there were many people – including military volunteers – who believed in the merit of homeopathic treatment, this preference had to be addressed. Accordingly, at least one group of homeopathic physicians visited President McKinley to ask that homeopathic practices be recognized by the United States army and navy. Not only was recognition forthcoming, but a number of homeopathic physicians received surgical commissions; one Illinois regiment alone had three homeopaths.[35]

A second issue concerned the medical role of women in this conflict. As a matter of official policy Surgeon-General Sternberg announced before the commencement of hostilities that no woman would serve as an army or navy nurse in Cuban battle zones; similarly, Red Cross nurses were to be barred from serving in the field. Sternberg made it clear that women in the battle zone were 'an encumbrance to an army mobilized for active operation'; another medical colleague echoed this sentiment, noting that army forces were 'preparing for active service, and [that] female nurses would be

too much of an impediment in operations in the field'.[36] Two
exceptions to this rule did exist, however. Female nurses were
permitted to care for troops in base or non-combat camp hospitals;
in this capacity their skills were appreciated. However, the desirability
of female nurses was very much grounded in a Victorian construction
of womanhood. Senior ranking military surgeon, Nicholas Senn,
compared male and female army nursing, noting that

> Nursing is a woman's place. It is her natural calling. She is a born
> nurse. She is endowed with all the qualifications, mentally and
> physically, to take care of the sick. Her sweet smile and gentle touch
> are often of more benefit to the patient than the medicine she
> administers. The dainty dishes she is capable of preparing, as a rule,
> accomplish more in the successful treatment of disease than drugs
> .... For the time being she takes the place of the absent wife, the
> loving mother or the dear sister at the bedside.[37]

Thus, based on these sentiments at least, the believed inherent nature
of women made them more suitable for certain nursing duties while
excluding them from the more masculine tasks associated with actual
warfare. Needless to say, perhaps, women physicians were also
considered problematic for military service; although Dr. Anita
Newcomb McGee was appointed an Assistant Surgeon to oversee the
selection of women nurses. Even when the United States entered
World War I the acceptability of women physicians for military duty
remained a contentious issue.[38]

In contrast, the final personnel-related issue actually encouraged
the entry of some women to the military. The fear of yellow fever led
to the creation of unique regiments composed only of people
considered immune from the disease, those who had survived an earlier
attack. Accordingly, women having acquired a lifelong immunity to
yellow fever were in demand as nurses; so too were African-Americans.
The identification of 'immunes' as ascertained by their previous
medical history, then, became yet another task for physicians during
this mobilization phase of the Spanish-American War.[39]

In the midst of this hectic personnel and camp-life activity,
another development in the preparation/mobilization phase of the
Cuban campaign was taking shape. Probably the single most
important potential benefit that the medical profession secured for
the treatment of wounded and sick troops during this war was the
hospital ship. Although some attempt had been made to equip ships
for medical service during the Civil War, it was during the Spanish-
American war that vessels were first to be fully outfitted as floating

surgical treatment centres. Over $1,000,000 was spent for the purchase and refitting of two commercial liners which were renamed the *Solace* and *Relief*.[40] The refitting and equipping of these two ships, as well as a third – the Bay State (funded through voluntary donations by the citizens of the state of Massachusetts) – allowed the accommodations of up to 500 patients each. Moreover, these vessels were better equipped than many hospitals in North America as, for example, the *Solace* boasted two operating room tables, modern appliances to accommodate aseptic surgery, and surgical instruments of the 'latest and most approved patterns, and of the best construction'. The *Relief* also housed its own x-ray facilities, dark room, bacteriology laboratory, microscopic and other equipment suitable for haematological analyses. Generally speaking, the medical complement consisted of about 20 personnel including four surgeons, four apothecaries, and a dozen or so nurses and attendants.[41]

It was probably with thoughts of innovations such as the *Solace* and the *Relief,* and the knowledge that the army surgeons selected for this campaign were familiar with sanitation procedures, details of tropical fevers and the latest development in bullet wounds and other potential war injuries, that Nicholas Senn, now Chief of Operating Staff, declared in his last letter before leaving for Cuba from Camp Chickamauga that the 'American people expect that the sick and wounded of this war shall receive the best possible attention, and in this they will not be disappointed. The Government, although sometimes necessarily tardy, is willing and anxious to do all in its power to alleviate the horrors of this war ....'[42] Certainly, Senn's reassurance to the American people can be viewed on one hand as a patriotic and rhetorical gesture, but on the other, considerable thought had in fact been devoted to precautionary measures to 'alleviate the horrors' of the Spanish-American war. The extent to which they were adequate and appropriate, however, could only be revealed in the trials of actual conflict.

Owing to the brevity of fighting in Cuba, the time it took to send information back to the United States, and then publish it in medical journals, meant that often clinical accounts were embedded in news of war activities. The 23 July issue of *the Journal of the American Medical Association,* for example, carried news of the Spanish surrender, details of warfare, the outbreak of yellow fever, and sanitary conditions in Cuba, all in the same brief editorial.[43] More specific details of combat conditions were provided by the first wave of invading soldiers and physicians. These accounts clearly relate how from the beginning of the actual campaign, medical and surgical personnel encountered difficulties. In one instance no regimental medical and surgical supplies were unloaded from ships because no horses or mules were available to transport them; later, these same transport ships were ordered out of the harbour, with the result that medical personnel could no longer communicate with them.

Eventually, a launch was procured to which medical supplies were transferred. Owing to these oversights, 'only a percentage' of what was originally an 'adequate' amount of medical supplies was available for actual combat use. The situation was eventually ameliorated with the arrival of the hospital ship *Relief*;[44] however, even the *Relief* could not discharge its duty, for owing to 'some official red tape' the ship was not given an anchorage at first.[45]

On land, events were not going any smoother. One army surgeon complained bitterly about the lack of a good ambulance or hospital corps, contrasting the reality of the Cuban situation with the 'magnificent hospital and ambulance-service on paper'. To buttress his point he noted how wounded American soldiers were 'carried, some in ambulances, of which at first there were but five, but most of them in the horribly rough, springless army-wagons. The sufferings of the poor fellows was pitiable indeed, exposed as they were in most cases to the blistering sun, for those in authority had not taken the trouble to put up the ordinary cover with which the wagons are fitted.' Furthermore, necessity often compelled surgeons to rig up makeshift hospital tents and do the best they could despite their lack of medical and food supplies; patients often lay on the wet Cuban ground protected only by their army-issued poncho, which was as effective 'as an ordinary sieve'.[46] Other difficulties arose owing to the rocky and muddy roads across which supplies, personnel, and wounded soldiers had to be transported.[47]

Another contemporary source also reported the sorry state of troops and surgeons. George Kennan, commissioned by the New York periodical *Outlook* to report on the Cuban battles and the work of the Red Cross, described the following conditions of a Santiago military hospital:[48]

> The hospital ... consisted of three large tents for operating-tables, pharmacy, dispensary, etc.; another of similar dimensions for wounded soldiers; half a dozen small wall-tents for wounded soldiers'.
>
> The resources and supplies of the hospital, outside of instruments, operating-tables, and medicines, were very limited.

There was tent-shelter for only about one hundred wounded men; there were no cots, hammocks, mattresses, rubber blankets, or pillows for sick or injured soldiers; the supply of woollen army blankets was very short and was soon exhausted; and there was no clothing at all except two or three dozen shirts:

That it was wretchedly incomplete and inadequate I hardly need say, but the responsibility for the incompleteness and inadequacy cannot be laid upon the field force. They took to the hospital camp from the steamers everything that they could possibly get transportation for. ... In loading the mules and wagons preference was given to stores and supplies that could be used in killing Spanish soldiers ...[49]

Kennan further described the scene once battle casualties arrived, commenting on the poor care that wounded soldiers received owing to their great numbers as compared with the small number of first aid personnel:

The tents set apart for wounded soldiers were already full to overflowing, and all that a litter-squad could do with a man when they lifted him from the operating- table was to carry him away and lay him down, half naked as he was, on the water-soaked ground. Weak and shaken from agony under the surgeon's knife and probe, there he had to lie in the high, wet grass, with on one to look after him, and no pillow under his head.[50]

Kennan's bitterness over these unfortunate and miserable circumstances is offset somewhat by his support for the surgical staff, who, in his eyes, performed admirably. He reported that the five-man team performed over 300 operations alone in 21 consecutive hours of service.[51] It was also during Kennan's sojourn in Cuba that the outbreaks of fever occurred which, according to one of his sources, affected about 5,000 soldiers in the island.[52]

While the pre-war fears concerning the effects of yellow fever were well-justified, those concerns about the believed disastrous impact of the new, Spanish ammunition turned out to be unfounded. Many surgeons reported how 'clean' wounds were from such Mauser bullets; in most non-fatal cases the point-of-entry and exit of the bullet were similar and often the intervening damage to tissue was minimal. One surgeon reported how it was 'very strange that among all these wounded men there is not a single example of the terrible havoc said to have been caused by this bullet'.[53] And another noted that in several cases the bullet passed through soldiers' skulls without any apparent injury to the brain; such minimally incapacitated men soon returned to duty within two to three days.[54]

Bullets lodged in the soft tissues often spelled death, but in many other instances, wounded men survived and had to undergo surgery to locate and remove them. In these cases, late nineteenth-century 'high-tech' medical techniques were employed to both the patient's and surgeon's advantage. Chief of Operating Staff Dr. Nicholas Senn explained how older diagnostic techniques of locating bullets using a metal probe had been superseded by the x-ray. All wounded soldiers on board the *Relief* had x-ray photographs taken which were then used by surgeons to trace the specific location of bullets. Senn also remarked how this 'large collection of skiagraph pictures [x-ray images] will furnish a flood of new light on the effect of the small calibre bullet on the different bones of the body'.[55] Similarly, a junior medical officer in charge of an x-ray unit observed that while the present war was the first occasion for the Army Medical Department to use this new technology, there were 'great possibilities' for the adoption of radiology in other military field work.[56]

The Cuban Campaign: Aftermath and Post-Mortem

Although a military success, the Cuban campaign was shrouded in much confusion and bitterness because of the many allegations and denials, criticisms, and subsequent defence of the military medical conduct there. The voices raised came from all quarters: the general public, the press, the military, and the medical profession. Coupled with this 'post-mortem' process was the problem of transporting the thousands of dead, dying, sick, and generally debilitated soldiers from Cuba back to their homeland – a procedure that was much more demanding and complicated than their transportation to Cuba, owing to their poor state of health. Furthermore, upon the troops' arrival in the United States, they would be isolated not only for their own benefit, but also for the apparent protection of other American citizens who began to fear outbreaks of epidemics of tropical diseases. To add further strain to the army medical community, its members had to aid in mustering out the soldiers. It was these convoluted and conflicting issues that constituted the aftermath of the Cuban campaign.

Before the troops in Cuba could return to America, those who were ill had to be separated from those who were apparently healthy. Eventually Surgeon-General Sternberg issued a set of instructions dealing with this problem in which he drew attention to the need for medically observing troops, disinfecting suspected 'personal effects capable of conveying infection,' and loading troopships in daylight under the supervision of surgeons. Concurrent with this action was the decision that Montauk Point on Long Island, New York become the main disembarkation centre, which would provide temporary troop accommodation, disinfection and isolation facilities for yellow fever victims and others, as well as other hospital care and treatment for wounded soldiers. Such precautionary measures were viewed in a good light and at least one physician editor anticipated that the transfer of troops would be accomplished without 'mishap to itself [the army] or to the country'.[57] The camp at Montauk also saw the mustering-out process which now included a physical examination of officers and enlisted men, a procedure also designed to facilitate the settlement of pension claims in a way equitable to both the claimant and the government.[58] There can be little doubt that the work load of the army surgeons, even in this final stage, continued to be onerous.

By the last few days of August, the once desolate, marshy plains of Montauk Point had become Camp Wikoff, 'now a great hospital' according to Lt. Col. Senn. Indeed the whole peninsula had evolved into a 'tented field' where all troops arriving from Cuba had to comply with quarantine regulations; not surprisingly, the area soon became overcrowded, with the makeshift general hospital accommodating between 1,000 to 1,500 patients.[59]

Assisting the army surgeons at Camp Wikoff (unlike the field hospitals in Cuba) were 50 Sisters of Charity and 60 trained female nurses. In a subsequent report, Senn observed that the hospital tents were 'going up like mushrooms' and that by 31 August, 2,000 patients were being cared for in the camp. Although prevalent diseases included malaria, typhoid fever, and dysentery with, on the average, about 10 to 14 deaths per day, Senn remarked on the generally healthful environment afforded in the camp.[60] In all likelihood Camp Wikoff suffered from many inconveniences, oversights, and deficiencies; however, given the rapid influx of patients and the limited time constraint in which to design, locate, and build the field hospital, it must be considered to have been an overall success.

The other theme of the Cuban campaign was the questioning of the army's conduct, especially as it related to the health of the troops. The views of George Kennan, the investigative journalist for *Outlook* magazine, were especially acute. In his account of the Cuban affair he asked whether the situation was inevitable or could have been avoided. Based on his observations in Cuba, Kennan starkly concluded that 'owing to bad management, lack of foresight, and the almost complete breakdown of the commissary and medical departments of the army, our soldiers in Cuba suffered greater hardship and privations, in certain ways, than were ever before endured by an American army in the field. They were not half equipped, nor half fed, nor half cared for when they were wounded or sick'.[61] Although many people shared Kennan's opinion, others did not; and between these opposing groups a great deal of friction arose in both the popular and professional presses.

The editors of America's major medical journals especially advanced a wide array opinions on the subject. Most support for the army medical department came from the *Philadelphia Medical Journal*, whose editor, Dr. George Gould, criticized 'amateur newspaper critics' who did not appreciate that war was not 'naturally a strictly hygienic business.' Similar criticism was aimed at 'malevolent' medical journals which had 'taken the cue to be abusive and will not be quieted'.[62] By the early fall of 1898, however, even Gould argued stridently and in a somewhat racist manner against the conduct of the Cuban campaign:

> We stand before the world in concealed disgrace; we were not able to conduct a really small business matter or transport troops and supplies better than a barbarian tribe. Wholly unprepared, we went into a needless and useless war for a worthless lot of corrupt semi-savages, and showed ourselves incapable of buying provisions, or of transporting our men and materials in a land gridironed with railroads and boundlessly rich; we then came home from easy victories over a pitiable enemy to see our highest officials quarrelling among themselves as to who is to blame, like a lot of school-boys. Finally, enraged at our national blundering, and stung by a dividing self-consciousness, the jingoes and yellows now seek to make a scapegoat of the medical departments... But the profession and its journals – those that are genuinely such – must see to it that the scapegoat theory shall be met by the truth.[63]

The *Boston Medical and Surgical Journal*, although more reserved in its criticism, called for an investigation into the many alleged problems. At the same time, the journal felt it unwise to 'dim the glory of a brilliant campaign with unreasonable and bitter complaints'.[64]

Augmenting these criticisms was the aggressive and continued attack mounted by the *Medical Record*. Perhaps because this journal was New York-based and therefore had the most immediate access to information concerning the affairs and treatment of the incoming troops, it was the most virulent in its position. From July to September 1898, numerous editorials lambasted the Army Medical Department in general, and Surgeon-General George Sternberg in particular. The way troops were maltreated both in Cuba and on their return to the United States represented a 'disgraceful object lesson', perhaps a consequence of an incompetent medical department which appeared 'in a very unenviable light'. Moreover, because such poor management reflected upon the entire American medical profession, it behoved Sternberg to initiate a full investigation to identify the responsible party or parties. Grounding its argument on professional embarrassment, the *Medical Record* pressed the point that 'the medical profession of the country demands that our good name and fame may be freed' from any unjust implication of guilt.[65] Clearly, and repeatedly, such editorials viewed the debacle in Cuba as reflecting upon the entire civilian American medical profession; no distinction was made between military doctors and their non-uniformed counterparts. The 'good name' of all doctors had to be cleared.

Not surprisingly, Surgeon-General Sternberg responded to such editorial pressure. In defending both his actions and those of medical men serving under him, Sternberg asserted that, generally speaking, the medical units sent to Cuba had been well-equipped; transportation and landing difficulties meant that supplies were not available when needed – circumstances over which he had no control. Sternberg assumed personal responsibility for any lack of female nursing care, for he continued to believe that female nurses were an 'incumbrance to an army mobilized for active operations'. Finally, he chastised colleagues who had based their opinions on information carried in newspapers.[66]

At first, support for Sternberg and the Army in general came from Nicholas Senn, who wrote from the hospital ship *Relief*.[67] Senn acknowledged there were problems with supplies, but that usually they were quickly coped with. Of the greatest significance for Senn's defence of the Army was the fact that most of the complaints had originated with newspaper correspondents and not from soldiers themselves. Indeed, to the contrary Senn noted that from the troops he dealt with he had 'heard nothing but words of praise for the hard working, self-sacrificing medical officers and the department they represented in the field'.

Despite this defence, only shortly afterward an article by Senn, published in the *Journal of the American Medical Association*, condemned military surgeons. In Senn's opinion full-time, professional army surgeons had become lethargic owing to the monotonous routine of army medical life, were not aware of up-to-date scientific techniques and, generally speaking, were able to lead a fairly relaxed life owing to their rank and comfortable salary. His observations were apparently based on his own experience with army surgeons during the Cuban campaign. Not only did Senn's commentary add yet another dimension to the aftermath of this conflict – a physician openly criticizing his medical colleagues – but it fueled a battle within his own profession. One physician attacked Senn's article as 'unprofessional and unethical, coming as it does from a member and ex-president of the American Medical Association'. Feeling that Senn had violated the spirit if not the letter of the Association's code of professional ethics, this physician suggested that if Senn were a regular army surgeon some of his comments would be punishable by court-martial. Another critique viewed Senn's commentary as absurd, worthless, tasteless, and surprising inasmuch as it appeared 'over the signature of one whose reputation as a surgeon and whose position as the predecessor of the surgeon-general of the army in the presidency of the American Medical Association will give his words, in the minds of many of his readers, all the weight of indisputable authority'.[68] Interestingly, Senn's critics did not challenge the content of his allegations; rather, they were concerned with the professionalism of his whistle-blowing. Again, it is clear that American physicians took this whole debate to heart collectively, for this was a matter of national importance and professional esteem. While there was a desire to debate the issue, some physicians wished to contain the matter within the confines of the profession. For American physicians to air their dirty laundry in print now could easily signal a return to the fractious old days of a preceding generation of medical discord, strife, and public ridicule.

Criticism of the army medical department, however, came from yet another former officer and medical surgeon. In a lengthy published letter William Cuthbertson charged that the medical department was both 'incompetent and inefficient'.[69] To corroborate his claims Cuthbertson listed a number of problems he had experienced while based at Camp Thomas in Chickamauga, Georgia, which included denied access to some medical supplies, lack of others, and poor hospital and sanitation conditions. More importantly, Cuthbertson criticized the nature of army organization. First, there was no high rank for senior medical army officers:

The Surgeon-General only ranks as Brigadier-General; the Deputy Surgeon-General as Lieutenant-Colonel and so on down the line. It goes without saying that men who are sufficiently endowed by nature with brains and ability to enable them to take on elevated positions in this profession cannot be induced to enter the army service, when the highest position they can attain is that of Brigadier-General. We have seen the melancholy spectacle of beardless boys among the combatants ranking men who had grown grey in the medical service.

To remedy this situation, Cuthbertson believed that all medical officers should be elevated a rank to ensure the army would 'attract men of large ability'. While the integrity of Surgeon-General Sternberg may have been challenged here, implicit in Cuthbertson's argument is the notion that the medical department had little clout in the army; by raising their ranks, medical officers could then exercise greater control over medical affairs. Cuthbertson went further to recommend that the medical department should be an autonomous unit within the army framework: it should be 'cut loose from the line, the Quartermaster's and all other departments, and only in the matter of issuing rations should the Commissary be drawn upon'. By adopting this approach, the medical department could and should provide its own transportation of all kinds and also would be able to be apprised of troop movements, engagements, and so. This second suggestion clearly focused on one of the main problems that plagued the surgeons during the Cuban campaign, namely ensuring that supplies were readily available to those personnel concerned, where and when they needed them.

Soon to augment these articles and letters of complaint was a presidential board of inquiry, directed by General Grenville Dodge. At its Chicago meeting[70], for example, four former army physicians gave testimony, all of whom complained about the difficulty of obtaining supplies form the Quartermaster's store. One physician, Dr. Schooler from Iowa, identified an added difficulty during the early period of mobilization, when 'half our nursing force was sick or in the guardhouse for insubordination' at Camp Thomas in Chickamauga. But on the positive side, Nicholas Senn testified that the hospital ship *Relief* was a 'model hospital ship' and that the nursing arrangements were as 'perfect as possible'. Senn also spoke highly of the hospital at Montauk Point and said that it was the 'marvel of this short war'.

Another official analysis of the conduct of the army medical department soon appeared toward the end of 1898 in the form of Surgeon-General Sternberg's *Annual Report.*[71] Of special interest are Sternberg's comments and explanations of the problems already identified by other members of the medical profession and American public. For Sternberg the breakdown of the health of the troops in the transit camps was to be attributed to three factors: first, the age limit of volunteers had been reduced from 21 to 16, a problem because 'military experience shows that young men under 21 years break down readily under the strain of war service; and every regiment had many of these youths in its ranks.' (It should be noted, however, that the average age for volunteers was 25.[72]) Second, Sternberg claimed that 'ignorance on the part of the officers of the principles of camp sanitation and of their duties and responsibilities as regards the welfare of the enlisted men' also contributed to the outbreak of disease. Finally, he attributed the epidemics in part to the debilitated state of the volunteers owing to drunkenness and venereal diseases.[73] Addressing himself to the lack of medical supplies during combat in Cuba, Sternberg admitted that a 'portion was not available for service at the time it was most needed' and explained away this situation by observing 'in general, no opportunity was afforded to land the medical property'. Such an evasive explanation was clearly not designed to comfort the medical men and troops who were once in need of the supplies. The generally vague nature of his report is exemplified by Sternberg's blaming volunteer medical officers for his difficulty in preparing accurate medical statistics of the war: they were 'ignorant of the methods of keeping the records, and many failed to appreciate the importance of what was frequently regarded as "mere paperwork", which had no practical bearing on the welfare of their men.'[74] Nevertheless, Sternberg did acknowledge that by and large his officers did 'meet the demands of the service'.[75] However, in his conclusion, Sternberg made only one recommendation: the addition of 88 men to the medical corps.

The publication of this *Annual Report,* the ongoing investigation by a presidential board of inquiry (the Dodge War Investigation Commission), and the publications in the popular and professional press, did not stem the flow of criticism. Certainly a doctor who again voiced his disaffection was Nicholas Senn, now returned as Professor of Surgery in Chicago's Rush Medical College. In a speech delivered to a National Guard group in Chicago in December of 1898 Senn invoked Aesculapius to criticize the army medical department:[76] 'he shook his massive hoary head in disapproval, not because of what they [the medical department] did, but of what they could not do'. Furthermore,

Esculapius has drawn his own conclusions from the lessons of the war, and now suggests to you and to the people of the United States and their representatives in Congress the absolute necessity of a complete reorganization of the Medical Department. He insists that the rank of our Surgeon-General should be that of a Major-General, that he should be clothed with more executive power, and that he should have his own commissary and quartermaster's departments. He is satisfied if these important changes in the organization of the Medical department are made, that there will be less suffering and deaths from disease should we again be called upon to cross swords with another nation.

One may infer from Senn's and William Cuthbertson's complementary analyses that organizational problems did exist in the medical department vis-a-vis the army as a whole. Underscoring these concerns was a letter sent to the Secretary of War from Dallas Bache (Assistant Surgeon-General), Charles Smart (Deputy Surgeon-General), and Louis LaGarde (Surgeon) requesting that the ranks of medical officers be upgraded because they 'desire their responsibilities to be recognized and to be endowed with as much rank, power and position as officers of corresponding age and experience in the other staff corps ....' Accordingly the Surgeon-General should have the rank of Major-General and that the senior of the assistant-surgeons should be raised to the rank of Brigadier-General.[77]

By the close of 1898 and during the early months of 1899, then, the cataloguing of botched medical activities slowly gave way to more sober analysis of their root cause. With the publication of Sternberg's report and the release of the Dodge Commission's report, a consensus began to form that the army medical department needed major reorganization with centralized power within the army, an overhaul of the army supply system, a complete upgrading of the army medical service with less red tape, an increase in the number of regular commissioned army surgeons who would have increased rank, and so on.[78] This proposed reorganization was, of course, not inconsistent with the general aims and ideals of scientific management and business efficiency being promulgated in the mid-1890s, which were also being applied to medical practice.[79] A move toward the official recognition of these suggestions was initiated by Congressman A.T. Hull, Chairman of the government's Committee on Military Affairs, who introduced a bill to reorganize the whole army, one part of which would have affected the medical department. Although the bill was defeated at this time, a major reorganisation of

49

the army along the lines of Hull's original plan did follow in 1901. Along with subsequent revisions, these changes included the establishment of the General Staff, which helped pave the way for a more efficient and modern army. The medical department also underwent changes when it formed separate corps for each of its constituent units, viz. medical, hospital, army nurse, dental, and medical reserve.[80] There can be little doubt that the impetus for this major reorganization came directly from the medical agitation following the Cuban campaign of the Spanish-American war. (However, even by World War I the relatively low rank of military surgeons remained a debated issue among American doctors.)[81]

Although a considerable part of this discussion has focused on the conduct of American physicians during and after the Cuban campaign, it is not intended merely as an apology for them. Their own publications clearly indicate that physicians attempted at every juncture to acquit themselves in as competent a way as conditions would permit. Thus, it seems unjust to find these doctors culpable of any great acts of medical incompetence. But of greater interest, perhaps, is that the Cuban campaign, and especially its aftermath, is also revealing when viewed against the background of the increasing professionalization of American medicine during the latter decades of the nineteenth century. As historians of American medicine have argued, the medical scene in the United States from the 1880s onward was vastly different from that of the three or so decades preceding. In this later period, strides were taken to reinstitute medical licensing; the extremes of sectarian medicine had subsided; steps were taken to rationalize medical education somewhat; the general hospital was well on its way to becoming transformed; and the American Medical Association was being reorganized to become indeed the voice of American medicine. In short, the practice and profession of medicine of the Civil War period was vastly different from that of the era of the Spanish-American War. And yet, while American physicians had begun to consolidate their professional goals in many spheres, as has been shown here their power remained relatively weak within the military environment. Hence, it seems much of the criticism and professional embarrassment that surrounded physicians' involvement during the Cuban campaign resulted as much from "professional" pique as anything else. Here was an arena that had been overlooked when expanding the domain of the American physician. That military surgeons were not accorded due respect and power was not only an insult in relation to the army situation, but also to the entire American medical scene. Hence, as many medical editorials observed, the confusion surrounding Cuban affairs reflected upon all American doctors.

Moreover, the literal mobilization of the American medical profession for warfare may also be viewed in a metaphoric way: It probably was no coincidence that the 'mobilization' of doctors in the American Medical Association began in 1899. From this date, the Association's journal developed into an especially aggressive and lobbyist organ on behalf of America's doctors. Simultaneously, the Association also organized committees such as the Committee on Medical Legislation and the Committee on National Legislation which were first steps in the 'establishment of permanent machinery for the advancement of its [the AMA's] political goals'.[82] Although the initial success of these committees was limited, their very establishment and mandate at this time reflects the recognition that doctors had to become politically astute, centrally organized, more business-minded, and aggressive in their tactical and strategic planning. Thus a sector of American physicians soon became engaged in educating their brethren about efficiency, economics, good accounting and so on. For example, Dr. Frank Lydston of Chicago, who earlier wrote on the likely tissue damage of the new bullets in the Cuban campaign, now wrote *about Medicine as a Business Proposition* (1900).[83] Accordingly, the cries for more power and increased status within the military at once both reflected and strengthened the rising prominence of physicians in civilian affairs.[84]

On one hand the clinical activities and aspirations of the military surgeon underscored how far the American medical profession had developed in one generation, while on the other hand his recent plight reminded doctors across the United States that there remained much to be done to consolidate their power in all medical spheres.

Notes

I would like to acknowledge the support of the Hannah Institute for the History of Medicine, Toronto, Canada.

1   See, for example, R.A. Alger, *The Spanish-American War* (New York: Harper, 1901); French Ensor Chadwick, *The Relations of the United States and Spain – The Spanish American War*, 2 vols. (New York: Charles Scribner's Sons, 1911); Walter Millis, *The Martial Spirit: A Study of Our War with Spain* (Boston: Houghton Mifflin, 1931); and Frank Freidel, *The Splendid Little War* (Boston: Little, Brown, 1958).

2   Examples of such works include Marcus M. Wilkerson, *Public Opinion and the Spanish-American War: A Study in Propaganda* (New

York: Russell & Russell, 1932); Joseph E. Wisan, *The Cuban Crisis as Reflected in the New York Press, 1895-1898* (New York: 1934); George W. Auxier, "Middle Western Newspapers and the Spanish-American War, 1895-1898," *Mississippi Valley Historical Review* 26 (1940), 523-34; Charles H. Brown, *The Correspondent's War: Journalists in the Spanish American War* (New York: Charles Scribner's Sons, 1967); and Gerald F. Lindeman, *The Mirror of War: American Society and the Spanish-American War* (Ann Arbor: University of Michigan Press, 1974).

3   David F. Trask, *The War with Spain in 1898* (New York: Macmillan, 1981), ix. See also a more popular account by G.J.A. O'Toole, *The Spanish War: An American Epic – 1898* (New York: Norton, 1984).

4   Graham A. Cosmas, *An Army for Empire: The United States Army in the Spanish-American War* (Columbia, Miss.: University of Missouri Press, 1971).

5   See, for example, Graham A. Cosmas, 'From Order to Chaos: The War Department, the National Guard, and Military Policy, 1898', *Military Affairs*, 29 (1965), 105-21; Cosmas, 'Military Reform After the Spanish-American War: The Army Reorganization Fight of 1898-1899', *Military Affairs* 35 (1971), 12-18; Marvin Fletcher, 'The Black Volunteers in the Spanish-American War', *Military Affairs*, 38 (1974), 48-53; Jerry M. Cooper, 'National Guard Reform, The Army, and the Spanish-American War: The View from Wisconsin', *Military Affairs*, 42 (1978), 20-23; and John B. Wilson, 'Army Readiness Planning, 1899-1917', *Military Review*, 64 (1984), 60-73.

6   Figures cited in James Bordley and A. McGehee Harvey, *Two Centuries of American Medicine 1776-1976* (Philadelphia: W.B. Saunders, 1976), 334.

7   Figures cited in Trask, *op. cit.* (Note 3), 335.

8   See Scheffel H. Wright, 'Medicine in the Florida Camps During the Spanish-American War', *Journal of the Florida Medical Association*, 62 (1975), 19-26; Donna Thomas, '"Camp Hell": Miami During the Spanish-American War', *Florida Historical Quarterly* (October 1978), 141-56; and Robert H. Moser, 'Plagues and Pennants', *Military Review*, 45 (1965), 71-84, especially 77-8. See also Alger, *op. cit.* (note 1), 411-54.

9   Edward F. Keuchel, 'Chemicals and Meat: The Embalmed Beef Scandal of the Spanish-American War', *Bulletin of the History of Medicine*, 48 (1974), 249-64.

10 Cosmas, *op. cit.* (note 4), 245-94. For discussions of later developments of army medical care during the Philippine aspect of the Spanish-American War, see Mary C. Gillett, 'Medical Care and

Evacuation during the Philippine Insurrection, 1899- 1901', *Journal of the History of Medicine and Allied Sciences*, 42 (1987), 169-85; and Gillett, 'U.S. Army Medical Officers and Public Health in the Philippines in the Wake of the Spanish-American War, 1898-1905', *Bulletin of the History of Medicine*, 64 (1990), 567-87.

11   *Ibid.*, 250. Other evaluations of Sternberg are available in two biographies; see Martha L. Sternberg, *George Miller Sternberg: A Biography* (Chicago: American Medical Association, 1920) and John M. Gibson, *Soldier in White: The Life of General George Miller Sternberg* (Durham, N.C.: Duke University Press, 1958).

12   Cosmas, *op. cit.* (note 4), 278.

13   For comparison purposes discussions of military medicine during the Civil War are: Richard H. Shryock, 'A Medical Perspective on the Civil War', *in Medicine in America: Historical Essays* (Baltimore: The Johns Hopkins Press, 1966), 90-108; George W. Adams, *Doctors in Blue: The Medical History of the Union Army in the Civil War* (New York: Henry Schuman, 1952); H.H. Cunningham, *Doctors in Gray: The Confederate Medical Service* (Baton Rouge: Louisiana State University Press, 1960); Horace H. Cunningham, *Field Medical Services at the Battle of Manassas (Bull Run)* (Athens, Ga.: University of Georgia Press, 1968); and William Q. Maxwell, *Lincoln's Fifth Wheel: The Political History of the United States Sanitary Commission* (New York: Longmans, Green, 1956).

14   Useful introductions to the development of American medicine in the period under study include: William G. Rothstein, *American Physicians in the Nineteenth Century: From Sects to Science* (Baltimore: Johns Hopkins University Press, 1972); John Duffy, *The Healers: The Rise of the Medical Establishment* (New York: McGraw-Hill, 1976); James G. Burrow, *Organized Medicine in the Progressive Era: The Move Toward Monopoly* (Baltimore: Johns Hopkins University Press, 1977); John S. Haller, *American Medicine in Transition, 1840-1910* (Urbana: University of Illinois Press, 1981); and Paul Starr, *The Social Transformation of American Medicine* (New York: Basic Books, 1982); and George Rosen, *The Structure of American Medical Practice 1875-1941* (Philadelphia: University of Pennsylvania Press, 1983); Rosemary Stevens, *American Medicine and the Public Interest* (New Haven: Yale University Press, 1971), chapter 3; Ronald L. Numbers, 'The Fall and Rise of the American Medical Profession', in Judith Walzer Leavitt and Ronald L. Numbers (eds), *Sickness and Health in America: Readings in the History of Medicine and Public Health* (Madison: University of Wisconsin Press, 1985), 185-96; and Gerald E. Markowitz and David Rosner, 'Doctors in Crisis: Medical

Education and Medical Reform During the Progressive Era, 1895-1915', in Susan Reverby and David Rosner (eds), *Health Care in America: Essays in Social History* (Philadelphia: Temple University Press, 1979), 185-205.

15   During the nineteenth century many medical journals flourished in America, but most were ephemeral, local, or sectarian in nature; for this study only those of national importance have been consulted. These journals are: the Boston Medical & Surgical Journal (*BMSJ*); the Medical Record of New York (*MR*); the Philadelphia Medical Journal (*PMJ*); and the Chicago-based Journal of the American Medical Association (*JAMA*). Additional information on the American Medical Association is available in James G. Burrow, *AMA: Voice of American Medicine* (Baltimore: Johns Hopkins University Press, 1963) and Morris Fishbein, *A History of the American Medical Association from 1847 to 1947* (Philadelphia: 1947). For other discussions on the development of American medical journalism see: James H. Cassedy, 'The Flourishing and Character of Early American Medical Journalism, 1797-1860', *Journal of the History of Medicine and Allied Sciences* 38 (1983): 135-50; and Elizabeth Knoll, 'The American Medical Association and Its Journal', in W.F. Bynum, Stephen Lock and Roy Porter (eds), *Medical Journals and Medical Knowledge: Historical Essays* (London: Routledge, 1992), 146-64.

16   'The Care of Wounded Soldiers', *BMSJ*, 139 (1898), 47-48.

17   'War', *PMJ*, 1 (1898), 745.

18   'Some Medical Questions of a Possible War', *JAMA*, 30 (1898), 737-38.

19   'The War and Modern Surgery', *BMSJ*, 138 (1898), 431-32.

20   'Care of the Wounded in Action in Battle-Ships', *BMSJ*, 138 (1898), 478-79.

21   'The Accident Neuroses of War', *BMSJ*, 138 (1898), 357-58.

22   'The Coming War in Cuba', *JAMA*, 30 (1898), 993. See also 'Yellow Fever and the War', *MR*, 53 (1898), 701-702.

23   The noted bacteriologist Edwin Klebs wrote that 'water does not act as a propagator of the disease [as] shown by the fact that an epidemic never follows a river downwards, but spreads upward ....' See 'Anatomic Researches on Yellow Fever', *JAMA*, 30 (1898), 881-84.

24   'The President's Call for Volunteers', *JAMA*, 30 (1898), 1120-21.

25   'Mustering in of Volunteer Medical Officers', *JAMA*, 30 (1898), 1132.

26   'Examination of Surgeons for the United States Volunteer Service', *JAMA*, 30 (1898), 1421.

27 R.S. Woodson, 'Special Sanitary Instructions for the Guidance of Troops Serving in Tropical Countries', JAMA, 30 (1898), 1266-68.

28 See, for example, 'The Prevention and Cure of Yellow Fever', *MR,* 54 (1898), 125; "Unsanitary Conditions of Cuba," *MR,* 53 (1898), 810; 'Yellow Fever and the War', *MR,* 53 (1898), 701-702; 'The Yellow Fever Situation', *PMJ,* 2 (1898), 188.

29 G. Frank Lydston, 'Probable Influence of the Modern Small Arms Projectile on Military Surgery', *JAMA,* 30 (1898), 1268-71.

30 Edmund Andrews, 'A Plan to Modify the Japanese Jinrikisha into a Wheeled Litter for Removing the Wounded in Battle', *JAMA,* 30 (1898), 1389-90.

31 The American artist Frederic Remington also designed a wheeled stretcher which he felt might be of use. See 'The Remington Litter-Carrier', *BMSJ,* 138 (1898), 481. For a complete discussion of the evolution of military ambulances, see John S. Haller, Jr, *Farmcarts to Fords: A History of the Military Ambulance, 1790-1925* (Carbondale: Southern Illinois University Press, 1992).

32 L.E. Cofer, 'A Portable Operating-Room for Field Service', *MR,* 54 (1898), 107.

33 Nicholas Senn, 'War Correspondence', *JAMA,* 30 (1898), 1526-29.

34 See 'War Correspondence', *PMJ,* 1 (1898), 1072-74; 1127-29; 'The Condition of the Volunteers in Camp Black and Camp Alger', *MR,* 53 (1898), 845; 'Soldiers' Food – Camp Life: Its Benefits and Hardships', *BMSJ,* 138 (1898), 622-24.

35 See 'Homoeopathists and the Medical Services', *MR,* 53 (1898), 775; 'Sectarianism in the Army', *PMJ,* 2 (1898), 639-40; 'Homeopathy in the Army and Navy', *PMJ,* 2 (1898), 986.

36 See 'Women Nurses Not Wanted By Army', *MR,* 53 (1898), 704; 'Report on the Condition of the Second Army Corps', *PMJ,* 3 (1899), 1007-11; 'The Medical Department of the Army', *MR,* 54 (1898), 213-14.

37 Nicholas Senn, *Medico-Surgical Aspects of the Spanish-American War* (Chicago: American Medical Association Press, 1900), 318-19.

38 'A Woman in the Medical Corps of the United States Army', *PMJ,* 2 (1898), 442; see also Kimberly Jensen, 'Uncle Sam's Loyal Nieces: American Medical Women, Citizenship, and War Service in World War I', *Bulletin of the History of Medicine* 67 (1993), 670-90.

39 'The So-Called Immunes', *BMSJ,* 139 (1898), 149; and Marvin Fletcher, 'The Black Volunteers in the Spanish-American War', *Military Affairs,* 38 (1974), 48-53.

40 'Cost of the Hospital Ships', *JAMA,* 31 (1898), 42. See also Haller, *op. cit.* (note 31), 49-51, 84.

41 'The U.S.A. Hospital Ship "Relief"', *JAMA*, 31 (1898), 312-13; E.S. Bogert, 'The Naval Ambulance Ship "Solace" – Her Purpose and Construction', *MR*, 53 (1898), 698-700; 'Another Hospital Ship', *MR*, 53 (1898), 775; 'Special War Correspondence', *PMJ*, 1 (1898), 1018; 'War Correspondence', *PMJ*, 2 (1898), 4-5; 'The Hospital Ships', *MR*, 54 (1898), 237-38; C.A. Siegfried, 'Hospital Ships. The "Bay State"', *BMSJ*, 139 (1898), 125-28; and Senn, *op. cit.* (note 37), 63-73.

42 Nicholas Senn, 'War Correspondence', *JAMA*, 31 (1898), 79-82.

43 'The War News of the Week', *JAMA*, 31 (1898), 190-91.

44 'Wounds and Disease at the Front', *JAMA*, 31 (1898), 250.

45 'War Correspondence', *PMJ*, 2 (1898), 142-43.

46 'War Correspondence', *PMJ*, 2 (1898), 307-309.

47 'Some of the Difficulties of the Campaign in Cuba', *PMJ*, 2 (1898), 445.

48 George Kennan, *Campaigning in Cuba* (1899; reprint edn Port Washington, N.Y.: Kennikat Press, 1971).

49 *Ibid.*, 131-33.

50 *Ibid.*, 135-36.

51 *Ibid.*, 135.

52 *Ibid.*, 213-14.

53 Robert E. Bell, 'The Effects of the Mauser Bullet', *BMSJ*, 139 (1898), 123.

54 'New York Academy of Medicine', *MR*, 54 (1898), 566.

55 N. Senn, 'Recent Experiences in Military Surgery After the Battle of Santiago', *MR*, 54 (1898), 145-50.

56 H. Lyman Sayen, 'X-Rays in the Army', *PMJ*, 2 (1898), 1305-1307. A special training manual was also produced for the first time as a result of experience gained in this conflict; see W.B. Borden, *U.S. Army X-Ray Manual* (Washington, 1900).

57 'The Return of Shafter's Army', *JAMA*, 31 (1898), 421.

58 'The Mustering Out of the Volunteers', *JAMA*, 31 (1898), 541.

59 Nicholas Senn, 'The Returning Army', *JAMA*, 31 (1898), 652-54.

60 Nicholas Senn, 'The National Cry', *JAMA*, 31 (1898), 654-56.

61 Kennan, *op. cit.* (note 48), 214-15.

62 'Criticism of the Medical Department of the Army', *MJ*, 2 (1898), 248-50; "War's Aftermath," *PMJ*, 2 (1898), 436-37.

63 'The Proposed War-Board Inquiry', *PMJ*, 2 (1898), 525.

64 'The Health of the Army', *BMSJ*, 139 (1898), 200-201; see also 'The Medical Department of the Army', *BMSJ*, 139 (1898), 147-48 and 'The Responsibility for the Conditions of Our Soldiers', *BMSJ*, 139 (1898), 225.

65 'The Army and the Quarantine', *MR*, 54 (1898), 161. See also 'The Wounded After Siboney', *MR* 54 (1898): 161-62; 'The Soldiers and the Medical Department of the Army', *MR*, 54 (1898), 233; 'Who Is To Blame for the Neglect of the Sick and Wounded?' *MR*, 54 (1898), 269; 'The "Medical Record" and the Surgeon General', *MR*, 54 (1898), 271; and 'The Responsibility of the Army Medical Department', *MR*, 54 (1898), 450-51.

66 'Yellow Journalism Rebuked', *JAMA*, 31 (1898), 319-20; 'The Medical Department of the Army', *MR*, 54 (1898), 213-14.

67 Nicholas Senn, 'War Correspondence', *JAMA*, 31 (1898), 361- 63.

68 See Nicholas Senn, 'The Qualifications and Duties of the Military Surgeon', *JAMA*, 31 (1898); 'Disparagement of the Regular Army Surgeons', *MR*, 54 (1898), 378; 'The Qualifications, Responsibilities, and Duties of the Regular Army Surgeon – A Reply to Dr. Senn', *MR*, 54 (1898), 498-99.

69 William Cuthbertson, 'Correspondence - The Medical Department of the Army', *JAMA*, 31 (1898), 421-23.

70 'The War Investigating Committee', *JAMA*, 31 (1898), 1258-60.

71 'The Work of the Army Medical Department During the Spanish War', *JAMA*, 31 (1898), 1356-60.

72 Trask, *op. cit.* (note 3), 157.

73 'Work of the Army Medical Department', 1357.

74 *Ibid.*, 1359.

75 *Ibid.*, 1360.

76 Nicholas Senn, 'Esculapius on the Field of Battle', *JAMA*, 32 (1899), 1-3.

77 'Higher Rank Desired by the Medical Corps of the Army', *JAMA*, 32 (1899), 256-57.

78 'Some of the Medical Lessons of the War', *MR*, 54 (1898), 485-86; 'The Investigating Committee and the Conduct of the War', *MR*, 54 (1898), 486; 'The Work of the Medical Department During the Spanish American War', *MR*, 54 (1898), 809-10; 'Someone Has Blundered', *PMJ*, 2 (1898), 1089; 'The Investigating Committee's Report', *MR*, 54 (1899), 249; 'The Army Medical Department', *MR*, 54 (1899), 251.

79 For background on the connections between 'scientific management' and medicine, see Thomas Goebel, 'American Medicine and the "Organizational Synthesis": Chicago Physicians and the Business of Medicine, 1900-1920', *Bulletin of the History of Medicine*, 68 (1994), 639-63; Susan Reverby, 'Stealing the Golden Eggs: Ernest Amory Codman and the Science and Management of Medicine', *Bulletin of the History of Medicine*, 55 (1981),156-71; Stephen J. Kunitz,

'Efficiency and Reform in the Financing and Organization of American Medicine in the Progressive Era', *Bulletin of the History of Medicine*, 55 (1981), 497-515; Markowitz and Rosner, *op. cit.* (note 14), 187-88; Roger Cooter, 'Medicine and the Goodness of War', *Canadian Bulletin of Medical History*, 7 (1990), 147-59; and Roger Cooter, 'War and Modern Medicine', in W.F. Bynum and Roy Porter (eds), *Encyclopedia of the History of Medicine* (London: Routledge, 1993), vol. 2, chapter 66.

80 'The Proposed Legislation as Regards the Medical Corps of the United States Army', *PMJ*, 3 (1899), 119-120; 'Reorganization of the Army Medical Department', *MR*, 55 (1899), 134; Graham A. Cosmas, 'Military Reform After the Spanish-American War: The Army Re-organization Fight of 1898-1899', *Military Affairs*, 35 (1971), 12-18; Maurice Matloff (ed.), *American Military History* (Washington, D.C.: Office of the Chief of Military History United States Army, 1969; 1973), 346-50.

81 See Jensen, *op. cit.* (note 38), 672.

82 Burrow, *op. cit.* (note 15), 56.

83 See Goebel, *op. cit.* (note 79), 644, n. 15.

84 Similarly, one of the effects of medical military service during World War I was the appreciation by American doctors of 'organized medical work' along cooperative lines. Donald L. Madison writes how surgeons 'participating in the highly organized medical work in the base hospitals of France considered how they might replicate the positive aspects of that experience with some permanently organized formed of civilian teamwork. New private group clinics, drawing on the wartime experience... would gain a foothold that would lead... to their wider acceptance and gradual growth.' See 'Preserving Individualism in the Organization Society: "Cooperation" and American Medical Practice, 1900-1920', *Bulletin of the History of Medicine*.

2

'The Malingerers are to Blame':
The Dutch Military Health Service
before and during the First World War

Leo van Bergen

Introduction

Military and medical history are two of the oldest branches of the discipline but so far there has been little interest in the synthesis of the two. Military historians have often failed to see the point in describing or analyzing medical help in wartime, and medical historians have often lacked interest in military subjects, or have been reluctant to engage in medical military history, for in doing so they would have to describe what some might regard as the less reputable side of the medical profession.[1] A medical doctor working in the army not only has to consider what is medically the right thing to do, but also – and especially in wartime – what is militarily the right thing to do. That these considerations do not always produce the same conclusion will be obvious. A medical doctor has to act according to what is necessary for the physical and mental health of his individual patient. A military man has to act according to what is tactically or strategically necessary. Looking into the history of military medical men, one might conclude that most of them were more concerned with military requirements than with the medical. This explains why – to bring me to my main subject – the history of the Dutch Military Health Service has been almost completely neglected.

It has often been said that following public outrage at the medical disasters of the Crimean War; the introduction of military conscription in most Continental countries; and the foundation of the Red Cross in 1863; healthcare for military men began to improve substantially, and continued to do so throughout the nineteenth and early twentieth centuries. I do not wish to dispute this – in regard to militarily strong countries such as Germany, France and Britain – but it leaves the questions of to what degree it was improved and did military medicine advance more in some countries than in others? Improvement does not necessarily mean that, afterwards, the situation was good or even satisfactory. For instance, during the Gallipoli campaign in 1915 the Royal Army Medical Corps was only prepared for a ridiculously small number of casualties. As a consequence one of the hospital-ships had to carry 600 wounded to Egypt: a journey of four days with just one doctor to attend them, and he was a veterinary surgeon.[2]

This incident makes one wonder about the condition of the military health service (MHS) in countries that had less experience of war, such as the Netherlands. Did expenditure on the Dutch MHS keep pace with military expenditure more generally? Was improvement of weaponry followed by improvement of medical care? What, in other words, was the fate of military medicine in the army of a declining military power, which had withdrawn from most of its prior commitments. That is, of course, except in the colonies, in which the Netherlands, as many other European countries, were still militarily active. But, as one Dutch military doctor stated, military healthcare was not necessary in such countries, for 'there are not many wounded in colonial wars'.[3]

The early years

The Dutch MHS was set up in 1814, shortly after the end of the French occupation. The foundation eight years later of the Royal Training college for military medical men was intended to secure a constant flow of medical men into the army.[4] This could hardly have been called successful in the early years, and sheer improvisation formed the basis of medical assistance during the Belgian uprising of 1830-1831. Every soldier or officer who had ever bandaged a wounded companion was proclaimed a 'health-officer'. Despite their lack of formal training, these men would later, under the protection of King William the III, rise to the top of the MHS and exercise considerable influence in the Dutch Red Cross (DRC). As a result, this humaniatarian society quickly saw a conflict between a conservative, medically-unqualified head and young, progressive and medically-qualified doctors who had to execute his orders. This conflict has never been satisfactorally resolved.[5]

When, in 1848, the Dutch liberal constitution was set up and a liberal cabinet came into power, a period of retrenchment in military expenditure began. The cuts were logical, although, as one might expect, they were contrary to the wishes of the military staff and the (in 1849) newly-crowned King William III. The Netherlands was no longer an important military power and, with the loss of Belgium, its territory had been reduced by almost 50 per cent. The retrenchment ended in 1852 but its legacy did not become apparent until 1870, when the Dutch army mobilised during the Franco-Prussian War. The short-comings of the MHS in 1807-1871 were, however, less a consequence of the cuts themselves, than of the way in which the remaining money had been spent. Up until 1870 the Netherlands, like Great-Britain and France in 1914, had prepared itself for a type of war that was no longer feasible. Sieges were out of date. Armies moved faster as a result of, for instance, the railroads. Firepower had grown immensely. However, this does not mean that all sections of the army kept pace with the rapidly-changing requirements of modern warfare. The Dutch MHS – like other military medical services – was cut disproportionately, losing one-third of its budget up until 1860, even though the costs of treating sick and wounded remained the same. The importance of a good medical service for maintaining morale and manpower had still to impress itself on the government.[6] Another reason for this state of affairs was Dutch complacency in the years before the Franco-Prussian War. The vast majority of the Dutch were convinced that their country would never embark on a war, at least on European soil. This tempered the call for an efficient military medical service: it was believed that there would not be that many sick and wounded to take care of.[7]

This was true not only of the general public but the army itself. Not even the MHS seriously contemplated that they might be involved in battlefield-action in the near future; nor did the majority of those involved in the Dutch Red Cross, founded by William III in 1867 on the advice of his minister of war (partly in order to make good the deficiencies in the MHS).[8] The balance of power, Dutch neutrality, and the supposed impregnability of 'Bastion Holland', seemed to guarantee a peaceful future. Thus, the MHS was ill prepared for its task in times of war. It was said that there was no money to keep the MHS prepared for war in peacetime, and that the MHS probably would never be needed in any case. Problems in times of peace – resulting from epidemics for instance – were to be solved with the cooperation of the civil health service.

Another factor which made for complacency in the MHS was that few of its members had been intent on a military career. Few showed any signs of enthusiasm for active service and the majority had fallen into the MHS because it offered a stable if unremarkable income. Being a doctor in the Dutch army, poorly payed as it was, was a way of eluding hunger and poverty in an increasingly competitive medical marketplace. Most military doctors belonged to the lower classes from which they tried to escape through study at the Royal Training college. It is, therefore, unsurprising that medically and politically speaking they were progressives. A number of them helped to raise the standard of social medicine in the Dutch civilian population, and/or were members of the Society for Hygiene. But, although an important segment of the MHS was interested in military medical reform – and constantly emphasised the threat of war, even in the Netherlands itself – the majority had little interest in reform or wider matters of military policy.[9]

The DRC suffered from a similar lack of support and a shortage of members. It tried to improve its position by seeking more and more cooperation and consultation with the MHS but there was an obstacle to this in the form of the Royal Decision of 19 July 1867, which had brought the DRC into being. This Decision appeared to allow cooperation with the MHS *only in times of war.* A new Decision in 1895 cleared the way to cooperation in peacetime but cooperation between the military and voluntary medical services existed in theory only, and the DRC did not begin to grow steadily until the beginning of the twentieth century, when it was enlarged to help civilian victims of disasters, attaining a membership of 30,000 on the eve of World War II. This peacetime work was undertaken not only because of the hopeless situation in which the DRC found itself but also, and more especially, because it would help prepare for their task in wartime. Although the DRC referred to it as 'peacework', it had more to do with the fact that it took place in time of peace, than that it helped to preserve peace. The above-mentioned conflict between a conservative board and some more progressive sections of the DRC still existed however, and as an organisation the MHS was in a terrible mess.[10] Nevertheless, because of its growth, the DRC became vital to the functioning of the MHS in the event of war. Indeed, the Dutch military medical officer D. Romeyn argued that the DRC should be transformed from an organisation for helping wounded and ill soldiers irrespective of nationality, into one for helping the MHS. The medical officers could do the medical work on the battlefield, the DRC could take care of all the other activities;[11] an arrangemant that was essentially the same as the one that developed between the British and German armies and their respective Red Cross Societies.[12]

The Great War

Romeyn's plea, on the eve of the Great War, for civilian medical assistance suggests that the MHS had improved little since the days of the Franco-Prussian war. The Netherlands apparently had not followed in the footsteps of Germany, which had the largest and best-equipped MHS of all European countries; a Germany that was politically seen as hostile, but at the same time admired ideologically and militarily. The severe criticism which the MHS received in the press as well as in the Second Chamber (which can be compared to the British House of Commons) shows this was indeed the case. It was argued that the situation of Dutch MHS was as pitiable as that of the DRC:[13] an impression confirmed by several articles on the MHS, by the Minister of War N. Bosboom, as well as by medical officers like Romeyn.

Already four years before the violent death of archduke Franz Ferdinand, a commission had been appointed to study the military health service and it had recommended improvements. Members of this commission included Miss G.J. Beynen, matron of the Red Cross-hospital in The Hague, the military doctor C.J. Prins, the right-hand man of MHS-general A.A.J. Quanjer, and Quanjer himself. According to Prins, Quanjer was not only the chairman but also the soul of the commission. That is why criticism on the MHS by press and politics was completely out of line when aimed at Quanjer. Quanjer was asked to advise, which he did, and that his advice was not taken, was not his fault.[14]

Romeyn went even further. In 1912 he had written that not one single member of the MHS was to blame for the faults of the service, for it was the MHS itself that had predicted the abominable situation, and had at the same time recommended a list of measures by which this situation could have been prevented.[15] As a consequence of the professionalization of the MHS at the end of the nineteenth century – military doctors from that moment on had to have a university degree too, as a result of which the Royal training college had ceased to exist – the MHS had to contend with a lack of personnel.[16] This shortage of staff was so great that it was incalculable, even before mobilisation. Already in the previous century it was decided that the MHS should consist of one inspector-general, three directing health-officers first class, fifteen directing health-officers second and third class, and ninety-six non-directing health-officers first and second class.[17] The army as a whole had expanded rapidly during this period, but not only was the number of appointments within the MHS never altered, they were also never completely filled. In the last few years the number of health-officers had even dropped and Reserve health-officers were unable to bridge the gap. Not only were they insufficient in number, they were also unfamiliar with the specific aspects of war surgery. Considering the morale of fighting men, Romeyn believed that 216 non-directing health-officers was the absolute minimum necessary to service the army.[18]

In view of this, it may come as no surprise that a commision for the improvement of the MHS was put together; its aim being to give an overview of the service and to decide if it was really necessary to give female nurses access to military hospitals. As a result of the experience gained in the Boer-War, in which the Dutch doctors and nurses were very much opposed to imperialistic Albion, it was decided in 1910 that this should take place. In practice however, it did not alter very much.[19]

In an article of March 1916, J. Rotgans, former as well as future member of the DRC-council, tried to clear the MHS, as well as the mobilisation-cabinet, of all blame. The shortcomings that had been revealed in August 1914 and the months thereafter, were: 'a result of mistakes made by a list of previous cabinets. In time and under the circumstances they grew to the magnitude that had made the discontent as rampant as it was.' Apparently the MHS had always been 'a unwanted child of the army leaders'. This is not so strange if one considers that medicine was seen as a very civilian profession, which smelled, as far as some combatant officers were concerened, of 'weakness and sentimentality'.[20] Furthermore, the hospital was thought to be a refuge for malingerers, simulators, shammers, slackers and loafers, present in every army when it is composed of men who had to don the military cloth involuntarily.[21]

Bosboom agreed wholeheartedly with the 'unwanted child'-remark, and he also had an explanation. In peacetime the Netherlands had a small army, mainly composed of recruits who were declared healthy. So in the Dutch army there there was little for a doctor to do. This was on the one hand accompanied by a belligerent European atmosphere, which, according to Bosboom, made necessary a strengthening of the military force, whilst on the other hand there was the wish to keep the military budget as low as possible in times of peace. The consequence was that every year there was a laborious debate over the war-department budget. Bosboom asked rhetorically:

Was it under these circumstances strange that the army headquarters primarily kept an eye on the things they thought important for the fighting-ability of the army, and that because of this the needs of an army unit the urgency of which was not daily apparent, came under pressure?[22]

Rotgans and Bosboom were certainly right in so far as on the rare occasions some extra money could be spent, it was not spent on medical care. So, in 1903, it was decided to postpone the building of a new military hospital in The Hague, which, in fact, was urgently needed. Instead the funds were used to pay for the changes in the army, which were a consequence of the militia-law of 1901. In later years new weapons for the artillery, modernisation and expansion of the barracks and improvement of the coastal-defence system were repeatedly preferred above improvements in the MHS. This was furthermore followed by an army-expenditure as a consequence of the militia-law of 1912.[23] Of course, none of the medical services of the fighting armies were ready for the task they had to accomplish in the dreadful war of 1914-1918. The Dutch MHS, however, was, as a consequence of the above cuts, not only unprepared for the expected war, it was not even prepared for the much simpler task that awaited it in practice. This task was described by Bosboom as 'the medical treatment of a large army, which had to be mobilised for a number of years, constantly renewing itself in the course of time, and, as a consequence of the continual expectation in which it existed, was also, from a psychological point of view, a completely different army than a peacetime army'.[24] The MHS had to see to it that, 'in cooperation with the army commander, the men were kept in an excellent physical condition, so that as few men as possible were absent from training'.[25]

Bosboom blamed the malingerers that the MHS did not succeed in ensuring that only a few soldiers did not attend the exercises. It was this group of men he had in mind when he wrote that 'from a psychological point of view' a mobilised army differs from a peacetime army. By feigning an illness or exaggerating a wound, the loafers and shammers – which Bosboom detested from the bottom of his heart – tried to avoid having to march. Bosboom described their attitude as a 'catching army disease', an 'evil that undermined army-discipline'. Unless nipped in the bud, it could easily become a psychic epidemic.[26] According to Bosboom, this army-disease had already obtained unacceptable proportions, so the military doctor had to be a policeman and a medical man at the same time. As a result some of the malingerers went to hospital, and some of the really sick were sent back to the barracks to march and exercise, which did not contribute to their speedy recovery. Furthermore, it was necessary to give some of the work to Reserve health-officers and even to cilivians, who had, quoting Bosboom, 'fewer problems giving in to the complaints of the loafers', because 'they sooner believed the so-called sick than their military collegues'. Apart from this, they were,'at least in the early wartime-days, not completely aware of the responsibility that rested on them from the military point of view'.[27] On top of this, in many cases 'no cooperation in the military interest could be expected from the civilian doctors; far too easily they handed out certificates, and this made controlling visits by military doctors inevitable, with loss of time and withdrawal from more important duties as a consequence'.[28]

According to Bosboom and Prins aproximately 90 per cent of the hospital-patients were malingerers, who on top of that did not even know how to behave themselves. A report published some ten years before the war even mentioned a sickness-percentage of $3^{1}/_{2}$.[29] Of course, all these figures hail from military die-hards, who detested anyone who tried in whatever way possible, to make military life somewhat less trying. Furthermore, doctors were probably more keen to weed out malingerers than their combatant colleagues, since the existence of malingering reflected badly upon them. By emphasizing this problem they could draw attention to the importance of an MHS, an importance so often ignored. A military doctor was not only a doctor but also a detective.[30] But even if horror and frustration made them slightly exaggerate the percentages, it is clear that malingering was a serious problem.

As this debate was going on, in July 1916 a commission was again established to look into frequent complaints made about the MHS. Amongst others the members consisted of the above-mentioned Quanjer, W.F. Veldhuyzen, of the Amsterdam Red Cross Committee, and P.P.C. Colette, who was also a member of the military court of justice, headcommissioner and, in later years, honorary-member of the DRC.[31] The first point of their conclusion was that 'simulators and malingerers wasted time that was badly needed for investigation of the really sick and wounded'. Although the report was published a half a year after his dismissal, it made Bosboom a happy man. The commission was also convinced that the loafers undermined the trust that had to exist between doctor and patient. They were therefore 'jointly responsible for diagnostic mistakes, made towards seriously ill patients'. Also, the addition that simulation and malingering were due to the spirit of the people – to deficiencies of national character – had Bosboom's wholehearted consent. All in all, the report confirmed that, while in office, Bosboom was right to defend himself and the MHS against the most severe criticism. Yes, the MHS was in urgent need of improvement, but this was neither the fault of the MHS, nor of its chief (Bosboom was probably referring to Quanjer rather than to himself).[32]

But Bosboom did admit that the MHS had its shortcomings, and they certainly could not all be attributed to malingerers. At the beginning of mobilisation, the Netherlands had 44 military hospitals for 48 garrisons, to which in 1915 the hospital in Venlo, near the German border, was added. Furthermore it was agreed that 21 civilian and twelve psychiatric hospitals would nurse military sick and wounded also. These numbers do not seem too large, but raw statistics do not tell the whole story. One has to bear in mind that of all the 'military hospitals' only twelve were originally intended for medical use. The 'military hospital' at Utrecht for instance, was a former monastery dating from the fourteenth century, of which a commission set up in 1912 by the minister of war – Colijn – described as 'Unsuitable and beyond improvement'. Roughly the same verdict had already fallen upon the The Hague hospital in 1879, without this leading to alterations.[33] Although, as always, there were exceptions to the rule, the rule certainly was that most hospitals did not meet the requirements of a military hospital at the beginning of the twentieth century. Prins pointed out that even the hospital in Venlo, built in 1915, did not have either a surgical-department or a seperate department for the infectious diseases. Most Dutch military hospitals were therefore obsolete and in urgent need of renovation. The only positive exception to the sorry state in which the MHS found itself was the supply of medical instruments, which were of good quality, although falling short of the quantity required. Moreover, of the hardly abundant staff only half were qualified. Partly because they were allowed to have a civil practice as well, the one-hundred regular doctors of the MHS were so busy that maintaining normal medical knowledge, let alone obtaining specialist know-how, was too much to be asked. Bosboom wrote in his memoirs, which were published in 1930, that:

> Such was the condition on the first of August 1914. That in many ways it fell short, I will not argue. The inspector for the MHS, (Quanjer) did so even less. He wrote a circumstantial account, recommending necessary improvements, which he had handed over

to me. Of course I knew that these improvements would be costly, and that therefore they could only be realized after some years. As a consequence we had to call upon the entire nation for help if the Netherlands was dragged into the war. I trusted that societies and individuals would not hesitate to place their equipment at the disposal of the army, in particular the MHS, and take over the care of the sick and wounded the MHS would not be able to treat.[34]

In 1913, as well as in 1914, the military doctors got a raise in salary to combat the lack of professionel personnel. But, of course, the 72,000 guilders by which the MHS-budget was raised in 1914 could not alter the situation in the short term; even though, after the mobilisation, a considerable effort was made to remedy the situation. The burden fell upon the voluntary sector, and appeals for assistance were responded to enthusiastically; after all, both male and female nurses could now make a 'military' career without having to leave the sickbay. After 1914, another 119 civilian hospital agreements were made for the nursing of soldiers; emergency barracks were built and special hospitals were equipped for jaw injuries and other specialised forms of treatment. Nursing-measures were agreed upon with the DRC, the Order of Saint John, the Order of the Knights of Malta and with the Committee for Immediate Assistance. These voluntary bodies would, for example, take care of sixty emergency hospitals. But even without these hospitals, some 20,000 sick and wounded soldiers could have been accommodated at short notice. The improvement and increase in the numbers of hospitals was constantly worked at, and due consideration was given to the quality and quantity of the MHS's equipment. In 1916 the DRC handed over two ambulance trains to commander-in-chief C.J. Snijders. Personnel increased in knowledge as well as in numbers and, at the end of 1916, the military hospitals had three times more qualified male and female nurses than in 1914. Furthermore, whereas, in 1914, there had been 200 military doctors and reserve-health officers, in 1917 there were 500; not including the civilians who were also were doing their part of that work. On top of that, a health-committee was set up, the chairman of which became Quanjer's hygienic advisor. Yet, in spite of all these efforts, Bosboom had to admit that 'in a few months time the mistakes of years could not possibly be set straight'.[35]

Rotgans saw a way out of the mess. In his 1916 article he advocated the improvement of medical care for soldiers, because a soldier who defended his country – especially in an army of conscripts – simply had the right to be looked after if he got shot. Besides that, if this improvement was not undertaken in peacetime, too great a sacrifice had to be asked from the civilian population in wartime, because of the requisition of civilian hospitals for instance. But an adequate MHS and Red Cross-society were not enough. Military healthcare had to be above strength, so that it would not only have a curing effect, but that it would also contribute to raising the fighting strength of the Dutch army. Rotgans was well aware that pushing the MHS to such untold limits would, to put it mildly, not be easy, especially in these days in which a war was likely to cost not hundreds, but tens of thousands of wounded:

> Even without regarding the duty of the state towards its wounded sons, it will not go unpunished if the value of healthcare for an army is underrated. The curing army (as Rotgans referred to it) has to develop in the same tempo as the fighting army. The insufficient recognition of this demand is severely felt nowadays. The more the work is in arrears, the more impossible improvement gets.[36]

Rotgans' judgement was that improvement without a radical change of the system would be impossible and that reorganization was inevitable. That the authorities, at first, had wanted to wait for a complete reorganization of the MHS until after the war, was understandable. Was not everybody convinced that the war would be over by the Christmas of 1914? But now it was clear that it could go on for years and the press, therefore, pushed for reorganization. Although a part of the Dutch army saw war as the engine of society – amongst them some military doctors – all in all few men wanted the Netherlands to join the war. But one could never know how it developed. If the Netherlands became involved, the MHS had to be ready and therefore reorganization could not be postponed. That was precisely why the DRC had called a reorganization-committee into being after a meeting in 1915 that had got completely out of hand.[37] Local committees were fed up with the authoritarian style of government of the central-committee; a committee that a critical medical doctor typified as being extremely conservative, militaristic and non-medical, very male and very aristocratic in the most negative sense of the word.[38] However according to Rotgans, who was a member of the central-committee of the DRC, the DRC had seen that it had to cut off its roots, not to take the life out of the organisation, but to give new life a chance to come in. The result of the DRC-reorganization was not however a more democratic style of government, but the complete subordination of the DRC to the

MHS. Submission to military doctors had already been the practice in the first years of the war, but it was now made statutory. This meant that the task of the DRC increasingly became that of the MHS. To the extent that it was not already the case, the DRC no longer offered impartial assistance to the sick and wounded of all nationalities, but preferentially to soldiers of the Dutch army. Not medical but military necessity prevailed.[39] Rotgans thought this reorganisation of the highest importance, not only for the DRC, but for Dutch military medical care as a whole. Now that the DRC was reorganised, the MHS could also be rebuilt on new foundations.[40]

To make the total reorganisation of military healthcare a success, certain measures were unavoidable. New hospitals had to be modern and spacious: a well equipped hospital was an inspiration for a mediocre physician and kept the good ones interested and in high morale. Wages had to be improved still further to make the profession attractive, for only then would the best doctors choose the military profession, a profession they had to become acquainted with in a very early stage of their medical education. To accomplish this, Rotgans thought it inevitable that the civilian health care should be militarised in its entirety. Only then would the physicians have the military attitude that was so badly needed, and only then would enough doctors be willing to enter the barracks. This could be achieved if military education started already during their medical education. Medical students would be free of conscription, but were obliged to serve for some time in the medical corps, from the lowest rank of stretcherbearer up to assistant health officer. For the student this had the advantage of going into society as a reserve officer of health, with the knowledge that one would never have to serve involuntarily, unless there was a general mobilisation.[41]

Rotgans estimated that with these measures the army would have about a thousand reserve-health officers at its disposal within ten years. Also, a lot of the students would be willing to become professionals. In peacetime, however , the professional corps would have to be contracted somewhat, to facilitate better wages. As far as nursing was concerned, Rotgans thought female military-medical conscription unavoidable. Women could serve either as a MHS-, or as a Red Cross-nurse.[42]

In spite of all this, it would still be necessary to requisition some of the civil hospitals in wartime. About two thirds of the nursing personnel, and one third of the doctors had to come to the rescue. The difficulties this would bring for nurses and doctors could be met by spreading them equally. Doubtless everybody would accommodate themselves to the circumstances and give up peacetime-privileges without complaining. Rotgans did not say which measures had to be taken to make the civilian patient give up what he called the 'priviliges of peacetime', such as expert care. Not the civilian, but the military patient was his sole concern. As Rotgans stated:

> Maybe after the war, many will be of the opinion that there will never be another war. As a consequence old habits will rear their heads, even more so than before 1914. I hope with all of my heart that this will indeed be the last war, and if the above opinion is well founded, then the army may disappear as well. However, as long as a fighting army is thought necessary, a curing army is necessary. As long as it is necessary to enlarge and strengthen the fighting army, the curing army should be enlarged and strengthened with the best men available from the Dutch medical world and with the best equipment, science and technology can produce.[43]

Rotgans did not see much point in minor improvements in the military-healthcare organisation. Total reorganisation was the only way forward.

Aftermath

What was the result of all this? As far as the MHS was concerned, not much: it fell victim to a large reduction of the ministry of war's budget in 1922; a reduction that was defendable militarily.[44] However, all-in-all, military healthcare would get sufficient attention. Under the leadership of a minimally expanded military-medical corps, more and more tasks were to be handed over to the DRC – although it is questionable whether this organisation could cope with them. As a result, the DRC had to live up to what was officially the MHS's task, even more than already was the case. It was now charged with taking care of the morale and manpower of the entire, national army instead of taking care of the sick or wounded soldier irrespective of the country he had fought for.[45]

Eleven years later the DRC was asked officially to take over completely the care of the sick and wounded in the evacuation-areas. The MHS and the DRC now were, essentially, one organisation. The hierarchical order of military medicine had also become a geographical order. The MHS would work in the direct neigbourhhood of the battlefield, the DRC in the hinterland. Among other things this meant that it was the MHS and the MHS alone that decided which sick and wounded soldiers were or were not taken to the hinterland for further Red Cross treatment. One of the main reasons for setting up the Red Cross – taking care of the wounded the MHS had to put aside because they were of no value to the army anymore – no longer existed.[46]

A mobilisation plan was set up in 1938, in which there was talk of 40,000 sick and wounded soldiers if the Netherlands should become the scene of warfare. To be able to accommodate such numbers, all the hospitals in the evacuation-areas had to enlarge their capacity by 25 per cent and then clear at least $^2/_3$ of the beds. This meant that some 60 per cent of the civilian patients had to leave the hospitals.[47] In Great-Britain, where a similar measure was taken, hospital-almoner C. Morris said: 'Surely never before has a nation inflicted such untold suffering on itself as a precaution against potential suffering. Why should it have been considered less disastrous for anyone to die untreated of cancer, appendicitis or pneumonia than as a result of a bomb?'[48]

However, criticism was unable to make the hospital-boards resist. They adhered to the measures, probably because only an at least partially militarised hospital was entitled to put the protective red cross-sign on its roof. So they were not to blame that the fantastic theory of the mobilisation plan had absolutely no value when it had to be put into practice on 10 May 1940. Not only had the German attackers no regard for the boundaries of the evacuation-areas, they had no intention whatsoever to fight at those places which the Dutch army-headquarters had two years earlier planned to fight. Also, the mobilisation plan was based on the premise that there would be a struggle of many months; instead, within five days, the fighting had ceased. The vast majority of hospital beds had not even been slept in.

Conclusion

Events during the two world wars highlighted what had been persistent weaknesses within the Dutch MHS. Indeed, in World War II it may have been a blessing that the Netherlands was defeated so quickly, considering the state of military healthcare and the problems experienced in mobilising the army in 1914-1918. With respect to the main task of the MHS – taking care of the strength of the entire army, and raising the fighting spirit – it can only be hoped that Dutch soldiers were not aware of its weakness. This weakness was a result of several dilemmas the MHS had to face. It was part of an army that kept on pressing for more and more funds because in its eyes it was too small and too ill-equipped to stand even the slightest change of holding back any aggressor, be it Germany, France, or

Britain. But the Netherlands was no longer the European power it had been some centuries ago. Budgetary restraint was unavoidable and, because the army regarded the MHS as less important than its combatant branches, most of the remaining resources were diverted to other parts of the organisation. This left the army with frustrated doctors who had to work in hospitals which were ill-equipped and under-staffed, and who were regarded by their superiors as second rate. Spotting malingerers was one way in which military doctors could prove themselves of true military stock, hence their virtual obsession with the 'problem' in 1914-1918.

Another way out was to show the military men that nursing and caring were not 'weak and sentimental'. Not only military doctors, but also the civilian doctors of the DRC, cultivated a military air and had few reservation about providing assistance to the MHS. For doctors in the MHS and the DRC, the needs of the army were paramount, not those of the individual soldier. Some even went so far as to suggest a complete militarisation of the medical education in order to prepare civilian doctors for their role in any future war.

But the Netherlands was not Prussia; The Hague not London; and King William III not Emperor Napoleon III. Most Dutch men did not want to engage in fighting and never thought that the Netherlands would ever engage in a war, at least not in Europe. However, the suggestions that were made to get the Dutch MHS out of its misery, were suggestions that suited militarily strong countries, countries that indeed fought wars. The Netherlands in the second half of the previous century, and the first of the twentieth, was anything but a warring country. Politics as well as military strategy were aimed at neutrality and peace, as befitted a declining military power.

Notes

1 See for instance: Fielding H. Garrison, *Notes on the History of Militairy Medicine* (Hildesheim & New York: 1970; 1st edn., 1922), 5, note 1: One of the greatest of modern medical historians, when approached on the matter, replied: 'The subject is distastful to me'.

2 Lyn MacDonald, *1914-1918. Voices and Images of the Great War* (London: Penguin, 1988), 76.

3 D. Romeyn, 'De toepassing van de conventie van Genève in den Zuid-Afrikaanschen oorlog en eenige noodzakelijke wijzigingen en aanvullingen in die conventie', *Orgaan van de Vereeniging ter Beoefening van de Krijgswetenschap*, 1902-1903, 517-614, 529.

4 D. de Moulin (ed.), *Rijkskweekschool voor Militair Geneeskundigen te Utrecht (1822-1865)* (Amsterdam 1988); J.A. Verdoorn, *Arts en*

Oorlog. Medische en Sociale Zorg voor Oorlogsslachtoffers in de Geschiedenis van Europa (Rotterdam 1995; 1st edn., 1972), 192.

5 Conversation with prof. dr. M.J. van Lieburg, 5-9-1990; J.H. Rombach, *Nederland en het Rode Kruis* (Amsterdam: De Bataatsche Leeuw, 1992), 36.

6. W. Bevaart, *De Nederlands Defensie 1839-1874* (The Hague: SMG, 1993), 116, 155, 160, 462-3, 470, 604-605. W. Klinkert, *Het Vaderland Verdedigd. Plannen en Opvattigen over de Verdediging van Nederland 1874-1914* (The Hague: SMG, 1992), 23-4; H. Hardenberg, *Overzigt der Voornaamste Bepalingen Betreffende de Sterkte, Zamenstlling, Betaling, Verzorging en Verpleging van het Nederlandsche Leger, Sedert den Vrede van Utrecht in 1713 tot den Tegenwoordigen Tijd*, part 2 (The Hague: Gravenhage, 1861), 442-3; 'De geneesher op het slagveld', *Onze Tijd*, 5 (1870), part 2, 310-323, 315-16.

7 Bevaart, *op. cit* (note 6), 160; N. Bosboom, *In Moeilijke Omstandigheden, Aug. 1914- Mei 1917* (Gorinchem: J. Noorduyn & Zoon, 1933), 175.

8 Het Roode Kruis en de Amsterdamsche linie', *De Nieuwe Militaire Spectator*, 1874, 188-205, 189.

9 Hoe zal men onze toekomstige officier van gezondheid voor de militaire dienst kunnen behouden', De nieuwe militaire spectator, 1867, 290-294; 'Hoe een toekomstig officier van gezondheid nu reeds over zijne betrekking denkt', *De Nieuwe Spectator*, 1863-1864, 102-105; 'Geneeskundige dienst', De nieuwe spectator, 1855-1856, 463-471, 464; A.H.M. Kerkhoff, 'De militair-geneeskundige dienst en de medische hervormingen in de negentiende eeuw', in De Moulin, *op. cit.* (note 4), 3-16; *Grieven der Geneeskundige Dienst in Nederlandsch-Indië* (1867), 3-5, 50-1; 'Open brief over de geneeskundige dienst in Nederlandsch-Indië', *Tijdschrift voor Nederlandsch-Indië*, 23 (1861), part I-3, 172-86, 173; E.S. Houwaart, *De Hygiënisten. Artsen, Staat & Volksgezondheid in Nederland 1840-1890* (Groningen:Historische Uitgeverij, 1991), 341-50.

10 Leo van Bergen, *De Zwaargewonden Eerst? Het Nederlandsche Roode Kruis en het Vraagstuk van Oorlog en Vrede* (Rotterdam: Erasmus, 1994), 154-160, 174-93.

11 D. Romeyn, 'Iets over ons Roode Kruis', *Het Reddingwezen in Vredes en Oorlogstijd*, 5 (1916), 263-71, 271; D. Romeyn, 'De commissaris van het Ned. Roode Kruis bij de divisieën van ons veldleger', *Het Redding wezen in Vredes en Oorlogstijd*, 4 (1915), 83-91, 88-9.

12 With thanks to Mark Harrison.

13 J. Rotgans, 'De militair geneeskundige dienst', *Algemeen Handelsblad*, 31-3-1916, evening-edition, second paper, 1, column 1-2; Bosboom, *op. cit.* (note 7), 187-196; C.J. Prins, 'De militair geneeskundige dienst van 1 mei 1910 tot 1 mei 1917', *Militair Geneeskundig Tijdschrift*, 21 (1917), 5-10, 9-10.

14 Prins, *op. cit.* (note 13), 5.

15 D. Romeyn, 'De geneeskundige dienst', *Wetenschappelijk Jaarbericht Krijgswetenschap*, 8 (1012), 460-77, 462.

16 De Moulin, *op. cit.* (note 4), 89.

17 In 1860 there was talk of one inspector, two dir. off. of first class, and five of the second class, 33 non-dir. off. of health first class, and 100 second and third class. *Inlichtingen Omtrent den waren Toestand der Militaire Geneeskundigen in Nederland* (1867), 22.

18 D. Romeyn, 'De geneeskundige dienst', *Wetenschappelijk Jaarbericht Krijgswetenschap*, 6 (1910), 412-34, 413-14; o.c., 1911, 428-48, 428.

19 *Ibid.*, 414.

20 Rotgans, *op. cit.* (note 13), column 2.

21 *Ibid.*, column 2.

22 Bosboom, *op. cit.* (note 7), 175.

23 *Ibid.*, 175-6.

24 *Ibid.*, 178.

25 *Ibid.*, 182.

26 *Ibid.*, 183.

27 *Ibid.*, 183.

28 *Ibid.*, 184.

29 D. Romeyn, *op. cit.* (note 18), 416-34, 425.

30 Thanks to Mark Harrison.

31 Bosboom, *op. cit.* (note 7), 196-7.

32 *Ibid.*, 199; J.P. Bijl, 'De militair geneeskundige dienst', *Wetenschappelijk Jaarbericht Krijgswetenschap*, 10 (1914-1919), 474-87, 485.

33 Bosboom, *op. cit.* (note 7), 176-7.

34 *Ibid.*, 177-178 (quotation: 178); E. Kraft, 'Militaire hospitalen', *Militair Geneeskundig Tijdschrift*, 20 (1916), 110-13.

35 Bosboom, *op. cit.* (note 7), 176, 178-82 (quotation: 182); Bijl, *op. cit.* (note 32), 477-82, 484-85; D. Romeyn, *op. cit.* (note 28), 424-25.

36 Rotgans, *op. cit.* (note 13), column 1-2 (quotation: 2).

37 *Verslag der handelingen van de vereeniging Het Nederlandsche Roode Kruis, XXV* (1917), 18.

38 'Tribunus', 'Noodzakelijke reorganisatie van het Nederlandsche Roode Kruis', *De Amsterdammer*, 3-10-1915, 1.

39 Van Bergen, *op. cit.* (note 10), 243-56.

40 Rotgans, *op. cit.* (note 13), column 1-2, 4.

41 *Ibid.*, column 3.

42 *Ibid.*, column 3-4.

43 *Ibid.*, column 4.

44 H. Amersfoort & P.H. Kamphuis, *Mei 1940. De strijd op Nederlands grondgebied* (The Hague: Staatsdrukkerij Uitgeverij, 1990), 54.

45 Van Bergen, *op. cit.* (note 10), 280-94.

46 *Ibid.*, 400-6.

47 *Ibid.*, 401-2.

48 H. Huizenga, 'Het ziekenhuiswezen in oorlogstijd', *Symposia gewijd aan de Vraagstukken betreffende de Bescherming Bevolking en Gezondheidszorg in Tijden van Oorlog en in Geval van Grote Rampen*, 22, (1954), 27-43, 32.

3

Almroth Wright at Netley:
Modern Medicine and the Military in Britain, 1892-1902

Michael Worboys

Almroth Wright held the post of Professor of Pathology at the Army Medical College, Netley, from 1892 to 1902.[1] In subsequent years he became one of the most famous, some would say infamous, medical scientists of his generation. He was the inspiration for the character of Sir Colenso Rigeon in George Bernard Shaw's play *The Doctor's Dilemma* and was the leading candidate to be the first head of the National Institute of Medical Research in 1913. However, by then he was already being seen as a flawed genius. His continuing advocacy of vaccine therapy in the face of the scepticism of most clinicians led many to doubt his judgement. Wright's outspoken opposition to women's suffrage and his controversial views on wound healing during the First World further cemented his reputation as an iconoclast. This characteristic emerged during his time at Netley, principally over his advocacy of anti-typhoid inoculations. Many of his biographers have projected his later frustrations on to the entire Netley period and suggest that he was generally held back the hierarchical organisation of an army institution and its conservatism towards laboratory medicine. In addition, Netley was geographically and professionally isolated on the south coast near Southampton. Thus, his creative powers were only able to bloom fully after he moved to St Mary's at the end of 1902.

Yet, while at Netley, Wright established an influential research school known as Wright's Men, and began to build a standing as an immunologist and bacteriologist that eventually led some to believe he would become the 'British Pasteur'. Ronald Hare, in an unpublished biography, argued that Wright's years at Netley were the most significant of his career and that he subsequently continued to develop the programme and style of research forged there.[2] In this chapter, following the lead of Hare and to some extent Cope, I argue that rather than being antithetical to research, the changing culture of the British army and Wright's particular situation was strongly supportive. The number of research programmes that Wright developed can be explained by a number factors. At one end of the spectrum, is the possibility that military medical demands set agendas for mission-oriented research, while at the other was Netley's potential as a green-field facility allowing Wright the freedom, time and resources to pursue curiosity-oriented research.

Wright and his 'Men' did more than research, they also turned ideas into action. The best known application to emerge from his laboratory was anti-typhoid inoculation, but beyond that Wright's men worked on vaccines, diagnostic methods and new therapies. However, I want to argue that Wright's department did more than pioneer clinical research and field trials, and to test the proposition that their work was congruent with, and perhaps anticipated, many of the features that Harrison was identified as typical of the changing role of medicine in twentieth century warfare.[3] Amongst the most important development was medicine's ability to improve 'manpower economy' and new vaccines and treatments certainly promised to keep soldiers at the front or return them there more quickly. Such measures were mostly aimed at the individual soldier rather than requiring the wholesale reform of army life. One way of viewing this programme is that it imported into the army many of the new approaches of civil public health, which had become more technical and aimed to promote personal health.[4] This approach contrasted with the sanitary approach, still dominant in military hygiene, of concentrating on environmental factors and social behaviour. As in civil society, the new policies and methods had the potential for increased surveillance and control of populations. In Wright's hands this meant that keeping records of individual soldiers and the properties of their blood serum was more important than measuring the temperature, rainfall, crowding, or topography of military stations. In this context, army personnel were potential 'recruits' for experimental investigation as individuals, being doubly subordinate to service discipline and medical authority, and collectively as control populations.

The article begins with a brief account of Netley before Wright that leads me to consider the character of 'research' at the School before the 1890s. I next look at the controversies surrounding Wright's appointment and at the research programme and style of work he fashioned at Netley. I then explore the relative importance of Wright's personality and leadership, as against the values and organisation of the army medical service and school, in the establishment and success of the Netley research school. Finally, I look at the introduction of anti-typhoid inoculations and argue, against the existing consensus, that the conditions of army medicine actually facilitated its development, and that its adoption was relatively rapid rather than being delayed by army bureaucracy. In writing about the controversies that surrounded the practice from 1897 to 1909, too many of Wright's biographers and friends have taken the eventual vindication of the procedure as their starting point, which leads them to develop a Whiggish account where anyone expressing any doubt about anti-typhoid inoculation was an enemy of medical science and its progress.

Netley Before Wright

The Army Medical School moved to Netley in 1860 and was sited within the new Royal Victoria Hospital.[5] The Hospital was a large and grand structure, built on the latest 'pavilion principles', with a frontage of over 400 yards, 138 wards and over 1000 beds. The association of school and hospital was typical of British medical education and Netley offered its postgraduate students opportunities to gain clinical experience from its 2-3,000 annual admissions. By the 1890s, the facilities had expanded to include a lunatic asylum, an infectious diseases' block and a women's hospital. The School took two cohorts each year for a four month course. From 1863 the course was also taken by recruits to the Indian Medical Service (IMS) and from 1871 by candidates for the medical branch of the Royal Navy. In the late 1880s, the student body comprised 50% army medical officers, 35% from the IMS and 15% from the Royal Navy. The quality of the intake varied depending on the market for medical graduates and the popularity of service life.

The core staff of the School were its four Professors, each of whom delivered a course in their appointed subject: Hygiene, Clinical and Military Medicine, Clinical and Military Surgery, and the Pathology of Diseases and Injuries Incident of Military Service. The School was home to many distinguished practitioners including the sanitarians Edmund Parkes and James Lane Notter, the surgeon Thomas Longmore, the physician Henry Cayley, and the pathologist William Aitken. From the start the course included practical laboratory work in hygiene, concentrating on water analysis, and in pathology, mostly microscopy. The School had a good reputation for teaching, though not always for the behaviour and dedication of its students who often seemed to be enjoying a sojourn on the Solent rather than an intensive training course in military medicine.[6] The staff were best known as the authors of textbooks, the most famous and widely used being Parkes's *Manual of Practical Hygiene*, first published in 1864. Although written for military medical officers the book was widely used by civil medical officers of health and became the defining document of British sanitary science. While incorporating the new germ theories from the early 1870s, later editions maintained the original structure based on Airs, Waters and Places. William Aitken was the author of a comprehensive medical textbook published in editions between 1863 and 1882, though in his final years he researched and published on the medical uses of alkaloids.[7] Aitken's studies seem to be nearest anyone came to pursuing 'research' at Netley before the 1890s, though Parkes kept the Army Medical Service (AMS) abreast of events, especially in bacteriology, in his synoptic annual reports of developments in the field of hygiene.

The absence of laboratory research from Netley before 1890 was entirely typical of English medical schools. These institutions were dominated by clinicians and lay governors who were, if not hostile to experimental medicine, unaware of its possibilities, or feared the expense and controversies it might create. Laboratory research was associated with vivisection, against which there was considerable public hostility, not only because of cruelty to animals but also because of worries about its brutalising effects of medical students and fears that experiments on animals would lead to experiments on patients.[8] As is now well documented, elite doctors valued 'clinical experience' more than formal learning or experimental instruction at the bench.[9] Indeed, clinical practice was seen as a form of 'research'. It provided a great store of empirical reference material and insights into the origins, processes and management of disease. In the 1880s, partly as a response to the growth of laboratory research, elite metropolitan clinicians formed the Collective Investigations Committee, which through questionnaires published in the *British Medical Journal,* surveyed clinical opinion on controversial questions.[10] The staff at Netley, as authors of textbooks, typified another feature of the nineteenth century medical 'art', its accumulation of knowledge from diverse sources and its synthesis into clinical wisdom.

In the late 1880s the School began to be criticised for failing to offer adequate clinical experience or appropriate training for overseas postings.[11] One problem was that the hospital was no longer receiving the number or variety of cases seen in earlier decades. The Pax Britannica and improving health in tropical stations meant that bed occupancy was down to 30-40 per cent at the end of the 1880s. The IMS, despite James Fayrer playing an increasingly influential role, began to query the expertise of the staff and its ability effectively to instruct in tropical diseases. While the senior staff were significant national figures, many were seen as belonging to an earlier era and good staff were difficult to retain as pay and status were low. Both issues came to a head over the replacement of William Aitken in 1892.

The first choice of the School was Francis Welch who had worked under Aitken in the 1870s and had then served overseas with the IMS.[12] However, Welch turned down the post because the salary offered was lower than that of his IMS rank. Negotiations saw no movement on either side, with the War Office unable to come up with the extra £150 per annum that would have secured the man their medical school wanted. Attention then turned to David Bruce (1855-1931), who had been assistant professor to Aitken since 1889.[13] Born in Australia, Bruce was educated in Edinburgh and himself trained at Netley in 1883. In the mid-1880s, while stationed in Valetta, he made an investigation of Malta Fever (or as it later became known – Brucellosis) in which he identified the micrococcus that caused the disease and showed that it spread from livestock, principally through goat's milk, to military personnel.[14] This work qualifies Bruce to be one of the very few British scientists, or more accurately British-based scientists, who should be in the Pantheon of Germ Discoverers.[15] Thus, he met the criterion of being up-to-date and was already teaching bacteriology at the School. However, Bruce was never a popular figure and may have been a poor teacher. Everyone agreed that he was devoid of any sense of humour and had a manner that was charitably described as brusque. The only extant explanation of why he was passed over was given by Wright, quoted in Leonard Colebrook's biography:

> Bruce he says was "nursing the chair", but [he] loved the bottle and
> the ladies and got himself much disliked so when the chair fell
> vacant everybody voted against him and the Director General had
> no one handy to put in.[16]

This cannot be regarded as a disinterested account as Wright once said that he was 'eternally grateful to Bruce for providing him with his one and only real impulse to hate'. Yet, animosity between the two men does not seem to have emerged until Bruce questioned the value of anti-typhoid inoculations in 1902.[17] That said, few found Bruce easy company, except seemingly Lady Bruce. Their marriage lasted nearly fifty years and she was his constant companion, being his laboratory assistant as well as his spouse.[18] They even died within four days each other in 1931.

Wright was appointed on the recommendation of Professor German Sims Woodhead, with whom he was then working at the Conjoint Laboratories of the Royal Colleges in London – one of the few research laboratories in London. The snub to Bruce must have been immense, especially as he carried on as Wright's assistant until 1894. Wright was six years younger, had no name in pathology, no army experience and little teaching experience, indeed, he had been turned down for the chair of pathology in Manchester for this very reason the previous year. Amongst the protests, one correspondent claimed that 'civilian science' had been preferred to 'army experience'. Insult was added to injury when Wright was appointed as a civil servant and did not take an army rank.[19] It seems that the School's hierarchy and the War Office bent all the rules to obtain their 'research scientist' and to respond to the criticisms made of Netley.

Wright and the Netley Research School

What kind of 'civilian science' did the new Professor of Pathology offer? Insofar as labels mean much, Wright was more of a physiologist than a pathologist, although 'Renaissance Man' may be more apposite. He had degrees in Modern Languages and Literature, as well as Medicine. He had also qualified in law, passed the Civil Service examinations, worked as a clerk in the Admiralty, undertaken part-time research at the Brown Institution and Cambridge, made two research visits to Germany and served two years as Demonstrator in Physiology at the University of Sydney. In Germany he had worked at Cohnheim's laboratory and then with Weigert and Ludwig. At Cambridge he had worked under C. S. Roy and then Michael Foster on diabetes. At the Conjoint Laboratories he was following up studies on the coagulation of the blood by Wooldridge, with whom he had worked in Leipzig.[20] At best Wright would have been seen as one of the new breed of patho-physiologists or experimental pathologists, so his qualifications to teach the Pathology of Diseases and Injuries Incident of Military Service were strictly limited.

There is no doubt, however, that Wright arrived at Netley with a research programme and that this owed everything to his prior work and socialisation and nothing to the 'diseases and injuries incident of military service'. As one former student observed, 'The Blood was the chief object of investigation. [Wright regarded] this as the only *tissue* that could be examined in a living state'.[21] Influenced by

Wooldridge's work on the properties on serum, he was trying to find ways to alter the internal environment of the body and measure the results of different interventions in the spirit of Claude Bernard. This whole approach was reflected in his lecture course which began with instruction of the Histology of Normal Blood and then moved on to the Pathology of the Blood. At one point the War Office actually asked him to say less about blood and teach a more orthodox pathology syllabus. His employers were equally annoyed about his final lecture to students on the 'Physiology of Belief', but he seems to have been allowed the freedom to teach his version of pathology. There are no syllabi for Wright's course, but those of his protégé and successor William Leishman in the 1900s focused on normal and diseased blood, and bacteriology. During the early 1890s, Bruce continued to teach bacteriology and others may have done so subsequently as Wright was always much more interested in the body's response to infections (immunology) than to the infective agents themselves (bacteriology).

The other feature of Wright's teaching was the stress he placed on the laboratory sessions and the acquisition of technique. This emphasis developed out of his experimental approach to the study of the blood as a 'living tissue' and his use of *in vivo* research methods. Students' memories of Wright's classes highlight the long laboratory sessions and the sense of camaraderie these developed. Many students literally became 'blood brothers' as they monitored each other's serum by new micro-methods, becoming both researchers and research subjects. The style of work is illustrated in Wright's laboratory notes from 1896 recording work on Malta Fever. He records the results of attempts to build up immunity levels to create an antiserum in the following subjects, all in a series of experiments:

Goat
Private Murphy
Monkey No. 11, No. 13, No. 14
Surg.-Maj. D. S. (David Semple)
Lt. R. N.
Sgt.-Maj. C. R.
AEW [Wright himself].[22]

Animals, patients, colleagues, and himself – any 'body' was a potential experimental subject to Wright. Self-experimentation was quite common in the late nineteenth century: Koch self-tested tuberculin for toxicity; Pettenkofer tried to show Koch's vibrio was not the cause of cholera by drinking a beaker of water supposed

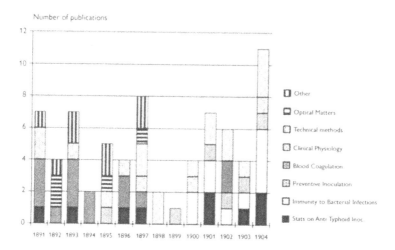

Table 1

Almroth Wright's Publications by Topic, 1891-1904

Source: L. Colebrook, *Bibliography of the Published Works of Sir Almroth E. Wright*, Heinemann, 1952.

containing the germs; Haffkine tried his anti-cholera vaccine on himself. None the less, the fact that Netley was isolated and that his pupils were under army discipline, would have made it easier for Wright to gain the consent and commitment of his colleagues and students to this style of work. Medical research in the twentieth century has often used social groups with circumscribed rights as control populations in medical trials, with military personnel, the mentally ill, the mentally deficient, and prisoners amongst the most common source of 'volunteers'.

To explore the sources and character of the Netley 'research school' it is necessary to look at Wright's output. Table 1 shows the number of Wright's publications in different areas between 1891, when he first began to publish, and 1904, his second full year at St Mary's Hospital. Two points stand out about his record: firstly the diversity of topics he published on, and secondly, that there was no lull in Wright's output during his Netley years. In fact, his rate of output and the foci of his work were erratic, with the only major gap occurring in 1898-99 when he served on the Indian Plague Commission. The high number of publications in 1904 followed his announcement of vaccine therapy.

After his arrival at Netley Wright continued to publish on the coagulation of the blood though the work did move towards diagnostic and therapeutic applications. His aim became that of finding substances that could be added to serum to improve clotting times, control bleeding and perhaps even produce a cure for haemophilia.[23] Inoculations of compounds were tried on animals and human subject, with their effects monitored with new haematological techniques. Interestingly, he does not appear to have worked on the obvious military application of controlling bleeding from wounds. He retained an interest in the topic throughout his time at Netley and was responsible for the entry on haemophilia in Allbutt's and Rolleston's *System of Medicine* in 1909. Teaching only two cohorts each year and without army duties to attend to, Wright was able to publish on colour perception, laboratory technique, serum diagnosis, serum therapy, diphtheria antitoxin, chilblains, colour vision, the emotions, diabetes and the modification of cow's milk for feeding to babies.

The first indication of the influence of army medical problems directly on his research agenda came when Wright wrote on scurvy in 1895 and then went on when opportunities arose to pursue clinical research. His ideas on the nature and cause of scurvy derived directly from his work on the coagulation of blood and how acidity levels and other factors influenced clotting times. His hypothesis was that scurvy was due to 'an acid intoxication' of the blood that was due to an insufficient intake of alkaline foods (green vegetables, tubers and fruits), or the consumption of an excess of mineral acids in the diet. Wright supposed that 'prophylaxis and treatment ... would consist in the administration of salts of oxidisable organic acids', which would restore normal alkalinity.

In 1897 Wright was able to treat one case of scurvy along these lines and in the summer of 1900 a further six cases, most of whom succumbed as a result of the siege of Ladysmith. These soldiers were all severe cases who had not recovered on the normal anti-scorbutic diet on the journey home from South Africa, often because of the consequences of other illnesses, such as typhoid fever. Wright's treatment was preceded by the measurement of the alkalinity of the blood, which in every case was low. Each patient was given controlled oral doses of sodium lactate or tartrate: four men recovered and three died, though none from scurvy as such. What impressed Wright and seemed to support his hypothesis was that in every case, except one where the patient died before the drugs could be absorbed, the alkalinity of the blood increased as acid intoxication was countered. In what later became his trademark, Wright was more impressed by heamatoalkilinity tests showing a return to normal blood pH than by clinical signs of recovery. The novel and important feature of this work which Netley allowed was a controlled clinical trial on a group of patients suffering from a disease brought on by similar conditions. The numbers of patients were small by modern standards, but Wright was never one for statistics and was happy to jump to conclusions because his claims were confirmed by observations on the common physiological milieu of the blood.

Wright's reductionist approach was evident in other research projects. In 1897-98 he published a number of papers on the serum diagnosis of infectious diseases, following the announcement of Widal's diagnostic test in 1896. Wright proposed technical changes which made the test easier and quicker, as well as extending it to Malta Fever.[24] He also introduced an important new principle for the treatment of infectious diseases, namely, to increase power and quantity of anti-bacterial chemicals in the blood. Indeed, this became the test for his preventive vaccinations as was clear in a publication in 1900 which measured the bactericidal properties of the blood of twenty members of that year's class.[25] It should also be noted that Wright's first publication on vaccine therapy was based on work at Netley – the treatment of six patients with boils – and published in the spring of 1902 before there was any hint of his departure.

According to Cope, the appointment at Netley was the turning point in Wright's career as its offered 'a stable position, the use of a good laboratory, suitable assistance and contact with patients in the adjacent hospital'.[26] In addition, Cope maintains that 'his routine duties were not heavy and allowed considerable time for research, while he had as pupils a group of intelligent postgraduates in whom he soon aroused that fiery urge for research he knew so well how to kindle'. Cope immediately describes a number of the key features of a successful research school outlined in Geison's summary of the historical literature on the topic.[27] The factors that studies have shown make for success, defined as establishing fertile and sustainable projects, were as follows:

'Charismatic' leader
Leader with research reputation
'Informal' setting and leadership style
Leader with institutional power
Social cohesion, loyalty, esprit de corps, 'discipleship'
Focused research programme
Simple and rapidly exploitable experimental techniques

Invasion of a new field of research
Pool of potential recruits
Access to or control of publication outlets
Students publish early under own names
Produced and 'placed' significant number of students
Institutionalisation in a university setting
Adequate financial support.

This list provides a mix of the personal and the institutional, which in the case of Wright's Men are difficult to prioritise. Wright became a leader, though this was a role he grew into as in 1892 his inexperienced and lack of reputation were issues in his appointment. There are mixed views about his 'charisma'. By the mid-1890s he was inspiring his students but it is worth noting that those who became 'Wright's Men' constituted only a tiny fraction of the candidates passing through Netley each year. The mature Wright was regarded as prickly, opinionated and far from easy to get on with, but that was the view of his many enemies rather than his friends and followers. Although a civilian, Wright would have had influence from his position in a hierarchical organisation and stories suggest that his department and classes operated a strict regime and long hours. Hare's observation that Wright's Men showed their leader 'loyalty and affection', may be unhelpful as these are sentiments that do not necessarily always go together in the military. Wright brought with him the research programme, though the opportunities and demands of military medicine led him to 'invade' new areas. The army also provided him with recruits, and the ability for these to be placed in key positions to take the reset programme forward. Lastly, the army provided the resources for his programme to flourish and by accident if not design, the time and freedom to pursue a large number of projects.

From Laboratory to Clinical and Field Trials

Wright's Men became known not simply for their research but also for the ways they took laboratory research to the clinic and the field, a trajectory for which the peculiarities of military medicine were critical. Their big project and success on this front was preventive inoculation. Wright first published on this topic in 1893, when he and Bruce reported on Haffkine's method of preparing anti-cholera vaccine. His own work only began in July 1896 after Haffkine suggested using live attenuated organisms to produce a vaccine against typhoid fever. According to Wright himself, he abandoned this line of research and switched to developing a vaccine using killed bacilli, after Richard Pfeiffer of Koch's Institute for Infectious Diseases in Berlin told him that he had obtained a specific immune response in a man inoculated with a heated (killed) culture of bacilli. Such vaccines carried fewer risks and were easier to standardise than attenuated live cultures, and this established Wright's approach to immunity as that of a physiologist rather than a bacteriologist. Working with David Semple, in July 1896 Wright began inoculating himself and 'volunteers' with different dilutions of heated cultures of typhoid bacilli, and used agglutination tests to measure any enhanced immunity produced. He used the serum of convalescent patients form Netley as his standard for the agglutinating power of immune blood and made this a proxy for the effectiveness of the vaccine. This work was first reported incidentally in a paper published in September 1896 on skin rashes and the first full details appeared in January 1897. Wright became involved in a priority dispute with Pfeiffer that remains unresolved, but there is no doubt that it was Wright who pioneered the large-scale development of anti-typhoid vaccination, and that his ability to do that depended heavily on his position at Netley.[28]

Most accounts of the history of anti-typhoid vaccination tell a story of Wright's struggle for the adoption of his vaccine against the indifference and open hostility of the Royal Army Medical Corps and the War Office. The assumption is that the army should have seen the value of preventive inoculation and that prejudice and hostility to medical research, typified by Wright's innovation, delayed the adoption of a life-saving measure. I want to turn this narrative round and argue two points: first, that such resistance to a new medical innovation was quite 'rational', and second, that Wright's campaign for the adoption of his vaccine succeeded exactly because of the opportunities provided by army medicine. Indeed, the speed with which anti-typhoid inoculation moved from first trials in 1897 to a standard, recommended procedure in 1910 was very rapid in comparison with other preventive vaccines. The key to its adoption was Wright's ability to institute field trials however sporadic, and this depended on the co-operation of sympathetic army doctors and their ability to persuade enough 'volunteers' to be guinea-pigs, no mean feat given the general hostility to all forms of vaccination.

The first trial of anti-typhoid inoculations was with a different control population, the staff of Barming Heath Asylum at Maidstone in Kent in 1897.[29] In the same year the Government of India, impressed by the success of anti-cholera vaccine, proposed to the Secretary of State for India, that Wright be seconded to the

Government of India for four months to offer anti-typhoid inoculations to any officer or soldier in India or embarking for service.[30] The proposal was turned down because medical opinion was split, but the letter from the War Office ended by stating that Lord Landsdowne's objection was 'to the formal authorisation of inoculation at public expense than to voluntary operations at private cost'. In 1898 Wright was appointed to the India Plague Commission and spent November 1898 to March 1899 travelling in the country. While there he used the loophole in Landsdowne's letter and persuaded the medical officers in various stations that voluntary trial of his vaccine were permissible. Neither the Government of India nor the head of the Indian Army knew of the trials, which were only made in certain stations. These seem to have been those headed by former students from Netley, in which Wright was allowed to make 'stump speeches' and persuade volunteers to come forward. The vaccines were provided by Wright having been made up and calibrated on trains, and he claimed later to have himself given two thirds of the 4,500 inoculations.[31] When the Government of India learned of the 'trials' they instructed them to be halted. Record keeping was poor or non-existent, but a clear impression grew up in certain section of the Indian Medical Service that the vaccine had worked. This came as much from clinical impressions as statistical returns, as those vaccinated, especially medical officers who ran a higher risk of infection, did not seem to succumb as readily and if they did go down with the disease they had a milder form.[32] In the spring of 1899, Robert Harvey, Principal Medical Officer to the Indian Army recommended dropping the ban on the vaccine with the following qualified endorsement:

> From experiments which have been carefully made, it has been conclusively proved to the satisfaction of those who are best competent to judge of the matter, that anti-typhoid inoculation, when properly carried out, achieves an immunity equal to or greater that which accrues to a person who undergoes and recovers from an attack of that disease.

The Government of India was more fulsome in a letter to the Secretary of State for India, Lord Landsdowne, in May 1899. This stated that 'we are very strongly of the opinion that a more extended trial should be made ... and we trust your lordship will permit to approve the inoculation at public expense, of all British officers and soldiers who may voluntarily submit themselves'. Policy was changed, leading to a further 5,999 men being inoculated in 1900 and 4,883 in 1901.

The policy recommended by the Government of India was also adopted for the whole army as after the outbreak of the South African War in October 1899, anti-typhoid inoculations were available on a voluntary basis to officers and troops. Wright's department supplied the vaccines and advice on when and how to vaccinate. The latter considerations had become an important matter for two reasons: firstly, many people reacted badly to the inoculation, suffering a local skin reaction and a short-lived bout of a flu-like illness, and secondly, Wright was now identifying what became known as the 'negative phase', a period immediately after inoculation when immunity was diminished before it became enhanced. This meant inoculation had to occur before than there was any chance of exposure, ideally before embarkation or during the voyage to South Africa, and that Wright's vaccine could not be used during an epidemic as it made men more vulnerable to infection in the short-term. A further complication was that Wright was now recommending a second booster inoculation for greater protection. This had to be made well after the first to avoid the negative phase, but itself produced a second 'negative phase' and further period of increased susceptibility.

Whatever the risks, the army authorities allowed inoculations to be given by medical officers who wanted to bother and to men willing to submit. Everything depended on the extent to which individual medical officers took up the cause, with inoculation rates of over 50% in some regiments, against an final average of under 5% for the War overall.[33] In the early months of 1900 a number of Parliamentary questions were tabled in that attempted to put pressure on the army to make the inoculations compulsory, but each was rebutted by the claim that its trial was still in progress. The practice did not become an issue until the summer of 1900 when William Burdett Coutts launched his attack on the performance of the army medical service in the War. His revelations focused on hospital conditions and how appalling conditions had led to outbreaks of typhoid fever. A Parliamentary debate followed and then Royal Commission was appointed which eventually reported in February 1901.[34] Anti-typhoid inoculation came to the fore when following a letter from Arthur Conan Doyle in the *BMJ* on 7 July 1900. He boldly stated that there was one mistake made in the campaign so far, 'Inoculation against enteric fever was not made compulsory'.[35] The following week Wright published an article in the same journal on the experience of typhoid fever in the beleaguered garrison in Ladysmith, which he treated as a control population.

Using data collected by Royal Army Medical Corps (RAMC) personnel, he showed that of the 12,214 men in the town, 1,705 or 17% had been inoculated.[36] The incidence of the disease amongst the non-inoculated was 1 in 7 and the mortality rate 1 in 32, the comparable figures for the inoculated were 1 in 49 and 1 in 213. Wright introduced many caveats, aware no doubt of opposition to the procedure within the RAMC, before concluding the results were 'encouraging'. The wider debate about typhoid fever continued in the medical press along more traditional lines, with debates about the type of disease, sanitary arrangements, dust and flies, and treatments, with most correspondents studiously choosing to ignore vaccination.[37] Indeed, in July the Director General of the Army Medical Service reportedly told an IMS dinner that while inoculations might reduce the incidence of the disease they increased the mortality rates.[38]

In November, antityphoid inoculations were strongly endorsed by Howard Tooth, who was Assistant Physician at St Bartholomew's, but currently serving as Physician to the Portland Hospital.[39] He reported statistics in favour of antityphoid inoculation that were more favourable than those from Ladysmith. His arguments were not damaged by the fact that four out of the hospital's five doctors had chosen to be inoculated and that clinical experience that it led to a milder disease. However, the most interesting part of his report was his observations that in a mobile campaign in unfavourable conditions, it was difficult to control fevers by 'sanitation only'. This was because of the difficulties in establishing latrines, providing clean water and in monitoring the behaviour of soldiers. Thus, he saw advantages in establishing 'artificial immunity in the individual soldier'. Working from the view that there was considerable variation in natural immunity amongst the population, from none to very high, like Wright, he saw inoculations as raising everyone to a uniform, high immunity 'standard'. On his return home in the spring of 1901, Tooth gave an address on typhoid fever to the Clinical Society of London, in which he again endorsed inoculations and called for it to be given a fair trial.[40] The discussion that followed showed clear differences of opinion on the matter. The two RAMC figures to speak, James, Director General of the AMS and W. J. McPherson, ignored inoculation while Sir Dyce Duckworth called for it to be made compulsory immediately. Wright continued to publicise results from India, Egypt and Cyprus, aided by the fact that the policy of voluntary inoculations always gave a control group and the fact that sympathetic colleagues were publishing their most favourable results. However, he had always to address possible 'fallacies', for example, that those taking the vaccine were a self-selected group, perhaps more hygienically aware and certainly with a higher proportion of officers. It was believed that inoculations were over-reported as many men were unable to distinguish smallpox and anti-typhoid inoculations. Wright's cause was not helped by his response to the side-effects of the vaccine. On the one hand he dismissed these as a price worth paying, but the other he said that he eventual hoped to be able to adjust the strength of the inoculation to each individual's immunological need, after measuring the existing natural bactericidal power of their serum. This implied that in many cases vaccination was probably unnecessary.

All this time, Wright was also assisting in drafting the Report of the Indian Plague Commission. Its delay was beginning to be remarked upon and there were reports of splits between its medical members, Wright and Ruffer, and the remainder over whether medical or lay authorities should administer anti-plague measures.[41] The Commission's report emerged in two stages, Chapter 4 on Haffkine's anti-plague vaccine appeared in May 1900 several weeks ahead of the main report.[42] Overall the recommendations were conservative and the Report attracted little or no attention in London. Haffkine's vaccine was given heavily qualified endorsement, being criticised mainly for not having the same sophisticated bacteriological and laboratory underpinning as antityphoid inoculations. Generally the Report supported the existing control policies, with the only dissent being a minority recommendation from Wright and Ruffer that the registration of deaths be made compulsory. Wright's imprint was also the recommendation that state-funded research laboratories be established. Wright published nothing more on the plague, though he did encourage Glen Liston, another Netley protégé, in his researches on the role of the flea in the transmission of the disease, which set both men against Haffkine and eventually William Simpson.

After the end of the South African War in May 1902, Wright pushed for anti-typhoid inoculations to be made a standard requirement for all troops posted overseas. He had the support of leading metropolitan doctors and the continuing sympathy of the Indian Government. The Medical Advisory Board charged with responding to the proposal considered three options: continuing the present voluntary policy, moving to compulsion, or suspending the practice. The Board asked a Sub-Committee to consider the matter and that group deferred to the opinion of David Bruce. His Report was unfavourable and highlighted many of the problems Wright himself had pointed to: uncertain statistics, the effects of age, preparation and dosage, the 'negative phase', and the need for further research and development. The Sub-Committee recommended suspending the practice pending further research and asked that Wright be asked 'to present to the Board a detailed scheme showing exactly on what lines and with what precautions he would propose that the system should be carried out'. They were also worried about the 'rights' of soldiers and public opinion lest a purported voluntary scheme would, in the context of military discipline, 'be in practice compulsory'.

Wright was angered by the decision, especially as the Board had accepted Bruce's opinion without allowing him to reply. Wright presented his own case in the *Lancet* in September 1902.[43] He claimed a reduction in the incidence of the disease of at least twofold and as high as 28-fold. Case mortality was also halved, which led to an overall minimum of a four-fold reduction in mortality. Wright did not do the calculations but on his figures, if anti-typhoid inoculations had been compulsory and all other factors had been equal, then there would have been 18,000 fewer cases and over 3,000 fewer deaths. Behind the scenes Wright wrote to the Secretary of State complaining about the decision to suspend inoculations and how it had been arrived at. A number of biographers have suggested that Wright then courageously resigned his post and applied for the post of Pathologist and Bacteriologist to St Mary's Hospital, which he gained and took in November. The actual sequence of events is somewhat different, he obtained the St Mary's post and seems to have contemplated retaining the post at Netley as well. This was possible as Netley had closed in that summer and the Army medical School was relocating to Millbank in London. The reasons for this were complex, but a major factor was the medical problems of the South African War and the sense that army medicine was out of touch with important new developments centred in London. However, the Secretary of State for War made it clear that Netley wanted a full-time Professor and that Wright had resigned his post. The controversy over anti-typhoid inoculations intensified in subsequent years, with the Royal Society, Royal College of Physicians, as well as the Medical Advisory Board being drawn in. In 1904, Karl Pearson, aided and abetted by Simpson, challenged the statistical basis of Wright's claims for the success of his vaccine.[44] The result of what became a very public and acrimonious dispute was that Leishman conducted a field trial on the 20,000 military personnel posted overseas between 1905 and 1909, in which half were inoculated and half not. This confirmed that the now improved inoculations gave an six-fold advantage, though this was only sufficient for the army to reinstate its voluntary policy.[45]

Conclusion

My claim in this paper is that during his decade at Netley, Almroth Wright established two major innovations: he created a research school and he pioneered clinical research, clinical trials and field trials. Each of these developments was the product of the interactions of Wright's ideas and drive, and the opportunities and constraints of military medicine. Wright arrived at Netley with a research programme that aimed to understand the impact of disease on the blood, and to use this to help in the diagnosis, treatment and prevention of disease. His new institutional environment led this programme to be directed towards two priorities of military medicine – infectious diseases and scurvy. That same environment also gave him the time, the research personnel and the patients to develop and test different methods. Indeed, Wright made little use of vivisection as he was able to find enough human guinea pigs, as his postgraduate students and patients 'volunteered' to be experimental material. There is no doubt that Wright inspired a generation of students to pursue medical research, but at the pressures to participate in research and clinical trials were stronger than in the civilian sphere. Indeed, Wright used his influence amongst former students and their authority to pursue field trials of his anti-typhoid inoculations. The AMS and IMS were opposed to these measures because they conflicted with the established environmental approach of military hygiene, but there was also unease about whether such trials, to use the modern jargon, were based on 'informed consent'. Wright was seen as rushing from very limited testing to full-scale trials with unproven methods, with soldiers who were possibly being coerced by 'enthusiasts' for Wright's methods into such trials. Military medicine and especially the exigencies of the South African War, gave him and his followers the scope to undertake sufficient testing to make an epidemiological and political case for further testing, if not full-scale adoption. Wright's claims, explicit and implicit, to improve efficiency by reducing morbidity and mortality, to make complex sanitary precautions less important, and to produce a resistant, immunologically standardised, soldier fell on deaf ears. However, these were exactly the attractions that were to become so important to military medicine in the twentieth century.

Notes

1   L. Colebrook, *Almroth Wright: Provocative Doctor and Thinker*, (London, Heinemann, 1954); Z. Cope, *Almroth Wright: Founder of Vaccine-Therapy*, (London, Nelson, 1966).

2   Contemporary Medical Archives Centre (CMAC), Wellcome Institute for the History of Medicine, PP/HAR/C.2. Ronald Hare, *Biography of Almroth Edward Wright*, (Typescript, no date), 3.

3   M. Harrison, 'Medicine and the Management of Modern Warfare', *History of Science*, (1996), 34, 379-410.

4   E. Fee and D. Porter, 'Public Health, Preventive Medicine and Professionalization: England and America in the Nineteenth Century', in A. Wear, ed., *Medicine in Society*, (Cambridge, Cambridge University Press, 1992), 261-75.

5   CMAC, RAMC 1091/1 M. A. Rundle, *A History of the Royal Victoria Hospital, Netley*, (Typescript of draft chapters, no date); 'The Royal Victoria Hospital, Netley', *Army and Navy Illustrated*, (1897), 3; 213-220; N. Cantlie, *A History of the Army Medical Department*, London, Churchill Livingstone, 1974).

6   *Army and Navy Gazette*, (17 August 1895) and (24 August 1895).

7   *Lancet*, 1892, ii, 60.

8   R. D. French, *Antivivisection and Medical Science in Victorian Society*, (Princeton, NJ, Princeton University Press, 1975).

9   C. Lawrence, '"Incommunicable Knowledge": Science, Technology and the Clinical Art in Britain, 1850-1914', *Journal of Contemporary History*, (1985), 20, 503-20.

10 W. Gull, 'An Address on the Collective Investigation of Disease', *BMJ*, 1884, ii, 305-8; T. J. Maclagan, 'On methods of therapeutic research', *BMJ*, 1884, ii, 260-1.

11 Editorial, 'The Government of India and the Netley Course of Instruction', *BMJ*, 1890, ii, 298.

12 Francis Henry Welch, Asst. Prof. of Pathology, Netley, 1871-76; d.25/10/1910.

13 J. R. Bradford, 'Sir David Bruce', Obituary Notices of Fellows of the Royal Society, (1932-35), 1, 79-85. Also see: E. E. Vella, 'Major-General Sir David Bruce, KCB', *Journal of the Royal Army Medical Corps*, (1973), 119, 131-44.

14 D. Bruce, 'The micrococcus of Malta fever', *Practitioner*, 1888, 40, 241.

15 Bruce finds a place in George Rosen's list. but is omitted from most lists of 'microbe hunters', probably because Brucellosis is still predominantly seen as an animal disease. G. Rosen, *A History of*

Public Health, (Baltimore, MD, Johns Hopkins University Press, 1993), 290.

16 Colebrook, *op cit.* (note 1), 31.

17 Bruce and Wright co-authored two articles in the mid-1890s. A. E. Wright and D. Bruce, 'On Haffkine's Method of Vaccination against Asiatic Cholera', *BMJ*, 1893, i, 227, 'A Note on the Staining Reactions of Leucocytes', *BMJ*, 1893, i, 400.

18 Z. Cope, *Journal of the Royal Army Medical Corps*, (1961), 107, 2-8. Cope makes the common observation that Lady Bruce did most of the laboratory work as her husband was too clumsy.

19 E. K. Campbell, *Lancet*, 1892, ii, 282 and 343.

20 J. Lister, 'On the Coagulation of the Blood in its Practical Aspects', *Trans. Medical Society of London*, (1891), 14, 413-25.

21 CMAC, PP/HAR/C.2. 'Wright's Laboratory 30 years ago', cutting from *New Zealand Medical Journal*, (December 1936).

22 CMAC, WTI/RST/g 5-8.

23 A. E. Wright, 'On the Methods of Increasing and Diminishing the Coaguability of the Blood *in vivo*', *BMJ*, 1894, ii, 57.

24 A. E. Wright, ''On the Technique of Serum Diagnosis of Acute Specific Fevers', *BMJ*, 1897, i, 139; A. E. Wright and F. Smith, 'On the Application of the Serum Test to the Differential Diagnosis of Typhoid and Malta Fever', *Lancet*, 1897, i, 656.

25 A. E. Wright, 'On a Method of Measuring the Bactericidal Power of the Blood for Clinical and Experimental Uses', *Lancet*, 1900, ii, 1556-60.

26 *Op cit.* (note 1), 7.

27 G. L. Geison, 'Scientific Change, Emerging Specialties and Research Schools', *History of Science*, (1981), 19, 20-40.

28 D. H. M. Grosöschel and R. B. Hornick, 'Who Introduced Typhoid Vaccination: Almroth Wright or Richard Pfeiffer', *Reviews of Infectious Diseases*, (1981), 3 (6), 1251-4.

29 *Public Health*, (1897-98), 10, 183.

30 Parl. Papers 1900, East India; Inoculation against Cholera and Typhoid.

31 A. E. Wright and W. B. Leishman, 'Results Which Have Been Obtained by the Antityphoid Inoculations', *BMJ*, 1900, i, 122-4.

32 The Army Medical Report for 1899 reports that during that year of the 4,502 men vaccinated, only 44 or 0.98% suffered from the disease, with nine deaths – case mortality of 20.4%. This compared with 25,851 non-vaccinated men amongst whom 657 or 2.54% suffered the disease, of whom 146 died – giving a similar case mortality of 22.2%.

33 A. E. Wright, 'On the Results Which Have Been Obtained by Anti-Typhoid Inoculation', *Lancet*, 1902, ii, 652-3.

34 *Hansard*, 29 June 1900. Report of the Royal Commission appointed to consider and report upon the care and treatment of the sick and wounded during the South African campaign, (London, HMSO, 1901).

35 A. Conan Doyle, 'The Epidemic of Enteric Fever at Bloemfontein', *BMJ*, 1990, ii, 49-50.

36 This data was based on self-reporting and Wright noted that it might be an overestimate as it was likely that many men would have confused typhoid fever and smallpox vaccinations.

37 *BMJ*, 1900, ii, 51, 114 and 1369.

38 *Lancet*, 1900, ii, 302.

39 H. H. Tooth, 'Enteric Fever in the Army in South Africa, with Remarks on Inoculation', *BMJ*, 1900, ii, 1368-9.

40 H. H. Tooth, 'The Recent Epidemic of Typhoid Fever in South Africa', *BMJ*, 642-8 and 770-3.

41 *Lancet*, 1900, i, 270.

42 *Report of the Indian Plague Commission*, British Parl. Papers, 1902, [Cd. 810], lxxii.

43 A. E. Wright, 'On the Results Which Have Been Obtained by Anti-Typhoid Inoculation', *Lancet*, 1902, ii, 652-3.

44 J. Rosser Mathews, *Quantification and the Quest for Medical Certainty*, (Princeton, NJ., Princeton University Press, 1995).

45 *Journal of the Institute of Public Health*, (1910), 18, 527.

4

'The Conquest of the Silent Foe':
British and American Military Medical Reform Rhetoric
and the Russo-Japanese War

Claire Herrick

From February 1904, to September 1905, 'the eyes of the world' focused on the conduct of the war between Russia and Japan in the Far East.[1] As the first 'modern' war of the twentieth century,[2] fought by 'two highly organised forces'[3], it attracted the close interest of other nations, eager to gain insight into the probable nature of future campaigns.[4] To this end, observers and attachés – military and medical – were appointed to the armies of both beligerents. It was hoped that the war would 'afford information of great value, both in its military and medical aspects'.[5] The performance of the medical services was of particular concern to the British, whose most recent campaign in South Africa had been fought in a colonial context, and to the Americans whose medical arrangements had been found wanting in the Spanish-American War of 1898.[6] For British medical observers, the expectation was that the war would be 'an object lesson to us in the probable working of our own arrangements in the event of a war with a continental power'.[7] It would also afford information on how British arrangements might 'compare in practice and results with the corresponding arrangements of other nations'.[8]

Wastage from disease was expected to be the main problem facing armies in future warfare.[9] Medical interest centred on the management of disease during the war, because, as the *BMJ* explained in February 1904, it was 'an axiom in the science of warfare that bacilli are far more deadly than bullets'.[10] This chapter is concerned with British and, to a lesser extent, American 'observations' of the medical aspects of the Russo-Japanese War, which centred almost entirely on the medical organization of the Japanese Army. But these 'observations' made by would-be reformers of the military medical services, not all of whom were medical men, were not objective accounts of the war in the Far East. Rather they were infused with the rhetoric of military medical reform prevalent in Britain in the second half of the nineteenth century, and heightened by the respective failures of the British and American medical services in the South African and Spanish-American Wars.

Military medical reformers, basing their 'observations' on 'official' reports, communications from correspondents and attaches in the Far East – which were often sketchy and incomplete – as well as on rumour and supposition, constructed a particular image of the war based around the overwhelming 'success' of the Japanese in the conquest of disease. The war was perceived and portrayed by reformers in terms of the 'lessons' which could, and more importantly for them, needed to be learnt by the military authorities of Britain and America.[11] Accounts of the war were prescriptive, more than descriptive, concerned with both the structural and conceptual organisation of the medical services. The events in the Far East were considered and interpreted in light of pre-existing concerns surrounding the 'fitness' and 'efficiency' of armies and their medical services, and the perception that these were no longer separate spheres. This reform rhetoric was directed at the apathetic attitude of the military authorities and the public towards military reform. Concern with military and medical preparedness for war was perceived by reformers to be ephemeral, linked only to immediate 'national crisis'.[12] The juxtaposition of the Japanese conquest of Russia *and* disease, with the failures of Britain and America can be seen as an attempt by reformers to bolster flagging enthusiasm and counter, especially in Britain, increasing resistance to ever-increasing spending on the military.[13]

In essence then, this chapter is concerned not with the medical history of the Russo-Japanese War, but with the selective reporting of events viewed through the eyes of those with the re-organization of military and medico-military structures in mind. Their vision built on a wider appreciation of the Japanese as a race, and amounted to a celebration of the military, medical and cultural attributes that were perceived to be lacking in the West.

The War in the Far East and the Cult of Japan

At the time of the Russo-Japanese War, the Japanese were regarded as a nation Western in ideals, if not in origin. Although the Russians were expected to win the war in view of the size of their army,[14] the Japanese were not seen as underdogs. They had been accorded 'special status' among non-Western nations, being perceived by the

West as an industrial and largely civilised nation.[15] According to the *Lancet*, 'Within the past forty years... Japan has changed from a medieval and feudal country to one imbued with all the advances of modern Western civilisation.'[16] The Japanese had remade 'their society in the image of industrial Europe'.[17] Learning from military advisers of France and Germany,[18] they adopted a conscript army, replacing their traditional reliance on the Samurai.[19] The success of the Japanese in assimilating Western military ideals was demonstrated by their unexpected and emphatic victory over the Chinese in the Chino-Japanese War of 1894-5.[20]

The 1902 alliance with Britain was symbolic of the growing status of Japan.[21] Their military preparations had been spurred by the inevitability of war with Russia, the cause of which lay 'in the basic conflict of two powers anxious to expand their interests and influence in the same region' – Manchuria.[22] Interest in the continued 'awakening' of Japan was sustained during the war against Russia. The opening gambit of the war, a surprise attack by the Japanese on the Russian Far East Squadron at Port Arthur on 8 February 1904, ensured the loss of Russian battleship superiority. It also ensured that the Japanese, rather than their Russian opponents, were the nation to watch during the war.

Reports of the war were characterised by an immense admiration for the Japanese, in particular, their ability to adopt and to improve upon the methods of Western nations was acknowledged.[23] They were revered as a 'nation of soldiers',[24] combining the tradition and ideals of the Samurai – known as *bushido*[25] – with the strategic and organisational skills assimilated from Western nations. Japanese soldiers were, in the words of E. Emerson writing in *The Contemporary Review*,

> possessed of the soldierly virtues of self-immolating bravery, manly fortitude and endurance, implicit obedience to orders and devotion to duty. With these ancient virtues of the fighting man they combine the modern winning qualities of good shooting and individual initiative.[26]

The lifestyle, discipline, education, and character of the Japanese peoples were singled out for praise.[27] According to the historian G.R. Searle, this 'extravagant cult of Japan' in Britain during the war, developed within the context of British fears of national degeneracy, and the associated 'quest' for national efficiency.[28]

Similarly, for medical observers of the war, it was the Japanese army which was of most interest. For the *BMJ*, the Japanese in their medical arrangements had 'taken as a model the British Army Medical Department'.[29] The concept of the war as a test, albeit at a distance, of British medical arrangements was short-lived. Dissatisfaction with reform of the British Army Medical Department (AMD) following the South African War placed a different emphasis on the war in the Far East. Rather than being a straightforward test of British military medical organisation, the war served mainly to expose its flaws. Accounts of the medical aspects of the Russo-Japanese War were both prescriptive and descriptive, emphasising the ways in which the Japanese had assimilated and, more importantly, improved upon the medical organisation of the British Army. Admiration of the Japanese military medical organisation was fuelled by the perceived stagnation of reform in the British AMD. A similar trend can also be identified within American medical literature.

Army Medical Reform

The outbreak of the Russo-Japanese War coincided with a period of army medical reform in Britain in the wake of the South African War. Reforms prompted by the war were being instituted. The Army Medical Advisory Board which served to advise the Secretary of State on medical, surgical and sanitary matters affecting the military services, was formed in November 1901, and consisted of both military and civilian medical experts.[30] The Army Medical School, formerly at Netley, and once regarded as an 'archaic school of instruction',[31] was in the process of being relocated to London, and renamed the Army Medical College.[32]

It was the publication in 1904 of the Esher Committee's recommendations for the reform of the War Office, which particularly concerned those interested in the organisation of the army medical service. The creation of an Army Council implemented as part of the Esher Reforms brought criticism from reformers of the AMD, because it contained no medical representative. That medicine had been placed under the authority of the Adjutant-General incensed those who had campaigned for the transformation of the AMD into an autonomous body, no longer subordinated to military authority. In combative mood in February 1904, the *BMJ* stated:

> We warn Mr. Arnold-Forster [Secretary of State for War] that the medical profession will not tolerate a reversion to the bad old system which has been the cause of so many misfortunes to the army and such terrible cost – not in money only, but in lives – to the country.[33]

Fear was expressed in the *BMJ* that there would be a reversion to the thinking, prominent in the nineteenth century, that the wounded were 'encumbrances', and that those who ministered to them were no more than 'camp-followers'.[34] An even greater fear was expressed that the 'terrible lessons of the South-African War' had been 'thrown away', allowing old military attitudes towards medicine to be perpetuated.[35] To this end, those seeking to reform the AMD resurrected the oft-quoted (and arguably misused) words of the archetypal anti-sanitarian Lord Wolseley as evidence of combatant contempt for medicine.[36] His decree that 'medical advice is a good thing – when it is asked for', was used as a symbol, not of nineteenth century, but of contemporary military attitudes towards medicine.[37] By the middle of 1904, it was suggested that without a seat on the newly formed Army Council, the medical service of the army had 'three arms without a head'. The article continued, 'This is not reform, but retrogression.'[38]

The *BMJ* was quick to place responsibility for the 'vast amount of preventable disease and great and needless loss of life' during war-time on military mismanagement expressed through neglect of the AMD.[39] Andrew Clark, Chairman of the Council of the British Medical Association, expressed the same sentiment in a letter to *The Times*.[40] What Clark criticised was the failure of the army administration to recognise the strategic importance of the medical services to the waging of war. As Clark argued: 'military history teems with instances in which the dispositions of the most skilful commanders have been defeated, not by the enemy but by epidemic disease'. Epidemics, 'so fatal to the efficiency of an army', could only be avoided 'if the army is organised and administered with constant reference to its sanitary needs'. Sanitation was regarded by reformers as a central feature of army medical reform, one all too often subordinated to changes in the structure and organisation of the AMD.[41] This was clear in the reforms instituted after the South African War which concerned new administrative structures, a new college for medical officers, and greater integration of civilian and military medical officers, rather than furthering and disseminating sanitary knowledge.[42] That a medical service organised for the prevention of disease both in terms of structure and sanitation was essential to the waging of modern warfare was a central concern for those of the medical profession interested in medical reform. Writers like Clark were keen to furnish a link between military mismanagement – expressed through failure to recognise the value of medicine – and disease as a cause of military inefficiency. This was evident in the *BMJ*'s statement that 'although the medical profession can do without the army, the army cannot do without the profession',[43] and was *clear* in British and American descriptions of the medical aspects of the Russo-Japanese War.

Aseptic Fighting

Throughout the second half of 1904, it was frequently asserted in the columns of the *Lancet*, that there was little definite information regarding the medical history of the war then being fought in the Far East.[44] This lack of reliable evidence, especially regarding the performance of the Russian Army,[45] presented conditions ideally suited to the aims of reform-minded British and American medical writers. Manchuria was commonly regarded as 'an especially dangerous' theatre of war,[46] 'a notoriously unhealthy country'.[47] Fitting in with this image of Manchuria were the rumours given credence in the *Lancet* of 'much sickness' – especially typhus and typhoid – amongst the Russian troops, in spite of "official" reports to the contrary.[48]

In connection with the Japanese army, by stark contrast, the *Boston Medical and Surgical Journal* wrote, 'Apart from occasional rumors(sic), we hear very little of epidemic disease, usually so fatal in time of war.'[49] Suggestions that disease amongst Russian soldiers was 'attributable to the character of the clothing, supplies and foodstuffs furnished by dishonest contractors',[50] or confusion in the categorisation of typhus and typhoid,[51] rather than poor medical organisation, were the exception not the rule. Selective credence given to rumour and official reports in conjunction with both armies was also extended to casualty statistics. Those of the Russians were 'not to be relied upon', but those of the Japanese were accepted without question.[52]

From such speculations on the relative performance of the Russian and the Japanese medical departments, the *BMJ* concluded that through her commitment to hygiene the Japanese would be able 'to neutralize the numerical advantage of her enemy's superior numbers'.[53] For the *BMJ*, in the dichotomy between Russian and Japanese performance 'there could not be a more striking illustration of the inevitable consequences of the fatuous and fatal system of treating the medical officers of the army as "camp-followers"'.[54]

It was not just the *BMJ* which fixed on the educative value of the alleged Japanese successes. For the *Boston Medical and Surgical Journal*, the role of the Japanese 'had been to demonstrate that disease may be prevented'.[55] This was in contrast to the American experience of the Spanish-American War, where 345 deaths from wounds and 2,565 deaths from disease were sustained.[56] The article continued: 'Certainly, the fact that any deaths occur from preventable disease must always be in a measure, a reflection on the medical management of an army.' The Japanese had shown the possibility of rendering war hygienic and 'humane'[57] through effective medical management of disease.[58] By making her army 'practically immune to epidemic disease',[59] Japan had ushered in the concept of 'aseptic fighting'.[60]

This dichotomy between the Russians and the Japanese in terms of medical 'success' in the war, was *clearly drawn* in the observations made by Louis L. Seaman, who had served as a surgeon in the United States Volunteers in the war against Spain. At the International Congress of Military and Naval Surgeons in St. Louis in November 1904, Seaman 'declared that the Japanese are the first people to recognise the true value of the army medical corps'.[61] Ever vigilant, Japanese medical officers, armed with microscopes and chemicals, were devoted to disease prevention, and had, according to Seaman, achieved a significant reduction in mortality from wounds and disease.[62] In comparison, he argued, the Russians were inadequately furnished with medicines and stretchers; their wounded transported in conditions of filth and overcrowding. Seaman had observed the daily workings of the Japanese medical department during the war with Russia, and it was this personal experience of the Japanese army on which his remarks were based. The foundations upon which he based his description of the Russian medical organisation is less clear.

By the end of 1904 therefore, the major lesson of the Russo-Japanese War seemed to be that of disease prevention; prophylaxis, rather than cure. The performance of the Japanese in disease management was juxtaposed with that of the Russians, and with that of the British and American armies. Casualty statistics were the one means of comparison between Russia and Japan, the baseline measurement being figures from the South African and Spanish-American Wars.[63] The focus for writers on the war was on the differences, not the similarities in the medical systems then existing. The seeming gulf between the Japanese and other nations was exploited by reformers in order to emphasize the failings of other nations, and to sustain efforts for army medical reform in those countries.[64]

As memories of the South African and Spanish-American Wars faded, so too did the impetus for reform and regeneration of military medicine in America and Britain.[65] Medical writers concerned with this growing amnesia sought to place the Japanese successes within a local context. For the British at least, with 'South Africa... forgotten, and Manchuria... a long way off',[66] writers sought to render the experience of the Russo-Japanese War more familiar.

The Medical Arrangements of the Japanese

For observers of the war in the Far East, the 'unique' performance of the Japanese in the matter of disease prevention[67] was not attributed to superior medical knowledge on their part.[68] Despite suggestions that the Japanese as a race were immune to certain diseases like typhoid,[69] attention focused on aspects of the Japanese medical organisation which differed from those of other nations. The focus was not on medical and surgical treatment.[70] As the *BMJ* explained,

> It is not that the Japanese are superior to us in the practice of the healing art, but simply that they apply the knowledge which they have learnt from Western nations more effectively to the necessities and emergencies of war.'[71]

Differences in the organisation of the medical service were perceived to be crucial to their performance, as were differences in the perception of, and the attitude towards the role of medicine, especially sanitation, within the army. The value of education – of medical men and combatants – was also identified as a significant contribution to the 'success' of the Japanese.

For observers the organisation of the medical services in the Japanese army was not unlike that of other nations, although there were minor differences in hospital provision.[72] What was different was the combination of reserve forces and medical aid to provide for rapid expansion of the regular army medical services in times of war, and the integration of civilian doctors into the medical service.[73] The Japanese were described as 'prepared for war in time of peace'.[74] Through reserve and voluntary relief their medical service had sufficient medical personnel who were trained in military procedure.[75] By contrast in Britain, civilian aid – once described as 'a screen to hide the nakedness of our real military medical service'[76] – was employed as a substitute, not a supplement to the RAMC.

For British writers, it was the apparent provision of a viable reserve of medical officers, not 'a mere paper scheme', on the part of the Japanese which attracted most attention.[77] This can be explained in terms of the perceived failure of the War Office to provide a scheme for the formation of a volunteer reserve force, a failure recognised at the time of the South African War.[78] In an editorial on

'The Future of the Volunteer Force', the *BMJ* described the medical branch of the volunteer force as one ten years behind the times, and inadequately organised.[79] Rather than organising an efficient reserve, the War Office had been – and according to the *BMJ* still was – content to rely on the civilian medical service in wartime; procuring civilian doctors to overcome a shortfall in military medical personnel.[80] The organisation of the Japanese was contrasted with the approach of the British: 'Organisation does not mean discussing how to muddle through with makeshifts; it implies arrangements to render makeshifts unnecessary.'[81]

It was not simply the makeshift nature of the British medical organisation that was criticised when compared to the supposed efficiency of the Japanese schemes. What was also questioned was the competence of civilian doctors brought into the unfamiliar context of an army at war.[82] According to one source, a force on active service required 'medical *officers* – men with knowledge and experience of military needs and procedure'.[83] Major M.M. O'Connor of the RAMC Militia, in a letter on 'The Military Medical Reserve Difficulty', summarised the problems facing civilian doctors on entering the army:

> It is a well-known fact (not to mention the impossibility of carrying on the routine work of a military hospital without a knowledge of the forms and customs of the army), that Tommy Atkins has and will pay more respect to a second lieutenant than he will to a civilian of the most exalted position.[84]

This preoccupation with the interface between civilian and military doctors betrayed a more general concern with the lack of overt militarism – symbolised by compulsory military service – within the British Army. Amongst critics of the AMD it was widely held that compulsory military training on the continent had enhanced the status of medicine within the armed forces.[85] Without this shared training professional status remained subordinate to military status. Japan, where doctors served with an infantry battalion for a number of years before receiving specialist training in medicine, was taken as a further example of the benefits of militarism. Concern with the lack of a medical reserve was also expressed by politicians. William Burdett-Coutts, who had played such a prominent role as correspondent for *The Times* in criticising the medical arrangements of the British Army during the war in South Africa,[86] maintained that the incorporation of civilian surgeons into the RAMC had an 'important bearing... upon the preparedness of the country for a great war'.[87]

For American writers also, the measured organisation of the Japanese medical service was a contrast to the American experience. Anita Newcomb McGee, doctor and supervisor of nurses at Hiroshima during the war expressed this in an article entitled 'How the Japanese Save Lives'. She wrote 'it is certain that the Japanese will continue to prearrange everything... while our Congress prefers trusting to luck for the health of its army rather than to a well-organised medical department'.[88] Where the Japanese had an elastic service, capable of expansion, the American medical department was 'lamentably deficient in numbers'.[89] It was, by implication, poor organisation, not poor medicine which had resulted in the failures of the Spanish-American War. Major Charles Lynch, American attaché in Tokyo, charged with investigating matters connected with the medical department, elaborated on this point:

> proof is not lacking that, in war, even exceptionally high skill in the general medical profession of a country cannot make up for ignorance of the problems which confront armies; and to rely to a very large extent on civilian practitioners, untrained in a military sense, can only result in disaster, with crippling of the army by much sickness and many deaths from preventable diseases.[90]

The folly of reliance on civilian doctors in the Spanish-American War was clearly expressed in the title of a paper by C.B.G. de Nancrede, 'Personal Experience During the Spanish-American War Showing the Disadvantages of Depending upon Untrained Civilian Physicians for Military Service in Times of War.'[91]

At the conclusion of the Russo-Japanese War, American writers speculated on the reasons for the success of Japan, with one eye on their own shortcomings. Theodore Roosevelt, American President and mediator in the Russo-Japanese War wrote 'The main reason why their medical department did well was that they had an ample supply of doctors who had been practised in time of peace in doing the duties they would have to do in war.'[92]

They prepared in peace for war,[93] and had medical officers trained in the specialty of military medicine.[94] The success of the Japanese was taken as a prescription for the reform of the American medical service. According to Roosevelt, what the American army needed was 'men who are not merely doctors', but those who were 'trained in the administration of military medical service'.[95] Such concepts were integrated into the Bill for the Improvement of the AMS, introduced by Roosevelt in 1906.[96]

The integration of civilian and military doctors, and relief organisations into a coherent system was not just taken as evidence of superior Japanese organisation and management. Rather, it spoke of significant differences in their perception of the position of medicine within the army. For American observers, that the medical officer within the Japanese army had definite rank and social position, was a state diametrically opposed to the position of medical officers within the American army. At the time of the Spanish-American War it had been suggested that the best doctors were not recruited into the army, because of the lack of high rank attached to medical positions,[97] a situation similar to that experienced by the British in the 1890's. Seaman, in 1904, argued that the difference in the performance of the Russians and the Japanese during the war was a direct consequence of the status of medical officers in the respective armies. He argued that

> it was impossible to escape the conclusion that the difference between the health conditions of the Japanese and the Russian armies was mainly due to the subordinate position assigned to the medical officer in the latter.[98]

It was not rank in itself which elevated the Japanese medical officer above those of other armies. High rank in the Japanese army conferred honourable status, respect and authority for both the medical officer[99] and for his profession within the army.[100]

In America, and in Britain (in spite of the formation of the RAMC in 1898), reformers argued that respect for the profession of medicine within the military was lacking.[101] In particular, sanitation was poorly regarded. Surgeon-General Sternberg attributed the high levels of typhoid suffered by the Americans in the 1898 war to 'the non-appreciation on the part of the regimental officers of what they were content to designate the 'fads' of the doctors relative to sanitation'.[102] Similarly, the failure to prevent enteric fever in the British Army, was assigned to 'the indifference of the community to army well-being and to those in high army quarters who have promulgated the teaching that sanitation is "a fad"', not to sanitary advisers.[103]

This perceived disregard for sanitary thinking contrasted with the image drawn of the Japanese. It was implied in the *BMJ* that 'the secret of the unprecedented freedom of the Japanese from disease is the ready compliance of officers and men with the sanitary rules laid down for them'.[104] In the Japanese Army, sanitation was 'a vital necessity, not a mere doctor's fad... an essential condition in the fitness of an army'.[105] According to Anita Newcomb McGee, this centrality was evident in the title of the Japanese army medical service, *Eisei-kimmu*, meaning sanitary corps.[106] She wrote:

> This is the body corresponding to our medical Department, but its key-note is struck by the very difference in the title. Sanitation, or keeping the soldier in good fighting condition, is its first object, and healing him after he drops from the ranks is the secondary consideration.[107]

The Japanese exhibited an attitude towards disease and its prevention which differed considerably from that of other nations. As McGee explained:

> In olden times it was thought cheaper to obtain a new soldier than to cure a sick or wounded one... But a progressing world demands that reckless and useless sacrifices of life shall stop, and at last, military commanders are beginning to appreciate the importance of keeping soldiers in fit condition. At least, the Japanese appreciate this.[108]

For reformers then, the Japanese as a nation were committed to the protection of life.[109] They recognised the real cost of disease, and the role of the doctor in reducing wastage from preventable disease. According to observers it was the Japanese who realised that without preventive measures 'the biggest battalions must in time shrink to a degree that will make them an easy prey to a more intelligently directed enemy'.[110] In other words, the Japanese had adapted to the needs of modern warfare with its heavy manpower demands, while other nations had not.[111]

It was implied by official observers that the Japanese had learnt the importance of disease prevention in their war with the Chinese,[112] where they suffered extensively from epidemic disease.[113] That Britain and America had failed to realise the same lesson from the South African and Spanish-American Wars was a further contrast between themselves and Japan. In February 1905, in a debate in Parliament on army reform, Sir Walter Foster discussed the military lessons which should have been learnt from the war in South Africa.[114] For him, the most important of these was the 'lesson... that from neglect... we lost an enormous number of men... mostly from a disease which of all diseases was the most preventable'.[115] For Foster, himself a qualified physician with knowledge of public health,[116] the most important duty of the medical officer lay in disease prevention. Invoking the importance of manpower economy, he argued that

> New artillery, rifles, long or short, would not by themselves save us,
> but men strong and vigorous, able to face their foe, were the best
> defence for a civilised nation.'[117]

For reformers of military medicine recognition of the strategic importance of disease and its prevention, was slow in permeating the military mind-set of countries other than Japan. In Britain, the *Medical Press and Circular* lamented such delays: 'We still fail to see any sign that the proportions of the problem of keeping the British Army free from disease are grasped by the War Office.'[118] A similar sentiment was expressed by the *BMJ* in a discussion of the role of the doctor in modern warfare.[119] According to this article, Wellington had understood the value of a medical staff for maintaining the troops 'in full vigour',[120] but this had long been forgotten by the military authorities:

> How little they have even now taken to heart the teachings of our
> terrible experiences in South Africa is shown by the readiness with
> which they fall back into the old ways as soon as any scare that
> galvanises them into an appearance of activity dies out.

The Japanese, by contrast, were perceived to be '*the* pioneers of preventive medicine in the field' (emphasis added).[121] They had recognised and given 'striking proof' of the value of medicine in the waging of war.

A similar dichotomy was outlined by McGee. For her, the aim of the Japanese was not just to win the war, but

> to conduct this war according to such high and humane principles
> that the whole world will recognise in Japan one of the most
> enlightened nations of the earth.... . Japan has learned much from
> the United States. Now the time has come when America should
> learn from Japan.[122]

Seaman went further. Where the Americans had been powerless to prevent 'sacrifice of life from preventable causes' in the war against Spain, Japan was 'empowered to overcome the silent foe'.[123] The Japanese were doubly victorious, having conquered both the Russians and disease. Seaman personified disease to enhance the significance of the latter 'victory'. For him disease was 'the hidden foe, always found lurking in every camp, the grim spectre, ever present, that gathers its victims while the soldier slumbers in hospital, in barrack, or in bivouac'.[124]

This emphasis on sanitation and disease prevention, he argued, placed the Japanese medical officer in the frontline of the army, a pre-emptive weapon, not a last resort. The Japanese medical officer was 'like a sentinel on duty', preventing danger and therefore equivalent to 'twenty men stationed in the rear to treat sickness after it had obtained a foothold'.[125] Echoing this sentiment Sir Walter Foster maintained that the Japanese put their medical officers everywhere, whereas 'Our system was to put the medical officer in the background and keep him there.'[126]

Medicine and Duty

Recognition of the centrality of disease prevention to military efficiency was not in itself sufficient to account for the uncommon success of Japanese preventive measures. Commentators on the medical aspects of the war drew attention to other factors determining Japanese performance, factors which, according to these reformers had been lacking in their own medical services and were consequently responsible for the ensuing failures. Cooperation of combatant ranks and officers in the fight against disease was identified as crucial by American and British observers alike. According to one American medical officer who had served in the Spanish-American War, doctors there had been 'powerless to prevent or cure disease unless the line officers follow his directions'.[127] Within the British Army, it was unclear where responsibility for outbreaks of disease lay.[128] As 'Progress' wrote in a letter to the *BMJ*, 'Army medical officers have always known what to do and how to do it, but it was not the duty of any person to carry out their recommendations.'[129]

According to Western observers, the importance of hygiene in the field was instilled into Japanese soldiers through education, both in peace and in times of war. In military and naval academies the study of hygiene was compulsory.[130] During the war a pamphlet titled 'Precautions on Individual Sanitation' was distributed to all men of the Japanese Army,[130] and regular lectures on health and first-aid, told 'of the awful results of not taking sanitary precautions'.[131] That reformers considered military training in hygiene to be the key to victory;[132] and health and fitness a weapon in itself,[133] was evident in rhetoric that the Japanese soldier was 'imbued with the idea that it is just as necessary to maintain his body in the best physical condition as to keep his rifle in a state of efficiency'.[134]

The military value of sanitary education to the Japanese was clear in the accountability for sanitation. Medical officers were responsible for ensuring that sanitary precautions were recommended to the commanding officer, who was in turn responsible for carrying out

112

those recommendations.[135] Ultimately, soldiers were responsible for their own welfare. According to one British observer Japanese soldiers were taught that it was shameful to succumb to illness, 'that disease is a far more dangerous enemy than the Russians'.[136] This notion of responsibility was present in the classification of illness. Illness was divided into three categories: first class illness or *itt_sh_* referred to wounds or illness resulting from hardship on service; second class illness or *nit_sh_* covered all ordinary diseases; third class illness or *sant_sh_* was 'disease or sickness brought on by the individual's own carelessness or disobedience of orders'.[137] Different degrees of shame applied to the three categories. As a result of this, at least for outside observers, every man in the Japanese army seemed determined to remain in a state of health. According to a distinguished Japanese officer, societal attitudes also had a part to play because 'people in Japan do not like sick soldiers, and they do not get the best of receptions if they leave the front in consequence of disease'.[138] Sickness and sick soldiers were culturally unacceptable – they were not *'bien vu'* in the Japanese Army.[139]

National characteristics were also recognised as being instrumental in the Japanese 'fight' against disease. The Japanese were renowned for their patriotism. Their passionate devotion to the nation and its defence, was admired[140] and in turn ridiculed in Britain,[141] primarily because of its perceived absence among the British.[142] This was identified as a factor in the Japanese obeyance of sanitary rules – 'Good hygiene was much promoted by the patriotism of the soldiers.'[143] Taken as an example of this dictum was the daily consumption of creosote pills as a prophylactic against intestinal disease. According to observers, these were dutifully consumed as 'patriotism was invoked in order that... [soldiers] might take them'. Such high morals were inspired by the following inscription on the box of pills: 'To defeat the Russians, take one pill three times a day.'[144] These pills were aptly known as *seiro-gwan* or Russian Punishers.[145] Significantly, for Western commentators the therapeutic value of this intestinal antiseptic attracted less attention than the patriotic fervour with which it was consumed.[146]

The want of such education and discipline within the British Army was expressed by a number of writers. For Captain E. Blake Knox of the RAMC, the only means to reform the sanitary arrangements of the British Army and to render the army free from disease was to make every rank pass an examination on the basic elements of sanitation.[147] Alexander Ogston, in his evidence to the Royal Commission on the War in South Africa, noted that even men of the RAMC had little understanding of sanitation: 'many of them looked upon it as a species of cowardice if they attended to such things as avoiding infection – a sort of shirking of duty.'[148] It was also maintained elsewhere that cleanliness was a character trait of the Japanese peoples, but a neglected art amongst the British.[149]

Another medical officer argued that the soldier needed to be taught 'to protect himself and those around him from the 'invisible poisoned bullets' often harboured on his own person.'[150] The dangers of disease had to be made explicit and intelligible to soldiers. In his lectures to officers and men, he likened a person with enteric to a 'magazine, which is full of high explosives... more dangerous to the general safety of the community than the magazine'. In this context, it was the duty of the soldier to further his health and, more importantly, the health of the army. Such teaching mirrored that of the Japanese.[151]

For British and American observers, Japan had shown that health was 'the normal condition of the soldier'.[152] The influence of this idea was evident in a series of lectures delivered by Surgeon-Captain F.F. Maccabe, of the South Irish Horse Regiment, at the Staff College in October 1906. Inspired by the 'state of ignorance in which our men were sent to the front' during the South African War,[153] these lectures taught that 'diseases are not irresistible'; they could be 'fought and defeated... by organisation, initiative and suitable strategy'.[154] Soldiers were instructed to 'declare war against these germs, regard them as enemies'.[155] In this 'fight' they were to be aided by the 'white army' within their blood.[156] The use of the military metaphor by Maccabe allowed the moral obligations of the soldier/potential sickman, to be outlined. As with war against a human foe, soldiers were expected to devote themselves to the contest; failure in the war with disease – sickness – was caused by 'ignorance and carelessness and ought to be avoided by all men who are worthy to be called soldiers'.[157] Sick men were not to be pitied, or sympathised with, but identified as men who had not done their duty, by themselves, or their fellow soldiers.[158] This was a further assimilation of Japanese attitudes.

But it was not only soldiers who needed to be educated as to their responsibilities. Accountability for disease prevention also rested with the government and military authorities. In a speech to Parliament Sir Walter Foster argued that

> whilst among the civil population death from enteric fever was a scandal to the local authority, every death from enteric fever in the

course of a war was a crime on the part of a government department.[159]

War Office apathy towards disease management, described in one article as 'lukewarm assent to sanitation'[160] was obvious to critics of the War Office. A prime example of this was the reduction to a minimum of a course of lectures in hygiene given to cadets at Woolwich and Sandhurst.[161] It was just such a 'scandalous disregard of modern science' which had resulted in the needless deaths of thousands of soldiers in the South African War.[162]

Critics of the existing medical organisation of the army argued that unlike the Japanese, the British had failed to appreciate the cost of disease, which acted as 'a heavy tax on military efficiency',[163] or the value of medical science in the promotion of military strength.[164] It was further argued that poor laboratory facilities,[165] and indifference towards science had hindered investigations into disease prevention in both the military and civilian context.[166] By contrast, the Japanese appreciated the value of science. At an early age, the Japanese were educated in the natural sciences.[167] Their attitude towards science was portrayed as being exemplary, in spite of evidence that the success of Japan in reducing wastage from disease was not due to any new medical or explicitly scientific knowledge. L.L. Seaman made much of the Japanese use of the monocular microscope. It was described as a 'superb weapon... against the Russians', more so than the murata rifle; and with its assistance 'war was made on bacteria'.[168] The microscope symbolised the rise of Japan and further highlighted the barbarity and degeneration of other nations. As the *BMJ* remarked:

> It is scarcely complimentary to our intelligence that a truth so readily grasped by a people to whom modern science is an acquisition almost of yesterday, should be practically ignored in the country which is the birthplace of hygiene.[169]

Here, the use of the term 'science' referred explicitly to sanitary science, or hygiene. Again, the performance of the Japanese was juxtaposed with that of the British and the Americans to highlight the perceived deficiencies of the latter. The level of sickness in war was an indicator of national fitness, of civilisation, of modernity; science was one aspect of this. As an article entitled 'Japanese Lessons' explained:

> Japan at the moment represents the spirit of modernity incarnated in a nation; a nation, moreover, which has definitely shaken off from the past everything but the driving power derivable from an intense sense of corporate duty. A nation thus equipped will be satisfied with nothing short of the best... whether it be in war, administration, or science.[170]

Conclusion

By the end of 1905, the lessons to be derived from the war in the Far East had been firmly outlined by British and American observers. Recognition of the ultimate danger of disease, and the identification of medicine as a powerful weapon against disease was uniformly praised. Dissemination of the importance of medicine through sanitary education, and a culture of individual and national responsibility were features absent in Western nations. Unfavourable comparisons of Britain and America on these criteria were central to the 'war' against peace-time inertia in their respective countries.

Whilst invoking disease as a powerful enemy of armies, reformers alluded to a worse fate, national degeneration. Reformers made use of existing failures – in the South African and Spanish-American Wars – and fears of future campaigns to further their own concerns in the absence of information 'neither so full nor so reliable as could have been wished'.[171] In a context where medical information was lacking, concerns of those observing the war determined what was perceived. 'Success' of the Japanese in the prevention of disease and conservation of manpower was effected through comparison with Anglo-American failures.

Accounts of the Russo-Japanese War seen through the eyes of British and American observers were more an account of their own inefficiencies and inadequacies, than of the medical history of the Russo-Japanese War. Statistics published after the war questioned the uniqueness of the Japanese performance, and by definition, the perspective of the observers. Colonel W.G. Macpherson in a report in January 1906 compared the wound and disease statistics of the Japanese Army with that of the British in the South African War. For him, the table did not 'bring out evidence of any marked immunity from disease' on the part of the Japanese.[172] On a more ironic note, post-war statistics hinted at the superior performance of the Russians in the prevention of disease.[173] This did little to change the war-time impressions gathered by outside observers.

By the end of the war, the image of the Japanese as conquerors of disease was firmly entrenched, building, at least in Britain, on the more general appreciation of the Japanese as a nation, and the associated critique of the decline of Western nations. The patriotism, discipline, and intelligence of the Japanese appealed to British and American observers, in their struggle for regeneration and revitalisation of both army and society. The success of the Japanese, both military and medical, was accentuated through juxtaposition with Russia and with British and American performances in former campaigns.[174] The Japanese had defeated the Russians; they had been victorious in the fight against disease; and they had overcome the ultimate foe – apathy of the military authorities. It was this latter success which observers hoped to emulate through their accounts of the Russo-Japanese War.

But the 'lessons' of the Russo-Japanese War were not just limited to the immediate post-war context. The dichotomy drawn by observers between the performance of Japan and the Western nations in disease management had wider relevance. The concept of the Japanese as leaders in disease prevention survived despite statistics to the contrary, and served as an example of what could be achieved. In October 1914, shortly after the declaration of the First World War, Sir William Osler delivered a lecture to officers and men encamped at Churn, on the subject of 'Bacilli and Bullets'. The following extract illustrates the resonance of the descriptions of the Russo-Japanese War:

> I am here to warn you soldiers against enemies more subtle, more dangerous, and more fatal than the Germans – enemies against which no successful battle can be fought without your intelligent cooperation. So far the world has only seen one great war waged with the weapons of science against these foes. Our allies, the Japanese went into the Russian campaign prepared as fully against bacilli as against bullets, with the result that the percentage of deaths from disease was the lowest that has ever been attained in a great war. What lesson shall we learn? Which example shall we follow – Japan, or South Africa with its sad memories?[175]

Notes

1 The war has been described as 'the most observed, chronicled, and discussed conflict until the First World War', David Walder, *The Short Victorious War. The Russo-Japanese Conflict, 1904-5*, (Devon: Reader's Union, 1974), 9.

2 And according to J.N. Westwood, *The Illustrated History of the Russo-Japanese War* (London: Sidgwick & Jackson, 1973), the first modern war.

3 'The War in the Far East', *BMJ*, 13 Feb., 1904, 384.

4 See, Keith Neilson, '"That Dangerous and Difficult Enterprise": British Military Thinking and the Russo-Japanese War', *War and Society*, ix (1991), 17-37.

5 'Treatment of the Wounded in the Russo-Japanese War', *Boston Medical and Surgical Journal*, 22 Sept., 1904, 335.

6 'An Arraignment of the Army Medical Department', *Journal of the American Medical Association*, 13 Aug., 1898, 360-1, noted that the press had called for an investigation into the conditions faced by the sick and wounded during the war.

7 'The War in the Far East', *op. cit.* (note 3), 384. Although the Japanese were not perceived to be as impressive a military nation as the Russians, their medical arrangements were, according to the *BMJ*, 'so much up to date as to be scientifically comparable with those of any nation', 'Japanese and Russian Military Medical Systems', *BMJ*, 9 Jan., 1904, 91.

8 This interest in the medical organisation of other nations was reflected in the contents of the *Journal of the Royal Army Medical Corps*, which had been founded as 'a medium for exchanging ideas with foreign medical corps', Colonel F. Smith, *A Short History of the Royal Army Medical Corps* (Aldershot: Gale & Polden Ltd, 1929), 61, and in other medical journals. See 'The Relative Sanitary Condition of Different European Armies', *BMJ*, 7 May, 1904, 1087-8.

9 G.J. Stoney Archer, 'A Lecture on Hygiene', *JRAMC*, v (1905), 741-7, gave figures from late nineteenth century wars to illustrate the fact that 'in all modern wars the losses by disease have been far greater than those sustained by the acts of the enemy', 741.

10 'The Medical Service of the Army', *BMJ*, 20 Feb., 1904, 446.

11 Notes on 'lessons' to be learnt from the war.

12 S. Squire Sprigge, *Medicine and the Public*, (London: 1905).

13 E.M. Spiers, *Haldane: An Army Reformer*, (Edinburgh: Edinburgh University Press, 1980), 48.

14 Westwood, *op. cit.* (note 2), 26. Although Russia had a system of

conscription, many exemptions were allowed. They had 4,500,000 men compared to 850,000 in the Japanese Army.

15 Michael Adas, *Machines as the Measure of Men. Science, Technology and Ideologies of Western Dominance* (London: Cornell University Press, 1989), 360.

16 'The Social Problem in Japan', *Lancet*, 19 March, 1904, 817.

17 Adas, *op. cit.* (note 12), 360.

18 Janet E. Hunter, *The Emergence of Modern Japan. An Introductory History Since 1853* (London & New York: 1989), 8. According to E. Emerson, 'Japan at War', *Contemporary Review*, lxxxvi (1904), 6-17, the army was developed upon French lines, until their failure in the Franco-Prussian War, 1870-1.

19 Hunter, *op. cit.* (note 18), 270.

20 *Ibid.*, 23.

21 Colin Holmes & A.H. Ion, 'Bushid_ and the Samurai: Images in British Public Opinion, 1894-1914', *Modern Asian Studies*, xiv (1980), 309-29, at 315.

22 Hunter, *op. cit.* (note 18), 22 and 24.

23 'Japanese and Russian Military Medical Systems', *BMJ*, 9 Jan., 1904, 91.

24 Captain F. Brinkley, 'Japan', *Encyclopedia Britannica* (New York: Encyclopedia Britannica, Inc., 1910-11), 11th edition, 205.

25 Holmes & Ion, *op. cit.* (note 21); G.R. Searle, *The Quest for National Efficiency. A Study in British Politics and Political Thought, 1899-1914* (London: Basil Blackwell, 1971), 57; Hunter, *op. cit.* (note 18), Chapter 12, 'The Role of the Military', 265-88.

26 Emerson, *op. cit.* (note 18), 16.

27 In medical journals a number of general articles on the Japanese appeared: 'The Physique of the Japanese', *BMJ*, 12 March, 1904, 622-3; 'Japanese Students', *BMJ*, 28 Jan., 1905, 205; 'The Japanese Art of Ju-Jitsu', *BMJ*, 4 Feb., 1905, 259-60; 'Japanese Lessons', *Medical Press and Circular*, 12 July, 1905, 39.

28 Searle, *op. cit.* (note 24), 57.

29 'The War in the Far East', (note 3), 384.

30 The board was made up of the Director-General and his Assistant, and nine other members. 'Army Medical Service. The Advisory Board', *BMJ*, 23 Nov., 1901, 1546.

31 R.H. Firth, 'Medical Science and Army Efficiency', *Nature*, lxxiv (1906), 613.

32 Sir William Taylor, 'An Address on the Work and Purpose of the Royal Army Medical College', *BMJ*, 6 Feb., 1904, 291-4; 'The Royal Army Medical College', *BMJ*, 6 Feb., 1904, 314-6; 'The Royal Army

Medical College', *BMJ*, 2 April., 1904, 802.

33 'The Medical Service of the Army', *BMJ*, 13 Feb., 1904, 381.

34 'The Medical Service of the Army', *BMJ*, 5 March, 1904, 561.

35 'The Medical Service of the Army', *BMJ*, 20 Feb., 1904, 445.

36 General Viscount G.J. Wolseley was the author of *The Soldier's Pocket Book for Field Service* (London: Macmillan & Co., 1886), (5th edition, first published 1869). In this he was critical of the medical staff of the Army, in particular the sanitary officer, who he described as a 'very useless functionary', 109. G.J.H. Evatt, a supporter of Army Medical Reform, writing under the pseudonym 'Justice', described Wolseley as the 'standard-bearer' of the anti-sanitary party, in *The Truth About the RAMC. A Memorandum Submitted for the Consideration of His Majesty the King on the Sanitary Condition of his Soldiers and the Care of the Sick and Wounded of His Majesty's Army* (Plymouth: Hoyten & Cole, 1901).

37 'The Medical Service of the Army', (note 33), 381.

38 'The Medical Service of the Army', *BMJ*, 25 June, 1904, 1504.

39 'The Medical Service of the Army', (note 33), 381.

40 'The Prevention of Disease in War', *The Times*, 22 Feb., 1904, reprinted in 'The Army Council and Military Medical Administration', *BMJ*, 27 Feb., 1904, 511.

41 Stephen A. Pagaard, 'Disease and the British Army in South Africa, 1899-1900', *Military Affairs*, l (1986), 71-6, has argued that reforms arising from the South African War were primarily organisational changes; little attention was directed to sanitation.

42 See, 'The Prevention of Waterborne Disease in the Army', *BMJ*, 12 Sept., 1903, 604.

43 'The Medical Service of the Army', (note 35), 446.

44 'The War in the Far East', *Lancet*, 2 July., 1904, 43, noted that 'We learn but little of the medical history of the campaign and what we do is rather conflicting'; 'The War in the Far East', *Lancet*, 16 July., 1904, 172; 'The War in the Far East', *Lancet*, 23 July., 1904, 250 notes that there are few official reports about the war.

45 In March 1905, Dr Marcou, Physician to the Troitsky Hospital, St. Petersberg, stated that after a year of fighting it was virtually impossible to learn the truth about the health, or otherwise of the Russian Army. See 'The Sick and Wounded of the Russian Army', *BMJ*, 11 March, 1905, 553. Later it was revealed by Colonel W.H.H. Waters, who was attached to the Russian Army to examine their medical arrangements, that he had been 'denied detailed information' about the Russian troops, see 'The Health of the Russian Troops', in *The Russo-Japanese War. Medical and Sanitary*

Reports from Officers Attached to the Japanese and Russian Forces in the Field (London: HMSO, 1908), 556-8, at 558.

46 'Disease in War', *Lancet*, 23 April, 1904, 1149. Quote from V.N. Okunev from a lecture on infectious diseases in war given at the Society of Investigators of Military Science.

47 *Lancet*, 7 Jan., 1905, 53.

48 *Lancet*, 15 Oct., 1904, 1105-6.

49 'Medical Lessons of the Eastern War', *Boston Medical and Surgical Journal*, 10 Nov., 1904, 523.

50 *Lancet*, 4 June., 1904, 1610.

51 Ethel McCaul, *Under the Care of the Japanese War Office* (London: Cassell & Co Ltd, 1904), 149-50.

52 'The War in the Far East', *Lancet*, 13 Aug., 1904, 487.

53 'Hygiene in the Japanese Army', *BMJ*, 12 Nov., 1904, 1332. The Russian Army outnumbered the Japanese army by the ratio of 3:1. See, Captain Ashley W. Barrett, 'Lessons to be Learned by Regimental Officers from the Russo-Japanese War', *Journal of the Royal United Services Institute*, lx (1907), 797-823.

54 'Hygiene in the Japanese Army', (note 50), 1332. The passage continued thus: 'We commend the contrast between the Japanese and Russian armies to the earnest attention of Mr. Arnold-Forster and the Army Council'.

55 'Medical Lessons of the Eastern War', (note 49), 523.

56 *Ibid.*

57 According to O. Eltzbacher, 'The Red Cross Society of Japan', *Contemporary Review*, lxxxvi (1904), 324-32, Japanese 'progress in humane sentiment has at least kept pace and probably more than kept pace with her marvellous progress in the art of war', 332.

58 It is interesting that the Russo-Japanese War was perceived to be a war of a similar character to those of the previous century, ie. highly destructive. 'Deaths in Battle During Last Century', *BMJ*, 2 July, 1904, 31.

59 'Medical Lessons of the Eastern War', (note 49), 523.

60 'Aseptic Fighting', *Medical Press and Circular*, 11 Oct., 1905, 387.

61 'Hygiene in the Japanese Army', (note 50), 1332; 'Major Seaman's Address Before the International Congress of Military and Naval Surgeons at St. Louis', *Lancet*, 28 Jan., 1905, 238-9.

62 Seaman, having discounted Russian statistics as unreliable, then accepted the reduction in wound and disease mortality by the Japanese as a fact without 'statistical proof', 'Major Seaman's Address', (note 61), 238.

63 The "success" of the Japanese in disease prevention was derived from

comparisons with the 13,000 deaths from disease in the British Army in South Africa, and the 4,965 deaths from disease – some 70% of all cases – in the American army during the war with Spain. 'The Medical Officer in the Field', *BMJ*, 25 Feb., 1905, 428-9.

64 In Britain, attitudes towards reform were displayed in attempts to rework the Army Medical Advisory Board, and in a scheme to abolish the naval medical service. See, 'The Army Medical Advisory Board', *BMJ*, 30 Sept., 1905, 824; 'The Army Medical Advisory Board', *BMJ*, 18 Nov., 1905, 1374; 'Royal Naval Medical Service. Proposed Abolition', *BMJ*, 11 Feb., 1905, 339.

65 As St. John Brodrick noted after the war, the medical service of the army was such that it 'excites the acutest criticism during a campaign and the most meagre public interest in peace''', Brodrick, 'Medical Science and Military Strength', *The Times*, 6 June, 1906, 7 col.b/c. A similar sentiment was expressed in 'The Army Medical Service and the Army Council', *BMJ*, 4 Nov., 1905, 1211-3.

66 'The Doctor in Modern Warfare', *BMJ*, 13 May, 1905, 1051.

67 That the performance of the Japanese was unique, was an idea expressed both during and after the war. Sir Walter Foster, *Parliamentary Debates. House of Commons*, 22 Feb., 1905, col.950. For L.L. Seaman, the results of the Japanese were 800% better than the average of history: 'This record is, I believe, unparalleled and unapproached in the annals of war', *The Real Triumph of Japan. The Conquest of the Silent Foe* (New York: D. Appleton & Company, 1906), 5.

68 According to the *BMJ*, writing after the war, 'observations... do not indicate that the Japanese possessed any more special arrangements for water analysis and scientific hygienic investigation than did our medical officers', 'Medical Arrangements in the Japanese Army', *BMJ*, 7 April, 1906, 819.

69 'Some Considerations Connected with the Relative Immunity of the Japanese from Typhoid Fever', *Lancet*, 20 May, 1905, 1365-6.

70 John Van Rensselaer Hoff, in an article on 'Medico-Military Notes in Manchuria', *Surgery, Gynaecology and Obstetrics*, iii (1906), 196-216, argued that one of the lessons of the war was that nothing new in medical or surgical treatment had arisen. Hoff served as Assistant Surgeon-General in the United States Army, and acted as military observer with the Russian Forces in the Far East.

71 'The Doctor in Modern Warfare', (note 66), 1052.

72 For evacuation of the sick and wounded in the Japanese army, a Bearer Battalion and a Sick and Wounded Transport Department were used. The latter was not comparable to any British unit. *Russo-*

Japanese War. Medical and Sanitary Reports, 7.

73 According to W.G. Macpherson, writing in *Russo-Japanese War.*
    Medical and Sanitary Reports, the medical service consisted of regular
    medical officers from the active and retired lists; reserve medical
    officers; civilian practitioners who joined the reserve; medical officers
    of red cross relief sections; and finally civilian doctors serving in
    hospitals at home, 10.

74 Eltzbacher, *op. cit.* (note 57), 332. These peacetime preparations
    were described by Sir Ian Hamilton in 'Report on the Medical
    Services in the Russo-Japanese War', 28 Nov., 1904. Wellcome
    Institute, Contemporary Medical Archives Centre (CMAC), RAMC
    446/2.

75 See W.G. Macpherson, 'The Medical Organisation of the Japanese
    Army', *JRAMC*, vi (1906), 250.

76 'Lord Wolseley's Army Corps', *BMJ*, 29 Jan., 1898, 322.

77 Although there had for some time been reserve forces to the AMD,
    these were only partially organised and insufficiently trained to carry
    out the work of the regular forces. For details of the organisation of
    the AMD during the Second Boer War see 'The Medical Services
    During the War', in L.S. Amery, ed. *The Times History of the War in*
    South Africa, 1899-1902 (London: Sampson Low, Marston and
    Company, Ltd., 1909), Volume 6, 499-543, especially 505-9.

78 Many articles on the question of a medical reserve appeared in
    medical journals during the war. According to William Coates, what
    was needed was a 'pre-arranged, well-organised and comprehensive
    scheme' of expansion. In the South African War expansion came via
    outside organisations 'ignorant of army routine and discipline', 'The
    Expansion of the RAMC in Time of War', *JRAMC*, iii (1904), 408.

79 'The Future of the Volunteer Force', *BMJ*, 7 Jan., 1905, 29-30, at
    29.

80 'The Efficiency of the Army Medical Service', *BMJ*, 26 Aug., 1905,
    446-7.

81 'The Future of the Volunteer Force', (note 76), 29.

82 *Parliamentary Debates. House of Commons*, 28 March, 1905, vol 143,
    col.1448-51, Sir Walter Foster criticised the lack of military doctors,
    and the use of civilian doctors in their place, col.1451; *Parliamentary*
    Debates. House of Commons, 7 Aug., 1905, vol 151, col.376, Mr
    Lambert asked whether there was 'a properly-trained medical
    establishment' for the army, and received the reply from Arnold-
    Forster that they would depend upon 'a large number of very highly-
    trained medical officers', which was later expanded to 'very highly-
    trained and highly competent **civilian** officers'. (My emphasis).

83 'The Future of the Volunteer Force', (note 79), 30.

84 Major M.M. O'Connor, 'The Military Medical Reserve Difficulty', *BMJ*, 12 Aug., 1905, 326.

85 W.H. Macnamara, *Notes on Medical Services in War* (London: Gale & Polden, 1895); V. Warren Low, 'An Introductory Address on the Relation of the Military Medical Service to the Civil Profession', *Lancet*, 10 Oct., 1903, 997-1001.

86 W. Burdett-Coutts, 'The Reform of the AMS', *The Times*, 8 Oct., 1901, 10 col.b. He had served as a special commissioner during the Russo-Turkish War.

87 *Parliamentary Debates. House of Commons*, 23 March, 1905, vol 143, cols.995-8, at col. 998. Burdett-Coutts served as M.P. for Westminster.

88 Anita Newcomb McGee, 'How the Japanese Save Lives', *Century Magazine*, (May 1905), 133-45, at 141. According to McCaul, *op. cit.* (note 51), Dr. McGee had undertaken the organisation of the American nursing service, during the Spanish-American War, 36.

89 McGee, *op. cit.* (note 88), 137-8.

90 Major Charles Lynch, 'The Medical Department of the Japanese Army', *Boston Medical and Surgical Journal*, 12 July, 1906, 51-7.

91 C.B.G. de Nancrede, 'Personal Experience During the Spanish-American War Showing the Disadvantages of Depending Upon Untrained Civilian Physicians for Military Service in Times of War; With Some Suggestions', *Military Surgeon*, xxvi (1910), 611-27, at 616.

92 'President Roosevelt on the Medical Profession', *BMJ*, 24 Feb 1906, 451-2.

93 Major Charles Lynch, 'The Medical Department of the Japanese Army', *Boston Medical and Surgical Journal*, 2 Aug., 1906, 118-21, at 120.

94 For Lynch, (note 90), 'the military surgeon... practices a specialty in medicine which... requires special study and constant practice', 52.

95 'The United States Naval Medical Service', *BMJ*, 13 Jan., 1906, 101.

96 'Army Medical Services', *BMJ*, 6 Jan., 1906, 40.

97 Cuthbertson, 'The Medical Department of the Army', 421-3.

98 'Hygiene in the Japanese Army', *BMJ*, 12 Nov., 1904, 1332.

99 Seaman, *op. cit.* (note 61), believed that the Japanese Medical Officer had complete authority in matters affecting the health of the troops; it was the authority not the rank conferred on the Japanese medical officer which was of importance, 144-5.

100 According to Captain B. Vincent's report of 17 May 1905, 'Medical Notes on the Japanese Army', in *Russo-Japanese War. Medical and*

Sanitary Reports, 133-7, the Japanese medical officer was 'proud of his profession, which is considered by the whole army to be a highly honourable one', 133.

101 'The Medical Service of the Army', *The Practitioner*, lxxiv (1905), 276-7.

102 'Some Remarks on Typhoid Fever Among the American Soldiers in the Recent War with Spain', *Journal of Tropical Medicine*, 15 June, 1899, 314.

103 F.H. Welch, 'Enteric Fever in the Army', *Lancet*, 11 Nov., 1905, 1428.

104 'Instruction in Hygiene for Army Officers', *BMJ*, 18 Nov., 1905, 1361.

105 'The Prevention of Disease in the Army', *Medical Press and Circular*, 1 Nov., 1905, 462.

106 *Russo-Japanese War. Medical and Sanitary Reports*, Appendix F of 'Translation of the Field Regulations of the Japanese Army', gives a vocabulary of terms used, 129.

107 McGee, *op. cit.* (note 88), 136.

108 *Ibid.* 137.

109 *Eisei*, meaning hygiene, or sanitation, has a more specific meaning when its component characters are broken down. The first means protect or defend, whilst the other means life. Therefore the work of the sanitary corps was to protect life. Thanks to Celia Russell for her help in the definition of this term.

110 'The Doctor in Modern Warfare', (note 66), 1051.

111 According to Mahito H. Fukuda, the adoption of western medicine, especially public health, as opposed to traditional individualistic regimes, was part of the Japanese policy *fukoku-kyohei*, meaning enrich the country, strengthen the army, adopted in the Meiji era. 'Public Health in Modern Japan: From Regimen to Hygiene', in Dorothy Porter, ed. *The History of Public Health and the Modern State* (Amsterdam: Rodopi, 1994), 385-402, at 388.

112 Lieutenant-Colonel C.J. Burnett, 'Sanitary Arrangements in the Japanese Army', 19 May, 1905, in *Russo-Japanese War. Medical and Sanitary Reports*. When questioning General Nogi about the performance of the Japanese Burnett wrote, 'He replied that during the Japanese-Chinese War they themselves had suffered most severely in consequence of the ignorance or neglect of the men to recognise the necessity of strictly observing the sanitary rules issued for their guidance', 450.

113 According to Seaman, *The Real Triumph of Japan*, in the war with China, the Japanese lost three men from disease to every one lost

from bullets, 4. Comparative figures for the Japanese in both wars were given in a lecture by Baron Kanehiro Takaki, Surgeon-General of the Japanese Navy during the Russo-Japanese War, in 1906. See 'The Preservation of Health in the Japanese Navy and Army', *BMJ*, 19 May, 1906, 1175-6.

114 Sir Walter Foster, *Parliamentary Debates. House of Commons*, 22 Feb., 1905, vol 141, cols.948-53.

115 *Ibid.*

116 Foster acted as Parliamentary Secretary to the Local Government Board, 1892-5, and during that time was instrumental in the improvement of the status of the Medical Officer of Health. 'Medical Members of Parliament', *BMJ*, 13 Jan., 1906, 95-6. At the time of the South African War he warned against the threat of epidemic disease, and had volunteered his services as an expert in sanitation. This offer was refused. Pagaard, *op. cit.* (note 38), 72.

117 Foster, *op. cit.* (note 114).

118 'Japanese Lessons', *Medical Press and Circular*, 12 July, 1905, 40.

119 'The Doctor in Modern Warfare', (note 63), 1051-2.

120 Lord Nelson was another officer reputed to have foreseen the value of medicine, as the following quotation from 11 March 1804, testifies: 'The great thing in all military service is health; and you will agree with me that it is easier for an officer to keep men healthy than for a physician to cure them'. Taken from the frontispiece of F.F. Maccabe's, *War With Disease* (London: Bailliére, Tindall & Cox, 1909), 5th edition, (first published 1906).

121 'The True Function of the RAMC', *BMJ*, 7 July 1906, 39-40. This post-war article asked the question "Why cannot the British Army follow the lead?"

122 McGee, *op. cit.* (note 88), 142.

123 'Major Seaman's Address', *op. cit.* (note 61), 238. In his The Real Triumph of Japan, Seaman dedicated the book to 'that vast army of American Dead, whose lives in war have been needlessly sacrificed through preventable disease, ignorance and complacency'.

124 Seaman, *op. cit.* (note 61), 1-2.

125 *Ibid.*, 7.

126 Sir Walter Foster, *Parliamentary Debates. House of Commons*, 22 Feb., 1905, vol 141, cols.948-53, at col.951. This was echoed by Treves: 'The medical energy of the British Army... in the field is at the wrong end of the column. It is in the rear to deal with the sick; it should be in the van to ward off the onset of disease', 'Army Medical Reform', *BMJ*, 16 June, 1906, 1431.

127 'Some Remarks on Typhoid Fever Among the American Soldiers in

the Recent War with Spain', *Journal of Tropical Medicine*, 15 June, 1899, 314.

128 'Sanitary Effort in the Army', *Lancet*, 23 Sept., 1905, 903.

129 'Royal Navy and Army Medical Services. Efficiency of the AMS', *BMJ*, 9 Sept., 1905, 610. Sir Gilbert Parker, M.P. for Gravesend, raised the question of the responsibilities of combatant officers for the occurrence of disease in their commands in a debate on 'Army Sanitary Re-organisation Scheme', *Parliamentary Debates. House of Commons*, 11 Aug., 1904, col. 231.

130 F. Treves, 'Army Medical Reform', *The Times*, 8 June, 1906, 9 col.e/f.

131 Surgeon Lieutenant-General M. Koike, 'Address Delivered Before the Japanese Medical Association at Tokio', *JRAMC*, vii (1906), 624-31, at 627.

132 Vincent, *op. cit.* (note 100), 136; 'Medical Notes from the Far East', *Lancet*, 11 Feb., 1905, 391-3.

133 The benefits of military training to individuals, society and the army were extolled in a number of articles: 'Manchester. Universal Military Training', *BMJ*, 3 Feb., 1906, 285; W.E.R. 'The RAMC Vol. Some Advantages of Joining the College Company', *The Manchester Medical Student's Gazette*, v (1905), 217-8.

134 'Medical Science and Military Strength', *BMJ*, 9 June, 1906, 1360.

135 Seaman, *op. cit.* (note 61), 143.

136 Vincent, *op. cit.* (note 100), 133

137 *Ibid.*, 136.

138 *Ibid.*

139 Lieutenant-General C.J. Burnett, 'Further Remarks on Sanitary Regulations in the Field', 1 July 1905, in *Russo-Japanese War. Medical and Sanitary Reports*, 453-6, at 456.

140 'Medical Science and Military Strength', *op. cit.* (note 134), 1360.

141 Emerson, *op. cit.* (note 18), 6.

142 'A Lesson in Patriotism', *Punch*, 6 July, 1904.

143 Earl Roberts in his speech on Imperial Defence bemoaned the lack of patriotism among the British: 'What we have to aim at is to get the people of this country to identify themselves with the Army, and to take an intelligent interest in what the Army may have to do. The peoples of other countries are, *Parliamentary Debates. House of Lords*, 10 July, 1905, vol 149, cols.13-15, at col.15.

144 Lynch, (note 90), 118-21.

145 Lynch, 'Medical Department of the Japanese Army', *Boston Medical and Surgical Journal*, 26 July, 1906, 96.

146 'Japanese Losses in the War', *BMJ*, 9 June, 1906, 1361.

147 W.G. Macpherson, 'Creosote as a Prophylactic in the Japanese

Army', in *Russo-Japanese War. Medical and Sanitary Reports*, 477-86.

148 Captain E. Blake Knox, 'Some Medical Notes on War', *JRAMC*, iv (1905), 440.

149 'Report of the Royal Commission on the War in South Africa', *JRAMC*, iii (1904), 100.

150 Stoney Archer, *op. cit.* (note 10), 742; Lieutenant-Colonel H.K. Allport, 'Training Soldiers in Personal Hygiene', *JRAMC*, iii (1904), 621.

151 Stoney Archer, *op. cit.* (note 9), 742.

152 This was also extended to civilian medical students. Sir James Crichton-Browne in his introductory address on 'Efficiency', at the Charing Cross Hospital in 1905 suggested that students should adopt certain character traits of the Japanese. Among these were 'patriotism and devotion to duty' and 'subordination of the individual interest to the common good', *BMJ*, 7 Oct., 1905, 877-8.

153 Seaman, *op. cit.* (note 91).

154 Maccabe, *op. cit.* (note 120), preface to the first edition, ix.

155 *Ibid.*, introduction by M.F. Rimington, Brigadier-General of 3rd Cavalry Brigade, xi.

156 *Ibid.*, 3.

157 *Ibid.*, 30.

158 *Ibid.*, Lecture 5, 'Health and Fitness', 83-92, at 92. This was a lecture given to recruits.

159 *Ibid.*, 85.

160 'Parliamentary Intelligence. The War Office and Medical Science', *Lancet*, 4 March, 1905, 610-11.

161 Barrett, *op. cit.* (note 53), 820.

162 'The Doctor in Modern Warfare', (note 66), 1051.

163 'The Prevention of Disease in the Army', *Medical Press and Circular*, 1 Nov., 1905, 461. Alexander Ogston in his evidence before the Royal Commission on the South African War went so far as to argue that in the British Army, 'bacteriology does not exist', 'Report of the Royal Commission on the War', *JRAMC*, iii (1904), 96-103.

164 'Sanitary Effort in the Army', *Lancet*, 23 Sept., 1905, 903-4, account of Presidential Address to Section of Naval and Military Hygiene by R.H. Firth at London Congress of the Royal Institute of Public Health. For details of the subjects concerning this section see *Journal of State Medicine*, xiii (1905), 122, & 187.

165 Firth, *op. cit.* (note 31), 612-4.

166 'Editorial. Review of Research Done by the RAMC in 1904', *JRAMC*, 219-21, here dissatisfaction was expressed about the Royal Army Medical College still not having been built. Failure to provide

adequate study leave for Army Medical Officers had also been
criticised, 'Reorganisation of the AMS', *The Times*, 30 Sept., 1901,
10 col.a.

167   Firth, *op. cit.* (note 31), 613, argued that the set-up of the British
      Army with reference to disease prevention was 'little better than... a
      hundred years ago', 613. Professor E. Ray Lankester, President of the
      British Association for the Advancement of Science (BAAS), in
      1906, was also critical of the failure to prevent disease through
      funding of scientific research: 'what is so spent is a mere nothing...
      Meanwhile, people are dying by thousands of preventable disease',
      'Presidential Address', in *Report of the Seventy-Sixth Meeting of the
      BAAS, York, 1906* (London: John Murray, 1907), 3-42, at 37.

168   'Japanese Lessons', *Medical Press and Circular*, 12 July, 1905, 39.

169   Seaman, op. *cit.* (note 61), 119.

170   'The Sanitary Function of the AMS', *BMJ*, 9 June, 1906, 1365.

171   'Japanese Lessons', (note 168), 39.

172   'Annus Medicus, 1905. The Naval and Military Medical Services.
      The Late War in the Far East', *Lancet*, 30 Dec., 1905, 1923.

173   Colonel W.G. Macpherson, 'Japanese Casualties, 1904-5', in *Russo-
      Japanese War. Medical and Sanitary Reports*, 304-9, 'Table Comparing
      the Wound and Disease Statistics of the Japanese Forces in the
      Russo-Japanese War with Those of the British Forces in the South-
      African War', 308.

174   See, John van R. Hoff, 'Medical Statistics and the Sanitary
      Department of the Russian Forces in the Far East', *Boston Medical
      and Surgical Journal*, 31 May, 1906, 599-607. In his report on 'The
      Health of the Russian Troops', *op. cit.* (note 42), Colonel W.H.H.
      Waters suggested that in spite of the poor conditions surrounding
      the Russian soldier, losses from disease were small, due to their
      superior physique, 558.

175   This was even extended to the characteristics of the Russians and the
      Japanese. According to Barrett, *op. cit.* (note 50), the Russians were
      'ignorant... slow, long suffering', whereas the 'Japanese are
      educated... cleanly in person and habits... stoical in their capacity
      for bearing pain... temperate, receptive of Western ideals', 799.

176   Sir William Osler, 'Bacilli and Bullets. An Address to the Officers and
      Men in the Camps at Churn', *BMJ*, 3 Oct., 1914, 569-70, at 570.

1

5

Pathology at War 1914–1918:
Germany and Britain in Comparison

Cay-Rüdiger Prüll

Introduction

As Jonathan Harwood has shown in his study of genetics in Germany between 1900 and 1933, scientific medicine is not culturally neutral but, rather, reflects differences in national styles of thought.[1] This chapter argues that such differences became especially prominent during the First World War, which was considered by contemporaries to be not purely a military or territorial conflict, but a battle of cultures. It was a 'Total War' in every sense of the term.[2]

When looking for national differences in medicine during the First World War, an examination of the history of the discipline of pathology is particularly fruitful. Dealing with fundamentals such as the causation and development of disease, the institutionalization of pathology during the nineteenth century was vitally important to the rise of scientific medicine. In the first decades of the twentieth century, pathology was one of the cornerstones of scientific medicine.[3] Comparing Germany and Britain in the First World War is an intriguing enterprise because of their very different traditions in pathology. In Germany, pathology was influenced by the work of Rudolf Virchow (1821-1902), who promoted experimental science and the use of the microscope in medicine and developed the principle of 'cellular pathology', which was based on the analysis of organs and tissues. Virchow advocated pathological anatomy and stimulated the foundation of institutes of pathology from as early as the 1850s.[4] Separated from clinical medicine, specialists examined routinely the causes of disease by analysing morphological changes of organs, tissues and cells. In the last third of the nineteenth century, however, this approach had to compete with bacteriology, the discipline which considered germs to be the origin of disease. In response to the bacteriologists' claims to have found the cause of a number of diseases by discovering various types of bacteria, many

German pathologists in the period following 1900 emphasised the significance of the human constitution and the 'inner' causes of disease. 'Constitutionalism' offered a chance to support Virchow's demand for experimental research on the development of diseases, but pathologists in Germany remained strong advocates of the morphological approach, which was also practised by Virchow throughout his life; that is, the post-mortem analysis of static pictures of organs, tissues and cells of the human body.[5]

In contrast, pathology in wartime Britain could not draw upon an easily visible network of institutions since the field had not yet been professionalized. Although Virchow's principle of 'cellular pathology' permeated into Britain in the last third of the nineteenth century, autopsies had been mostly in the hands of clinicians. "Morbid anatomy" was looked upon as the main area of pathology, but only gradually did it attain a certain degree of independence. The 'pathologist' of the nineteenth-century London voluntary hospital did his work in the hospital's post-mortem theatre in the hope of gaining a post as a clinician,[6] and the conviction that pathology was a mere servant of clinical medicine led to the development of a distinctive branch of pathology – 'clinical pathology'. This sub-discipline began to began to take shape around 1900, when, as a result of the success of bacteriology, many laboratories were set up in Britain. It dealt with the study of body fluids and tissues.[7] In the years before the First World War both branches of pathology – in contrast to German morbid anatomy – maintained close contacts with the clinic, even if they were not yet professionalized. Unlike Germany, British pathology was institutionalized also in the Army, namely the Royal Army Medical Corps (RAMC). Physicians had the opportunity to attend courses and be trained in bacteriological work and the pathological aspects of tropical diseases. The routine and research work of the pathological laboratories of the military hospitals was supervised by the Pathological Department of the Royal Army Medical College in Netley. The latter had close contacts with the pathological departments of the medical schools and hospitals, but this education had only limited effect and, in 1914, only 59 trained pathologists belonged to the RAMC's active services.[8] There was no distinct pathology department in the RAMC until 1921.

Did these two traditions of western pathology influence the reaction of the German and British pathologists to the challenges of the First World War? More generally, does the example of pathology show war to have any significant impact upon the development of scientific medicine in Britain and Germany?[9] When answering these questions four parameters will be taken into consideration: 1) the objectives of pathology, 2) the organization of pathology, 3) its activities and findings, and finally with respect to cultural history – 4) attitudes toward death and autopsy.

The Objectives of German and British Pathology

Immediately after the outbreak of the First World War, the German pathologist Ludwig Aschoff (1866-1942), head of the pathological institute at the University of Freiburg, organized what was then called *Kriegspathologie* ('war pathology').[10] He outlined his approach at the so-called 'War Pathology Meeting' held in Berlin in 1916. The meeting was held in order to clarify the general objectives of pathology during the war and Aschoff intended to combine two major areas of the discipline.[11] First, practical routine work had to be implemented to meet the new military requirements, which meant conducting autopsies on a routine basis in order to ascertain cause of death and to draw up mortality statistics. In addition, various diseases which the pathologist rarely encountered in peacetime were to be researched. Of particular importance was the effect of vaccination on those involved in the war and on direct war injuries; the impact of projectiles on the human body and questions involving wound treatment and the rising number of traumatic infections were other areas that urgently needed to be investigated. In addition, pathologists were to examine special forms of injury relating to the war, such as those resulting from falls, burial under rubble, and gas poisoning.[12]

Secondly, the war pathologists' main point of interest, according to Aschoff, was to be 'constitutional pathology' and, hence, the substantiation of the theoretical concept of 'Constitutionalism'. Aschoff, in his objectives for war pathology, referred to the examination of organs, tissue, and cells in terms of the morphological programme of Virchow's 'cellular pathology'. Furthermore, he wished to propel research into the cause of disease by studying the *Habitus* (the body's disposition) and the overall constitution of the individual, thus integrating holistic aspects into pathology. He aimed to create a 'secure foundation for the constitutional doctrine', most likely because he felt the time was ripe for this once-in-a-lifetime opportunity

> to perform autopsies on such a great number of individuals in their best years of youth and manhood, some of whom had no previous illnesses of note, their death having set in rapidly following gunshot wounds.[13]

The focal point of pathology was no longer the sick individual but rather the comportment of the healthy organism of the able-bodied male and how it adapted to the war situation. The crisis of war was exploited for this purpose and, as a result, autopsies, to be conducted immediately after the subject's death, became a crucial measure for eliciting information about normal anatomy and physiology. In the future, post-mortem examinations were to be conducted on all soldiers that had been killed.[14] Weight, dimensions, and altered condition of the individual organs were to be registered and compared; constitutional anomalies were to be looked for and the influence of war on their development was to be analysed.[15]

At the meeting in 1916, Aschoff had invited all those 'German and Austrian colleagues who were active in some way as pathological anatomists in the service of the Army'.[16] Among the 47 pathologists who gave lectures or took part in the discussion, 13 of 27 full professors from pathological institutes of the universities in the German-speaking countries were present.[17] Hence, the activities generated by war pathology were supported by a vast number of the Reich's expert representatives. Aschoff was able to win these colleagues over to his own ideas; thus, it seems reasonable to suggest that Aschoff's aims were shared by most German pathologists at that time. They believed that it was important keep the morphological tradition of German pathology with its methods, which should prove theoretical ideas about constitutional pathology.

Unlike German 'war pathology', the discipline in Britain was not constricted by theory and followed a more pragmatic programme. Military pathology in Britain was organized by Colonel Sir William Boog Leishman (1865-1926), a well-known specialist in tropical medicine, whose orientation was very different from that of Aschoff. Leishman clarified his views on the tasks of pathology during the First World War in a co-edited publication in 1923; they effectively sum up the general course of military pathology in Britain:

> It remained for the war itself to demonstrate the importance of the services which modern pathological knowledge was in a position to offer in aid of the common aim – the maintenance of the health of the troops and the effective treatment of the sick and wounded.[18]

Leishman, after all, only applied *this* doctrine when dealing with the objectives of British pathology. At first, British pathology intended to provide a service for clinicians that was supposed ultimately to benefit the patients: the health of the troops and the effective treatment of the ill and wounded soldiers were a core objective of pathology. The focus on the dominant illness, mainly infectious diseases, in the First World War, is in keeping with this pragmatic interest. According to Leishman's statement, the work of the pathologist in the field – in terms of diagnostics and therapy – must be chiefly of a bacteriological nature. For Leishman, opening the human body was of minor importance. In his statements concerning the organization of the 'pathological service', autopsy is mentioned only twice.[19] Morbid anatomy was subordinate to clinical pathology.

Leishman's aim was not so much to gain knowledge by working on the deceased but, rather, to provide direct assistance in the treatment of the living. However, he never formulated a more detailed, theoretical concept of the work of the British pathologists in the First World War. As the organizer of British pathology, Leishman had as much power as his German counterpart, Ludwig Aschoff, and just as Aschoff's work epitomised German 'war pathology', Leishman's was typical of British pathology.

The Organization of German and British Pathology

German 'war pathology' was established mainly because of Ludwig Aschoff's tremendous dedication. The program was created, following a conversation between Aschoff – aflame with national fervour[20] – and the head of the Army Medical Corps, Otto von Schjerning (1853-1921), in the main headquarters of the German army in Luxembourg in September of 1914.[21] As von Schjerning's consulting army pathologist, Aschoff was the head of the organization. The various Institutes of pathology in the German universities, founded since the 1850's, and their directors, formed the operation's backbone. A chief pathologist was to be assigned to each army and the entire army was to be provided with pathologists, and a graduated system of dissectors in the field and home-based military hospitals on all fronts of the war. Organs, organ segments, or organ specimens that had been obtained upon autopsy were to be forwarded to the appropriate army pathologists by the medical examiner in each case in order to be viewed and registered as instruction material in Berlin, Munich, and Vienna, and to be sorted out for war pathology exhibits. The co-ordination of this work among the individual pathologists was done by Aschoff himself in collaboration with an expert from the Kaiser Wilhelm Academy in Berlin.[22]

William Boog Leishman attained his position in a different way, for he organized British military pathology only when wartime pressures on clinical medicine forced him to do so. Following the outbreak of hostilities, the British military did not consider employing pathologists as a primary goal, but the unexpectedly high occurrence of tetanus, gas gangrene, and severe forms of blood poisoning after the initial battles changed the situation. On 3 October 1914 Leishman was dispatched to France to be with the troops of the British Expeditionary Force.[23] A few months later he obtained the title of 'Adviser in Pathology' and his work dealt with everything in respect to the practice of pathology. His tasks were various: 1) visiting and inspecting mobile and hospital laboratories along with co-ordinating their work, 2) working as an advisor regarding to the hiring of staff for these laboratories, 3) working as an advisor with regard to building new laboratories and procuring laboratory equipment, 4) organizing the distribution of laboratories and pathologists according to local need, 5) advising the "Medical Store Departments" concerning the procurement of laboratory equipment, reagents and technical equipment, 6) working as an advisor regarding all matters dealing with the use and replenishment of sera and vaccines, 7) working as an advisor for troop and work contingents concerning tropical diseases and parasitic illnesses, 8) assistance in checking the sanitary conditions on the front, 9) planning for the collection of pathological specimens.[24]

Due to his various obligations in the army, Leishman's work could only be accomplished by delegating the tasks and creating a network of army pathologists. To meet this objective, he was granted an assistant later on in the war, when an 'Assistant Adviser in Pathology' was hired for every army and base unit. The assistant advisers were responsible for the laboratories in their Army Area and also had an advisory function. Remarkably, in the course of the war, a gradual professionalization process can be noted: although the task of the local consultant was at first in the hand of a non-specialist, this office was increasingly being given to pathologists. Finally, by the end of 1917, 97 pathologists were employed in France. They were all responsible to the superior Adviser in Pathology, namely Leishman.[25] In contrast to Aschoff, he was integrated in a huge, complex network in the military medical service.

The Activities and Findings of German and British Pathology

The work of German 'war pathology' essentially comprised four areas: 1.) work in the autopsy room, 2.) the conducting of microscopic examinations and bacteriological analyses in the laboratory, 3.) work directly on the front, including the collection of soil specimens as part of the search for pathogens 4.) research in the field of morbid anatomy mainly in the universities of the homeland and, 5.) army pathologists travelled and gave lectures at evening events for war-physicians as a means of education for colleagues of other disciplines. They also met with representatives of the Central Powers at international meetings of their brothers in arms for the purpose of exchanging opinions.[26] War pathology collections of dissected material and autopsy-reports were scheduled to be set up for later evaluation in Berlin (*Kaiser-Wilhelm-Akademie für militärärztliches Bildungswesen*; collections were housed in the Pathology Institute of the University of Freiburg until the spring of 1916[27]), Munich (*Militärärztliche Akademie*), and Vienna. In 1921 there was a register of as many as 70,000 autopsy reports and over 6,000 dissected specimens in Berlin. In Germany, as of 1916, 21 representatives from the field of pathological anatomy at German universities were available as army pathologists. In addition, there were 30 medical specialists in the homeland, among them 15 professors and six lecturers (*Privatdozenten*) from major hospital institutions.[28]

British pathology between 1914 and 1918 did basically the same work as German pathology and four areas of work can be distinguished: 1) laboratory work in 'clinical pathology', e.g. microscopical examinations and bacteriological analysis, 2) the performance of autopsies. Work in both of these fields was done in the 'mobile laboratories' and in hospitals (and their laboratories) in the rear area of the front, 3) research performed in special research centres, 4) cooperative work with clinicians in research committees with the duty to publish the results. Similar to the German example, British professionals in the research institutions and hospitals in the homeland were mobilised for action.[29] As in Germany, the organisation of British pathology in the First World War was a massive undertaking: between 1914 and 1918, there were 25 mobile laboratories in service, 18 were operating on the Western Front. At the end of 1917, 75 pathologists on the English side were employed in all 85 hospitals in France.[30]

The work of German and British pathologists during the First World War followed closely their respective outlines, and different priorities were clearly evident in both countries. While German pathology focused mainly on traditional morbid anatomy, British pathologists did their work chiefly in the field of clinical pathology. This also had consequences for the relationship between pathology and clinical medicine.

Morbid Anatomy

The activities of German 'war pathology' were essentially based on the methods of pathological anatomy. The latter influenced the process of obtaining knowledge and the approach to particular problems in this field. The dominance of morphological thought in accordance with Virchow's legacy was taken up by Aschoff as of 1914 by limiting his military medical project mainly to autopsies. This is true of war pathology in general: of the 17 contributions on war pathology printed between 1914 and 1921 in the renowned professional journals *Virchows Archiv für pathologische Anatomie und Physiologie und für klinische Medizin* and *(Zieglers) Beiträge zur pathologischen Anatomie und allgemeinen Pathologie*, the post-mortem examination was of paramount interest as the basic method for gaining knowledge.[31] The volume edited by Aschoff in 1921 presenting the results of 'war pathology' was entirely devoted to 'pathological anatomy'.[32] This had consequences for the theoretical foundation of the acquisition of knowledge, for, in ascertaining the status of an organ, any changes at the moment of death were recorded. The development of disease processes usually was not investigated by performing continuous measurements on the basis of animal experimentation, but rather by a painstaking description of a sequence of individual pictures of the condition of the organ in terms of morphological 'momentary snapshots'. An exemplary experimental design of such a study by the pathologist, Roman Adelheim (1881-1938), is cited here:

> We did not preserve the deaths that occurred soon after the gas attack for a post-mortem examination since it was not possible to take away the bodies due to the fire of the Germans. As a result, only the later stages of death could be subjected to a post-mortem examination, namely deaths that were 2, 3, and 4 times 24 hours following poisoning. In order to avoid repetitions, we broke down our ... material into 3 groups: Group I, 7 corpses (death 2 x 24 hours after poisoning); Group II, 4 corpses (death 3 x 24 hours after poisoning); Group III, 2 corpses (4 x 24 hours after poisoning). In addition, there was still one case ... which met with death as a result of freshly disseminated pulmonary tuberculosis 7 weeks after poisoning.[33]

Probing into the cause of the death of those taking part in war brought important findings at first: the soldier in the field generally did not fall ill in a different way than did the civilian and many illnesses were not intensified as compared with peacetime.[34] However, the war could also aggravate symptoms that had already appeared in peacetime.[35] Furthermore, illnesses could be studied which the physician only rarely encountered in peacetime.[36]

The morphological approach described here was, however, mainly used for elaborating results for the field of constitutional pathology. Ludwig Aschoff's ideas about the concept of disease were decisive in this respect. In his talk held in 1915 entitled 'Disease and War', he categorically made a distinction between 'diseased states' and 'diseases'; for Aschoff, a diseased state meant 'a hopeless life of suffering against which the body seems to be denied any succour'. He drew a line between such 'inherent frailties of the body' and 'diseases in more narrowly defined terms' which he said were characterised by 'positive achievements as opposed to the mere stagnation of suffering'. Accordingly, illnesses can be eliminated by regeneration or reparation as well as by inflammatory processes. In the following statement, Aschoff interprets inflammation by equating it with a defensive war and, using military vocabulary, describes it as a defensive reaction to attack.[37] To him, war was a 'natural necessity' that took care of selection according to one's constitution. The carrier of a disease, he believed, may suffer damages from the disease; nevertheless,

> the unconsciously, or better yet, consciously tested adaptability of his constitution remains effective from generation to generation..... That which cannot be used succumbs, that which is useable remains and, in so doing, helpfully diminishes the risk of physical and moral disease in subsequent generations....[38]

Aschoff's notions coincided with the concepts of many of his colleagues in the field. In 1919, the full professor (*Ordinarius*) of pathology in Jena, Robert Rössle (1876-1956), emphasised the importance of the impression made by 'splendid human material' in conjunction with the significance and the results of war pathology. He contrasted the healthy young soldiers on the front who had been strengthened by the catharsis of the war to the 'urban, degenerate human material' that the pathologist usually encountered.[39] In a number of additional contributions, 'constitutional anomalies' were examined on the basis of post-mortem examinations that had been conducted during the War. In 1921, the pathologists Richard Hermann Jaffé (1888-1937) and Hermann Sternberg from Vienna suspected that sudden inexplicable deaths and casualties on the front as well as suicides had been caused by '*status thymicolymphaticus*' (characteristic: a particularly high parenchymal content of the thymus gland). The reason for accidental death, they felt, could be 'the inappropriate reaction of a mentally and physically inferior person to a momentary hazard'.[40] The expected conclusion was: 'Those with *status thymicolymphaticus* represent an inferior human race; they often succumb to the hazards of daily life whereas the majority of people withstand them without a problem.'[41]

German 'war pathology' was, thus, closely linked to the theoretical concept of constitutional pathology. The latter, in turn, was linked to racial hygiene and ideas about degeneration. 'War pathology' used the method of static morphological research, whereas animal experimentation was maintained only to a limited extent. Ultimately, the reason for dispensing with animal experiments on such a large scale was due to the unfavourable situation in procuring material during the war, yet it was due even more to the German tradition in the field of pathology that proved to be a hindrance for any dynamic functional research.

Autopsies were also performed in the British army, and the dissected specimens collected for pathology museums, but on a much smaller scale than in the German army.[42] This is illustrated by the work of the research centre for 'pathological anatomy', namely the central morgue in Etables-sur-Mer in northern France. The director of this institution as well as of the central laboratory, the pathologist Thomas Henry Gostwyck Shore (1887-1961), performed several thousand autopsies between 1914 and 1918. Each day the findings would be discussed with the medical and surgical physician of the military district. Because of the huge supply of material, Shore was also able to prepare specimens, and he developed a procedure for drying osseous specimens that kept them as white as possible. These specimens were passed on to the War Collection of the Royal College of Surgeons in London which grew immensely in the course of the war.[43] As of 1915, a 'Medical History Committee' even worked on viewing and collecting those specimens from the military hospitals that were particularly impressive and which could be useful for drawing up a 'Medical History of the War'. The potential result of this collecting work was shown in 1923 to be as follows: 2000 wet specimens showing the nature and the sequence of the wounds and diseases of modern warfare were supplemented by 600 dry specimens of bone injuries. As part of the collection there were, in addition, drawings, x-ray images, and 150 wax models which were supposed to demonstrate the results of facial plastic surgery. Although there were tremendous efforts to produce a large number of specimens, the British activities were somehow not as efficient as the German ones.[44]

Clinical Pathology

Clinical pathology was the most important domain of British pathology and 'mobile laboratories' were designed to ensure the medical management of the troops at the front. A laboratory comprised an enclosed truck with a built-in lab for carrying out routine bacteriological examinations as well as research. The clinical pathologist's daily work involved visiting field hospitals and regimental aid posts where he would personally take specimens of sputum, blood, urine, and stool of the ill patients as well as material from infected wounds of the injured. He also performed autospies: the specimens being examined in the laboratory and the findings wired to the appropriate agencies. Vaccines would also be made in these laboratories and, because of their varied work, clinical pathologists were in close contact with colleagues from other specialised disciplines, as well as with their patients, whom they were able to observe directly.[45] Furthermore, there were pathologists in hospital laboratories of the rear area: they dealt with direct treatment of the patients just as the mobile clinical pathologists. They also did bacteriological work, could observe the patients over a longer period of time and apparently had even closer contact with their colleagues in the clinical field.[46]

British military pathology in the First World War was mainly clinical pathology, and in the official history of 1923 – which presents the work of military pathology during the war – at least 20 of 23 papers dealt with bacteriological problems. Only one paper, by contrast, was dedicated to morbid anatomy.[47] Similarly, the 1913/14-1918/19 volumes of the *Journal of Pathology and Bacteriology* contain 21 articles on military pathology, of which at least 14 are on problems of bacteriology or clinical pathology; only four deal with topics in the field of morbid anatomy.[48] Professionals in research institutions and hospitals also did mainly clinical pathology: in both routine treatment and in research, pathologists combated general infectious diseases and those incurred through wound infections. One protagonist of this method is Carl Hamilton Browning (1881-1972), who was the first director of the Bland Sutton Institute of Pathology, founded in 1914 at the Middlesex Hospital in London.[49] His goal was to produce an antiseptic substance that, while exerting bactericidal action, would not induce any tissue damage. In his work, Browning incorporated the new knowledge about the mode of action of the leukocytes and, like Ludwig Aschoff, described his views by using military metaphors although not trying to justify his position by an abstract theory of illness or to deduce it from his findings:

> he great importance of not damaging the tissues lies in the fact that the tissue elements themselves make a brave fight against the infecting microbes, as Metchnikoff's brilliant experiments proved. These tissue elements which combat infection are the leukocytes of the blood and other tissue cells, microscopic soldiers, which carry on an incessant warfare against the bacteria....[50]

Two substances that exhibited both of the properties mentioned above, namely bactericidal action and preservation of tissue, were developed in Browning's laboratories: flavin and brilliant green. In assessing their action, he again made use of military terms without losing sight of the ultimate, practically visible goal of healing the wounded.[51]

Since research could only be conducted on a small scale by the clinical pathologists in mobile laboratories and the hospitals, during the war there arose an increasing need to centralise research in various geographic areas and to employ researchers who would be relieved of the daily routine work of military pathology. One example of such a research centre is linked to the name of the pathologist and bacteriologist, Sir Almroth Wright (1861-1947). He established a laboratory in Boulogne that served chiefly for research in the field of treating war wounds. The central aim of this laboratory was to develop a vaccine against wound infection.[52] Research was done also to support increasing criticism against the common antiseptics. In keeping with his earlier work, strengthening the organism's resistance was of foremost interest for Wright. Since the common antiseptics would have weakened the organism's defences, thereby also reducing the effectiveness of his vaccine therapy, Wright recommended a new agent, namely hypertonic saline, with which the wound would be soaked so as to generate an unobstructed flow of blood serum which would, in turn, promote the destruction of bacteria.[53]

Although Wright's proposals were controversial, his theoretical notions were of both direct and indirect benefit. The direct benefit was the useful propaganda for rapid cleansing of wounds and rapid surgical intervention. The indirect or long-term benefit of his proposals was the promotion of physiological thinking and intellectual controversy about the ideal antiseptic. Looking back, Wright's work must be viewed as a stepping stone along the road toward the discovery of the effective substance, penicillin, in 1928 by his assistant, Alexander Fleming (1881-1955).[54]

Wright's work was in the tradition of British pathology as a whole, since his scientific research ultimately focused on the therapeutic measures for the ill and/or wounded soldiers. Wright also moulded British military pathology in the First World War: among his students were Leishman and Leishman's successor, in April 1918, S. Lyle Cummins.[55] Although Wright applied the ideas of constitutional pathology when contemplating the defensive mechanisms of the entire individual, he did not intend to prove theories about the healthy or unhealthy constitution of the dead. Instead, he aimed at the therapeutic application of certain ideas on the living soldier.[56]

German pathology also did bacteriological work. It was devoted mainly to tetanus, gas gangrene and typhus.[57] But its intention was mainly to conquer lost terrain, since the field of bacteriology was occupied by the hygienists. Neither before nor during the First World War, did German pathologists get a foothold in this field, thus they could not participate in the successes of hygienists: beyond the already mentioned 17 papers in *Virchows Archiv* and *Zieglers Beiträge* there are only six other papers dealing with bacteriology. In the volume on "war pathology" (1921), only 165 of 582 pages were devoted to bacteriology. Moreover, problems were seen almost entirely from morphological point of view in the respective parts of ofthe work.[58]

Working together with Representatives of other Disciplines

German pathology often encountered problems when representatives of the discipline had to work together with colleagues from other fields. This is especially true of the relationship of pathology to internal medicine, surgery and hygiene. There was competition between pathologists and bacteriologists concerning the examination of material from operations, and surgeons were blamed by Aschoff for relying too much on the measures and results of the bacteriologists.[59] This was also true for contacts with colleagues of internal medicine, who – as the army pathologist, Siegfried Gräff (1887-1966), put it in 1921 – would rely far too much on the 'humoral sciences' bacteriology and serology. Moreover, the colleagues of internal medicine would expect the pathologist to give information about functional aspects of the development of diseases, which would overstrain the discipline.[60] But the static, morphological bent of German pathologists was not the only hindrance to cooperation; intraprofessional relationships were also complicated by the German professorial system, since each individual pathologist or clinician tended to defend his domain against incursions by his colleagues. This is also illustrated by an event that was celebrated as a tremendous success by Aschoff: in 1916, the army pathologists got nearly the same rank as army hygienists and thus had a superior position compared to the consulting surgeons of the armies.[61]

British pathology sometimes suffered from interdisciplinary problems as well. The diary of James Henry Dible (1889-1971), pathologist to No.1 General Hospital (since Autumn 1915) and head of No. 7 Mobile Laboratory (from 1916 to 1919), illustrates the ignorance of clinicians and army officers concerning clinical pathology.[62] In 1916, one of the clinical pathologists, Philip Henry Manson-Bahr (1881-1966), presented a lecture to clinicians in Cairo, where he promoted the mutual interest of both clinicians and pathologists.[63] But there were no such difficulties as on the German side: since the beginning of the war, pathologists in Britain were forced to work together with representatives of other fields. Problems of current interest were handled by committees that were especially set up in cooperation with the Medical Research Committee (later Council), founded in 1913, and which were directed to specific needs. Their task was to combat a certain illness, the cause and occurrence of which had first to be researched by scientific work. These committees met occasionally and set up work programmes in which the tasks were assigned to individual scientists. After results had been obtained, these had to be published on leaflets, which were distributed to medical officers at the respective war theatre.[64] Cooperation was so important, that the plan to build central laboratories at the greater hospitals on the Western Front was dismissed: it was feared, that the contact between pathologists, patients and physicians would be disturbed.[65]

On the whole, British pathologists had a much more pragmatic attitude to their work than their German colleagues. Clinical pathology dealt with the treatment of the living patient and offered the opportunity of a better cooperation between clinicians and pathologists. This was even true of morbid anatomy, being of relatively negligible significance in the British case. The objectives regarding to museum activity were also extremely pragmatic. Hence, British pathological anatomy during the First World War adhered also to the objectives of clinical pathology; namely, by contributing as effectively as possible to the elimination of the soldier's illnesses at the front. The transport of specimens from the Western Front to the homeland was organized mainly by physicians and surgeons, namely Thomas Renton Elliott (1877-1961) and Sir John Bland-Sutton (1855-1936).[66]

Notions of Death and Resistance to
Post-Mortem Examinations in World War One

Since pathological anatomy understands death as an instrument for gaining medical knowledge for the benefit of the living, it follows that such aspects are also significant for the history of war pathology. It is commonly held that resistance to autopsies stems from 'superstitions' and religious beliefs which have remained basically the same from Antiquity to the present day, and that such sentiments manifest themselves in essentially three ways. The first of these is the desire to care for the deceased: everything is done to facilitate the transition from life on earth to life in the realm of the dead. The second is the desire to protect the living: since the deceased is still thought to be 'alive' until the soul has departed the body, one must protect oneself from potentially evil influences. The third is the belief that death and dying embrace a potential for magic and religious ritual and that, for such rites, the integrity of the human corpse is of fundamental significance. Thus, with just a few exceptions, popular beliefs have tended to consider autopsies as a form of desecration.[67]

For these reasons, working with an abundance of corpses of soldiers killed in action became a problem for those involved in war pathology. Although it cannot be substantiated that the soldiers were repulsed by the idea of an autopsy, the presence and the reinforcement of such notions in war make it seem very likely that such a repulsion existed.[68] Hence, if someone carried something with him that had belonged to an innocent murder victim, it was purportedly supposed to help against the hazard of war. Also, hammering coffin nails or inserting a needle, with which one had sewn a corpse into a shroud, into the wooden parts of the top of the barrel of one's rifle was supposed to bring good luck.[69]

Superstitions relating to dying, death, bodies and burial, corresponded to the complex of beliefs described above, and existed in Britain and in Germany.[70] In keeping with tradition, it was regarded as important, at least, to bury one's comrades. That burial grounds were destroyed during armed conflicts was a matter of the utmost sensitivity, as the letter of a German soldier documents:

> The crosses and gravestones destroyed on the cemetery, not even the
> dead have peace under the earth; the graves have been unearthed –
> at such sites, one is struck by the entire misery of the war....[71]

Another matter was the mutilation of bodies. In the wartime correspondence of German and British soldiers, one can find many passages that show that the damage to physical integrity was regarded with horror.[72] In the British Army, attempts were made to bury the fallen soldiers right after battle, not only for reasons of hygiene but also to maintain reverence.[73] The mutilation of the human body was not simply taken for granted, since transcendental notions were associated with the body.[74] Other myths, some of which – as with the Germans – made use of an aggressively negative image of the enemy, reveal the loathsomeness of destroying a corpse or handling it disrespectfully. The opponent would be accused of disregarding customary rites and traditions.[75] Hence, some British soldiers believed that the Germans had factories for recycling corpses. The Britons believed that the blockade by their Navy had generated such a scarcity of fat in Germany that bodies had to be transported from the battlefields back to the homeland and be sent to appropriately equipped companies. The fat that would thus be obtained would then be processed into nitro-glycerine, candles, industrial lighting, and shoe polish.[76] Yet, the deeply-rooted horror of abusing traditional rites when handling mortal remains was not only directed toward the enemy but was also of a general nature. Similar events were thought to occur even on one's own side. In the British Army it was said that a 'destructor' – located at the training camp of Etables-sur-Mer – disposed of and incinerated body parts left over from autopsies conducted by British pathologists. It was also rumoured that soldiers had been executed here.[77]

This rumour illustrates a certain uneasiness regarding the dismemberment of the body after death.[78] Remarkably enough, there are no signs that the British pathologists regarded resistance to autopsies as a particularly serious problem, which was probably a reflection of the fact that autopsies were less frequent in the British than in the German army, and of less significance to the development of British pathology. A crucial point which explains why post-mortem examinations were not that central in the British Army was that the fundamental attitude toward the individual and his rights was different from in that in the German forces. This is illustrated by an article in the *Journal of Royal Army Medical Corps* written in 1915, which states that: 'The patient died, and permission for the autopsy was fortunately obtained.'[79] Apparently, the patient's rights were taken into consideration whenever the situation of war made this possible. This was true also with respect to the last wishes of the dying and the dead and the dealing with their belongings.[80]

In contrast, direct signs of resistance to autopsies can be found in the statements by German pathologists. The army pathologist, Hugo Häßner, wrote in 1916:

> Just thinking about the horrifying disfigurement that a shell can cause and how the suture following our examination is capable of restoring, at least to some extent, the shapes from before and eliminating the disfigurement, then I dare say that, far from any bias I may have as a specialist in pathology, the relatives are most certainly indebted to us.

> Another question is: Are we acting in the interests of and according to the will of the deceased himself? Without a doubt! Whoever has given his life for the Fatherland and, in so doing, has made the greatest sacrifice that men can make, will also be willing to have doctors examine the fatal wound on his body so that the observations made and the experience gained may serve the welfare of hundreds of comrades. Definitely the pinnacle in camaraderie and Christian love for one's neighbour [is attained] even in death![81]

The ardour with which post-mortems were performed was garbed in the language of Christian nationalism, which emphasised the willingness with which soldiers sacrificed themselves in the name of God and country. Even pathology, to some extent, was thought to be a 'holy' profession because of the assistance it provided to soldiers. Pathologists also tried to naturalise post-mortem examinations by requesting that members of other professions – as well as soldiers themselves – attend post-mortem examinations.[82] However, pathologists were aided by the very fact that the wartime situation masked their activities in forward areas: events at the front were known to civilians only through official reports. Thus, pathologists could perform autopsies on soldiers' corpses without seeking prior approval from the relatives and, hence, could proceed with dissection immediately after death. This accelerated the procedure and satisfied the needs of constitutional pathology as to authenticity of the material. As a result, frequent remarks that the body had been subjected to autopsy 'in a fresh state' can be found in the scientific papers of German war pathologists.[83]

Conclusion:
Germany and Britain in Comparison

In this chapter I have tried to show that, even in times of war, medicine remains embedded in social and cultural conditions and processes.[84] Pathology, in both Britain and Germany, reflected the political and cultural crises occurring in these countries during the First World War. At the beginning of the war, the basic structures and the organization of German "war pathology" and British military pathology were of a centralised nature with Aschoff and Leishman as leading figures who were fully in command. German "war pathology" was, however, organised in a far more hierarchical way than its British counterpart, reflecting the dominant political ethos of that country. Ludwig Aschoff was answerable only to the chief of the army medical corps. In turn, whenever the chief of the army medical corps gave new instructions, the Freiburg pathologist passed them on to his own colleagues who were either directly or indirectly his subordinates, or to other directors of the pathological institutes who were also involved in military activities. The latter were themselves part of the professorial system that corresponded to the hierarchical political system of Wilhelmine Germany, and these pathologists, themselves, often deputed these tasks to those on the lower rungs of the academic ladder.

The initial contact of the representatives of pathology with the military in each of the two countries corresponded to the attitudes and working methods of the respective pathologists during the war. While Ludwig Aschoff took the initiative on his own and turned to the military with a plan that was at least firmly outlined, his counterpart, William Boog Leishman, did not act until requested to do so. Thus, while German pathologists had their own clearly distinct agenda, their British colleagues thought of themselves as part of team, providing pragmatic assistance to the medical services as a whole.

The different pathological and cultural traditions in both countries and had also important consequences for medical work in the field. In the crisis of war, German pathology readily reverted to the well-tried concept of static, non-functional morphological routine work and research. The autopsy was of primary importance, whereas the examination of disease processes was neglected. Rather than applying routine diagnostic methods as a form of assistance in clinical medicine, research on the constitution of the young, healthy soldier was the predominant interest. The theoretical underpinnings of German pathology were less concerned with the individual than the interests of the German people as a whole, namely the health of the nation. With this perspective, therapeutically valid findings could only be attained with great difficulty; thus, 'war pathology' represented a step backwards rather than forwards.

British pathology, in contrast, adhered firmly to clinical research and was, thus, more directly concerned with the treatment of the living patient. Pathology in wartime Britain continued to be shaped by its traditionally close links with clinical medicine. When the war broke out, Leishman logically concluded that it would be his objective to contribute to diagnosis and therapy of war wounds and war infections. British pathology, accordingly, concentrated chiefly on bacteriological work involving the diagnosis, treatment and prevention of disease. The clinical pathologist was in direct contact with body fluids and body tissue as a result of collecting them with his own hands, and he became actively involved in discussions about such issues as antisepsis and asepsis. Another field of therapeutic activity was inoculation, an issue that German pathology also studied but to a lesser degree. Constitutional pathology and its way of thinking influenced British military pathology only in practical, useful measures and did not aim at proving theoretical constructs; the functional, dynamic approach was far more important. Thus, the term 'pathology' was understood more broadly than in Germany where it was basically put on a par with 'pathological anatomy'.

British pathology stressed the need for cooperation between pathologists, clinicians, and patients. William Boog Leishman was involved in a number of committees concerning a wide variety of topics. The measures that had to be taken were not implemented by pathologists alone but were always discussed and decided together with members of other clinical disciplines and/or the warring powers on the Allied side. The organization of British pathology as a discipline, therefore, corresponded strongly to the social and political culture of the country. Indeed, a recent study has shown that the education of girls and boys in nineteenth-century Britain placed strong emphasis on the discursive element, whereas in the hierarchical-structured German Empire there was no education that would have promoted independent reasoning.[85] At least until 1920, Liberalism dominated political attitudes in Britain,[86] whereas the German Empire, collapsing in 1918, was ruled by conservative thinking. In Germany, the relationship between pathologists and representatives of other disciplines was characterised mainly by competition between the 'leaders' of their respective fields.

In order to carry out their program for constitutional pathology, German pathologists had to take advantage of the war situation and had to conduct a large number of post-mortems. The battlefields – much more than in the case of British Pathology – had to be converted into 'experimental laboratories' and, therefore, popular resistance to autopsies had to be overcome.[87] Although religious and other forms of opposition to autopsies existed in Britain as well, the conflict never arose on such a scale as in the German army. British pathologists concentrated more than their German colleagues on the living patient and on the treatment of his ailments; they did not see the war as an opportunity to attempt autopsies on a large-scale. As a result, a more difficult conflict was spared.

In a period in which the discipline of pathology was still fundamental to the development of medicine as whole, the directions taken by British and German pathologists during the war show that modern medicine had evolved along distinctly national lines. These different traditions – which were revealed starkly by the upheavals of the First World War – corresponded closely to the different political and cultural-historical situations in their respective countries. War did not bring benefits as such for the development of pathology in Germany and Britain, but served only to strengthen national medical traditions, which had their roots in the nineteenth century. Indeed, the continued reliance on these traditions during the war had important consequences for the subsequent development of pathology and medicine in both countries. In Britain, clinical pathology became professionalised in the period between the two world wars and, due to its practical side, was able to contribute to the development of new therapeutic agents such as penicillin.[88] In Germany, however, pathology remained reliant on theories taken from constitutional pathology and which were enshrined, in 1920, in the establishment of the journal *Veröffentlichungen aus der Kriegs- und Konstitutionspathologie* (*Publications on War- and Constitutional Pathology*). In 1936, under the main influence of Ludwig Aschoff, the journal was published under the title *Veröffentlichungen aus der Konstitutions- und Wehrpathologie* (*Publications on Constitutional- and Military Pathology*). The 'war pathology' of the First World War, and its founder Ludwig Aschoff, thus had a formative influence on the development of German pathology into the interwar-period and, ultimately, under the Third Reich.[89]

Notes

1 J. Harwood, *Styles of Scientific Thought. The German Genetics Community 1900-1933* (Chicago, London: University of Chicago Press, 1993).

2 Cf. R. Koselleck, Krise, in O. Brunner *et al.* (eds), *Geschichtliche Grundbegriffe*, Vol.3. (Stuttgart: Klett-Cotta, 1982), 617-650; R. Cooter, 'War and Modern Medicine', in W.F. Bynum and R. Porter (eds), *Companion Encyclopedia of the History of Medicine*, Vol.2 (London/New York: Routledge, 1993), 1536-73, especially 1561-64;

W.L. Bühl, Krisentheorien, *Politk, Wirtschaft und Gesellschaft im Übergang* (Darmstadt: Wissenschaftliche Buchgesellschaft, 1988), 1-10.

3   A recent overview on the history of pathology and its problems is: R.C. Maulitz, 'The Pathological Tradition', in Bynum & Porter, *op. cit.* (note 2), Vol.1, 169-91.

4   Concerning Virchow, see: E.H. Ackerknecht, *Rudolf Virchow. Arzt, Politiker, Anthropologie* (Stuttgart: Enke, 1957); M. Vasold, *Rudolf Virchow. Der große Arzt und Politiker* (Stuttgart: DVA, 1988). The institutionalization of German pathology is described in: I. Hort, *Die Pathologischen Institute der deutschsprachigen Universitäten (1850-1914)* (MD Thesis, Cologne, 1987); J. Pantel, A. Bauer, 'Die Institutionalisierung der Pathologischen Anatomie im 19. Jahrhundert an den Universitäten Deutschlands, der deutschen Schweiz und Österreichs', *Gesnerus*, xlvii (1990), 303-28.

5   About constitutionalism: D.v. Engelhardt, 'Kausalität und Konditionalität in der modernen Medizin', H. Schipperges (ed.), *Pathogenese. Grundzüge und Perspektiven einer Theoretischen Pathologie* (Berlin, Heidelberg etc.: Springer, 1985), 32-85, especially 32-8; J. Probst, *Zur Entwicklung der Konstitutionslehre zwischen 1911 und 1980* (MD Thesis, Freiburg i.Br., 1982). Concerning the Virchow-heritage and German pathology: C.-R. Prüll, 'Die Grundkonzepte der Pathologie in Deutschland von 1858 bis heute und der Fortschrittsbegriff in der Medizin', *Gesnerus*, lii (1995), 247-63.

6   R.C. Maulitz, *Morbid Appearances. The Anatomy of Pathology in the early Nineteenth Century* (Cambridge: Cambridge University Press, 1987); George Cunningham, *The History of British Pathology* (Bristol: White Tree Books, 1992), 26-58.

7   W.D. Foster, *Pathology as a Profession in Great Britain and the early History of the Royal College of Pathologists* (London: The Royal College of Pathologists, 1983) 1-18; *idem, A Short History of Clinical Pathology* (Edinburgh, London: Livingstone, 1961).

8   W.B. Leishman, 'Organization of the Pathological Service', in *idem* and W.G. MacPherson (eds), *Medical Services Pathology (History of the Great War. Based on official Documents)* (London: His Majesty's Stationery Office, 1923) 1-31, especially 2/3.

9   Cooter, *op. cit.* (note 2), 1536-73; See also: D.E.H. Edgerton, 'Science and War', R.C. Olby, G.N. Cantor *et al.* (eds), *Companion to the History of Modern Science* (London/New York: Routledge, 1990), 934-45.

10 About the German 'war pathology' in general, see: C.-R. Prüll, 'Die Sektion als letzter Dienst am Vaterland. Die deutsche "Kriegspathologie" im Ersten Weltkrieg', W.U. Eckart, C.

Gradmann (eds), *Die Medizin und der Erste Weltkrieg (Neuere Medizin- und Wissenschaftsgeschichte. Quellen und Studien, Vol.3)* (Pfaffenweiler: Centaurus, 1996), 155-82;

11   Cf. *Kriegspathologische Tagung in Berlin am 26. und 27. April* 1916 (Centralblatt für Allgemeine Pathologie und Pathologische Anatomie, Supplement of Vol.27) (Jena: Fischer, 1916); L. Aschoff, 'Über die Aufgaben der Kriegspathologie', *ibid.*, 1-9.

12   *Ibid.*, 2-5.

13   Both quotations: *ibid.*, 3.

14   H. Häßner, *Pathologische Anatomie im Felde, Virchows Archiv für Pathologische Anatomie und Physiologie und für klinische Medizin* [hereafter *VA*], 221 (1916), 309-32, especially 309.

15   Aschoff, *op. cit.* (note 11), 1-9.

16   *Ibid.*, 1.

17   *Op. cit.* (note 11), Contents, iii-iv.

18   Leishman, *op. cit.* (note 8), 5.

19   These were short remarks about autopsies performed by the pathologists of the 'Mobile Laboratories' and about those done in the 'central mortuary' in Etables-sur-Mer in northern France. See: *ibid.*, 21, 23.

20   In respect of Aschoff's nationalistic attitudes, see: *idem, Bismarck. Lecture, given at the Bismarck-celebration of the city and university of Freiburg i.Br.* (Freiburg: Troemers Universitäts-Buchhandlung, 1915); *idem, Rede, gehalten am 13. Mai 1916 bei der öffentlichen Feier der Übergabe des Prorektorats der Universität Freiburg i.Br.* (Freiburg: Günther, 1916); Kaisers Geburtstag. Lecture, given at the 'Vaterländischen Abend' in the theatre of the city of Freiburg, 27 January 1916, (Freiburg: Wagners Hof- und Universitäts-Buchdruckerei, 1916).

21   Cf. Ludwig Aschoff to his wife Clara, Luxembourg, Headquarter, 19 September 1914, *idem, Ein Gelehrtenleben in Briefen an die Familie* (Freiburg i.Br.: Schulz, 1966), 222-3; F. Büchner, 'Ludwig Aschoff zum Gedenken an seinen 100. Geburtstag (10.1.1866 bis 24.6.1942)', *Verhandlungen der Deutschen Gesellschaft für Pathologie*, 50 (1966), 475-89, especially 476; *idem*, Gedenkrede auf Ludwig Aschoff. Gehalten bei der Gedenkfeier der Universität Freiburg am 5. Dezember 1943, Feldpostbrief der Medizinischen Fakultät der Universität Freiburg/Brsg. No.4, 1-24, especially 18. About Aschoff's life in general, see also: E. Seidler, *Die Medizinische Fakultät der Albert-Ludwigs-Universität Freiburg im Breisgau. Grundlagen und Entwicklungen* (Berlin, Heidelberg, New York etc.: Springer, 1991) 207-10, 270-2, 333/34.

22 Aschoff, *op. cit.* (note 11), 8-9.

23 Leishman, *op. cit.* (note 8), 25.

24 *Ibid.*, 7-8.

25 *Ibid.*, 8-9,15.

26 Prüll, *op. cit.* (note 10), 163-4.

27 Aschoff, *op. cit.* (note 21), 279.

28 C. Kliche, *Die Stellung der deutschen Militärärzte im Ersten Weltkrieg*
    (MD Thesis, Berlin, 1968), 18/19; L. Aschoff, 'Über die Bedeutung
    der Kriegspathologie', *Deutsche Militärärztliche Zeitschrift*, 47
    (1918), 81-87, especially 81; *idem*, 'Vorwort', in *idem, Pathologische
    Anatomie (Handbuch der Ärztlichen Erfahrungen im Weltkriege
    1914/1918*, ed. by Otto v. Schjerning, Vol.VIII (Leipzig: Barth
    1921), V. R. Rössle, 'Allgemeine Pathologie und Pathologische
    Anatomie: Bedeutung und Ergebnisse der Kriegspathologie',
    Jahreskurse für ärztliche Fortbildung, 10 (1919), 15-46, especially 16.

29 See, for example: J.W.H. Eyre, 'Work in the Bacteriological
    Department, 1914-1919', *Guy's Hospital Reports* (War Memorial
    Number), 70 (1922), 257-71; W. Fletcher, Report upon the
    Bacteriological Examination of one thousand Soldiers convalescent
    from diseases of the dysentery and enteric groups, *Journal of the
    Royal Army Medical Corps* [hereafter: *JRAMC*], 30 (1918), 51-75.

30 A.C.H. Gray, 'Mobile Laboratories', in *ibid.*, 257-71, especially
    270/71; Leishman, *op. cit.* (note 8), 12-15, 21-22.

31 Following the order of appearance: F. Henke, Pathologisch-
    anatomische Beobachtungen über den Typhus abdominalis im
    Kriege, Beiträge zur pathologischen Anatomie und zur allgemeinen
    Pathologie [hereafter: *Zieglers Beiträge*], 63 (1916), 781-88; Häßner,
    op. cit. (note 14); L. Aschoff, 'Über das Leichenherz und das
    Leichenblut, *Zieglers Beiträge*, 63 (1916), 1-21; L. Frankenthal,
    'Über Verschüttungen', *VA*, 222 (1916), 332-45; E. Miloslavich,
    'Hirnhypertrophie und Konstitution', *Zieglers Beiträge*, 62 (1916),
    378-402; C. Sternberg, 'Zur pathologischen Anatomie des
    Paratyphus', *Zieglers Beiträge*, 64 (1918), 278-96; H. Beitzke, 'Über
    Heilungsvorgänge bei der Ruhr', Zieglers Beiträge, 64 (1918), 436-
    53; W. Groß, 'Frische Glomerulonephritis (Kriegsniere)', *Zieglers
    Beiträge*, 65 (1919), 387-422; K. Nicol, 'Pathologisch-anatomische
    Studien bei Fleckfieber', *Zieglers Beiträge*, 65 (1919), 120-47; H.
    Koopmann, 'Die pathologische Anatomie der Influenza 1918/19',
    VA, 228 (1920), 319-44; T. Fahr, 'Zur Frage der Kriegswirkung auf
    Ernährungsverhältnisse, Morbidität und Mortalität', *VA*, 228 (1920),
    187-99; E. Billigheimer, 'Kasuistische Beiträge zur Pathologie des
    Peritoneums', *Zieglers Beiträge*, 66 (1920), 515-21; R.H. Jaffé, H.

Sternberg, 'Kriegspathologische Erfahrungen', *VA*, 231 (1921), 346-438; H. Groll, 'Anatomische Befunde bei Vergiftung mit Phosgen (Kampfgasvergiftung)', *VA*, 231 (1921), 480-518; H. Bettinger, 'Die Ödemkrankheit auf Grund der Kriegserfahrungen des pathologischen Institutes Halle', *VA*, 234 (1921), 195-209; O. Lubarsch, 'Beiträge zur pathologischen Anatomie und Pathogenese der Unterernährungs- und Erschöpfungskrankheiten', *Zieglers Beiträge*, 69 (1921), 242-51; R. Adelheim, 'Beiträge zur Pathologischen Anatomie und Pathogenese der Kampfgasvergiftung', *VA*, 236 (1921), 309-60. Only those papers were counted as contributions to "war pathology", which were written by field pathologists and/or were based on the examination of soldiers killed in action or deceased prisoners of war.

32 Aschoff (ed.), *op. cit.* (note 28), vii-viii.

33 Adelheim, 'Pathologische Anatomie und Pathogenese der Kampfgasvergiftung', 310.

34 See, for example, in the case of appendicitis: G. Herxheimer, Die Atmungs- und Verdauungsorgane und ihre Erkrankungen. Das Zentralnervensystem und seine Erkrankungen, L. Aschoff (ed.), *Pathologische Anatomie*, 18-25, especially 20.

35 See, for example: H. Beitzke, Fortschreitende Phthisen, in *ibid.*, 63-6, especially 65.

36 C. Sternberg, Mischinfektionen, in *ibid.*, 192-6, especially 193.

37 L. Aschoff, *Krankheit und Krieg. Eine akademische Rede* (Freiburg i.Br.: Günther, 1915), 7-8,12 ff.

38 *Ibid.*, 29, 32. Concerning Aschoff's attitudes in World War One see: H.-P. Schmiedebach, 'Sozialdarwinismus, Biologismus, Pazifismus – Ärztestimmen zum Ersten Weltkrieg', in J. Bleker and *idem* (eds), *Medizin und Krieg. Vom Dilemma der Heilberufe 1865 bis 1985* (Frankfurt/M: Fischer, 1987), 93-121, especially 103-108.

39 Rössle, *op. cit.* (note 28), 19, 34.

40 Jaffé & Sternberg, *op. cit.* (note 31), 434.

41 Jaffé & Sternberg, 'Die Drüsen mit innerer Sekretion', in: Aschoff (ed.), *op. cit.* (note 28), 36-44, especially 40.

42 See, for example: F.W. Mott, 'The Microscopic Examination of the Veins of two Men dead of Commotio Cerebri (Shell Shock) without visible external injury', *JRAMC*, 29 (1917), 662-77. Mott, who worked in the Pathological Laboratory of the London County Council in the Maudsley Hospital in London, examined the whole body of the deceased, even if he had special interests.

43 T.H.G. Shore, M.D., F.R.C.P., 'Obituary', *British Medical Journal*, 2.12.1961 II (1961), 1502/03, 1790.

44 Sir A. Keith and S.G. Shattock, 'The War Office Collection of
    Pathological Specimens', in Leishman & MacPherson (eds), *op. cit.*
    (note 8), 574-8. See also: R. Richardson, 'The Preparation of Dry
    Museum Specimens of Bone for the War Office Collection', *Journal
    of Pathology and Bacteriology* [hereafter: *JPathBact.*], 21 (1916-1917),
    491-2, especially 491; P. Turner, Some Experiences of the Work of
    General Hospitals in France, *Guy's Hospital Reports* (War Memorial
    Number), lxx (1922), 157-82, especially 169.

45 Gray, *op. cit.* (note 30), 257-71; Leishman, *op. cit.* (note 8), 9-12;
    J.T. Wigham, Adrian Stokes (1887-1927), *JPathBact*, 31 (1928) I,
    121-5, especially 122; A.E.B. (Arthur Edwin Boycott ?) and H.C.
    (Hector Cameron ?), Major Sydney Domville Rowland (1872-
    1917), *JPathBact.*, 21 (1916-1917), 453-6, especially 455.
    Concerning autopsies and 'Mobile Laboratories', see: W.C.B. Meyer,
    J.W. Dew, A. Stokes, 'A Note on four Post-mortem Examinations in
    which Rupture of the Intestine was found, although the Course of
    the Projectile was extraperitoneal', *JRAMC*, 26 (1916), 100-102.
    Stokes did all autopsies and examined every organ, see: *ibid.*, 100.

46 Turner, *op. cit.* (note 44), 167; T.K. Boney, L.G. Grossman, C.L.
    Boulenger, Report of a Base Laboratory in Mesopotamia for 1916,
    with special reference to water-borne diseases, *JRAMC*, 29 (1917),
    409-23; O. Richards, 'The Development of Casualty Clearing
    Stations', *Guy's Hospital Reports* (War Memorial Number), 70 (1922),
    115-23, especially 115, 121.

47 See: Leishman, *op. cit.*, (note 8); also: Sir A. Wright, 'The Physiology
    of Wounds', 32-77; A. Stokes, 'Gas Gangrene', 78-96; M.
    Robertson, 'Bacteriology of anaerobic Infections', 97-118; W.H.
    Tytler (with A. Fleming), 'Infection of Wounds by Microbes other
    than sporebearing Anaerobes', 119-41; Sir K.W. Goadby, 'Latent
    Sepsis in Wounds', 142-63; S.L. Cummins, 'Tetanus in its Statistical
    Aspects', 164-87; Sir F.W. Andrewes, 'The Pathology and
    Bacteriology of Tetanus', 188-210; Sir W.B. Leishman, 'The Enteric
    Fevers', 211-64; J.C.G. Ledingham, 'Diarrhoea and Enteritis', 265-
    76; C.C. Dobell (with D. Harvey), 'Amoebic Dysentery', 277-318;
    Sir F.W. Andrewes, 'Bacillary Dysentery', 319-46; A. Balfour,
    'Typhus Fever', 347-82; M.H. Gordon, 'Cerebro-spinal Fever', 383-
    412; J.G. Adam, 'Influenza', 413-66; S.L. Cummins, 'Tuberculosis',
    467-84; J.W. McNee, 'Trench Fever', 485-512; A. Stokes,
    'Spirochaetal Jaundice', 513-26; Sir J.R. Bradford, 'Acute Infective
    Polyneuritis', 527-32; Sir D. Semple, 'Gingivitis and Vincent's
    Angina', 533-40; R. Muir (with J.S. Dunn), 'War Nephritis', 541-
    65; S.P. James, 'Encephalitis Lethargica', 566-73; Keith & Shattock,

'The War Office Collection of Pathological Specimens', 574-8. All articles in Leishman & MacPherson (eds), *op. cit.* (note 8). The paper by Keith and Shattock is the only one dealing with morbid anatomy.

48 See: J.L. Smith, J. Ritchie, J. Dawson, 'Clinical and Experimental Observations on the Pathology of Trench Frostbite, *JPathBact.*, 20 (1915-1916), 159-90; M. Robertson, 'Notes upon certain Anaerobes isolated from Wounds, *ibid.*, 327-49; H. Henry, 'A Report to the Medical Research Committee from a Base Hospital Laboratory in France', *JPathBact.*, 21 (1916-1917), 344-85; C.G.L. Wolf and J.E.G. Harris, 'A Report to the Medical Research Committee. Contributions to the Biochemistry of Pathogenetic Anaerobes I. The Biochemistry of Bacillus Welchii and Bacillus Sporogenes (Metchnikoff)', *ibid.*, 386-452; H. Drummond and J. Fraser, 'Some experimental Observations on perforating Wounds of the abdominal Viscera', *ibid.*, 457-72; E. Emyrs-Roberts and E.M. Cowell, 'Gas Gangrene of Muscle, with a special Reference to its Morbid Anatomy and Histology', *ibid.*, 473-90; Richardson, 'The Preparation of Dry Museum Specimens of Bone for the War Office Collection', *ibid.*, 491/92; C.G.L. Wolf and J.E.G. Harris, 'A Report to the Medical Research Committee. Contributions to the Biochemistry of Pathogenetic Anaerobes IV. The Biochemistry of Bacillus Histolyticus', *JPathBact.*, 22 (1918-19), 1-21; H.W.C. Vines, 'Report to the Medical Research Committee (From the Cerebro-spinal Fever Laboratory Cambridge). Some Observations on the Agglutination Reaction of the Meningococcus among Carriers', *ibid.*, 56-73; J.W. McLeod and R.E. Bevan-Brown, 'The Technique of Blood Culture', *ibid.*, 74-84; S.M. Cone, 'Histological Observations on normal Nerves and war-injured Nerves with the 'Neurokeratin' Stain', *ibid.*, 105-11; C.G.L. Wolf, 'A Report to the Medical Research Committee. Contributions to the Biochemistry of Pathogenetic Anaerobes V. The Biochemistry of Vibrion septique', *ibid.*, 115-28; R. Donaldson, 'Character and Properties of the 'Reading' Bacillus, on which a new method of treatment of wounds has been based', *ibid.*, 129-51; H.W.C. Vines, 'Strains of Meningococci hyper-sensitive to Agglutination', *ibid.*, 197-209; R.H. Malone and C.J. Rhea, 'Studies on streptococci recovered from sick and wounded soldiers in France. A brief review of previous papers on streptococci, with a report on the types isolated from twenty-five selected cases', *ibid.*, 210-21; R.H. Malone, 'A simple Apparatus for isolating single Organisms, *ibid.*, 222-3; A. Distaso and H.A. Scholberg, 'Agglutination Results with certain dysentery

organisms placed against homologous and heterologous Sera', *ibid.*,
257-61; C.G.L. Wolf, 'A Report to the Medical Research
Committee. Contributions to the Biochemistry of Pathogenetic
Anaerobes VI. The proteolytic Action of Bacillus Sporogenes
(Metchnikoff) and Bacillus Welchii', *ibid.*, 270-88; C.G.L. Wolf, 'A
Report to the Medical Research Committee. Contributions to the
Biochemistry of Pathogenetic Anaerobes VII. The Biochemistry of
Bacillus Proteus', *ibid.*, 289-307; J.H. Mueller, 'Comparative
Toxicity of Triphenylmethane and Flavine Dyes for Tissue and
Bacteria', *ibid.*, 308-18; R.S. Adamson, 'A Report to the Medical
Research Committee. On the Cultural Characters of certain
anaerobic Bacteria isolated from War Wounds', *ibid.*, 345-400.
Similar to the German case only those papers were counted as
contributions to military pathology, which were written by
pathologists in active service and/or were based on the examination
of soldiers killed in action or deceased prisoners of war.

49   See Charles Hamilton Browning, Obituary, *British Medical Journal*
     (1972), 382.
50   C.H. Browning, 'Flavine and Brilliant Green', *The Middlesex
     Hospital Journal*, 20 (1917-1918), 22-25, especially 24.
51   *Ibid.*, 24-5.
52   Leishman, 'Organization of the Pathological Service', 16/17.
53   W. Chen, The Laboratory as Business. Sir Almroth Wright's Vaccine
     Programme and the Construction of Penicillin, A. Cunningham and
     P. Williams, *The Laboratory Revolution in Medicine* (Cambridge:
     Cambridge University Press, 1992), 245-92, especially 269-72; Sir
     Z. Cope, *Almroth Wright. Founder of Modern Vaccine-Therapy*
     (London & Edinburgh: Nelson, 1966), 64-70.
54   Although W. Chen describes Wright's defence of vaccine therapy and
     of his prestige as the most important reason for the latter's campaign
     against surgical antiseptic wound treatment, in my opinion there is
     no contradiction to the positive results of Wright's work. For a much
     more positive assessment of the history of british vaccine therapy,
     see: M. Worboys, Vaccine Therapy and Laboratory Medicine in
     Edwardian Britain, in J.V. Pickstone (ed.), *Medical Innovations in
     Historical Perspective* (Houndmills, Basingstoke/London: Macmillan,
     1992) 84-103, 224-34. Concerning Wright and his scholar Fleming,
     see the works already quoted and moreover: G. MacFarlane,
     Alexander Fleming. The Man and the Myth (London: Oxford
     University Press, 1984); I. Pieroth, *Penicillinherstellung: Von den
     Anfängen bis zur Großproduktion* (Stuttgart: Wissenschaftliche
     Verlagsgesellschaft, 1992); R. Hare, 'New Light on the History of

Penicillin', *Medical History*, 26 (1982), 1-24; *idem*, 'The Scientific
Activities of Alexander Fleming, other than the Discovery of
Penicillin', *Medical History*, 27 (1983), 347-72; P. Neushul, 'Science,
Government, and the Mass Production of Penicillin', Journal of the
History of Medicine and Allied Sciences, 48 (1993), 371-95; Sir Z.
Cope, *The History of St. Mary's Hospital Medical School or A Century
of Medical Education* (Toronto, Melbourne, London, Cape Town:
Heinemann, 1954); P. Keating, 'Vaccine Therapy and the Problem
of Opsonins', *Journal of the History of Medicine and Allied Sciences*,
43 (1988), 275-96.

55 Cope, *op. cit.* (note 53), 7.
56 See: *ibid.*, 76-82.
57 See, as an example, the bacteriological work of Aschoff: F. Büchner,
op. cit. (note 21), 479; *idem*, (note 21), 18-19; Kaneyoshi Akazaki,
Ludwig Aschoff and Japan, in: *Recent Advances in RES Research*, 16
(1976), 165-75, especially 170; Aschoff, *op. cit.* (note 11), 83-4. See
furthermore: *idem*, *Über die Gasödeme (Veröffentlichungen aus der
Kostitutions- und Wehrpathologie, Issue 42, Vol.9)* (Jena: Fischer,
1938); *idem*, 'Die Störungen der Heilung durch Infektion der
Wunde', *idem* (ed.), *op. cit.* (note 28), 541-76. Concerning
bacteriological work of German 'war pathology' in general:
*Sanitätsbericht über das Deutsche Heer, 3 vols., Vol.II, Der
Sanitätsdienst im Gefechts- und Schlachtenverlauf im Weltkriege
1914/1918* (Berlin: Mittler & Sohn, 1938) 247.
58 See note 30; Aschoff (ed.), *op. cit.* (note 28), vii-viii; W. Hoffmann
(ed.), *Hygiene (Handbuch der Ärztlichen Erfahrungen im Weltkriege
1914/1918*, O.v. Schjerning (ed.), Vol.VII, (Leipzig: Barth, 1922).
59 L. Aschoff, 'Die Störungen der Heilung', 558. See furthermore: Kurt
Wolff, *Statistisches und Bakterioskopisches zur Gasödem-Frage
(Veröffentlichungen aus der Kriegs- und Konstitutionspathologie, Issue
10, Vol.3/Issue 1)* (Jena: Fischer, 1922), 1-48.
60 S. Gräff, Typhus abdominalis (Eberth), in Aschoff (ed.), *op. cit.* (note
28), 77-92, especially 84, 90-2.
61 See, for example, the discussions between Aschoff and the hygienists
Flügge, Wassermann, Kolle and Hahn concerning the development
of a vaccine for gas gangrene in spring 1917: L. Aschoff to his wife
Clara, Berlin, 11 April 1917, Aschoff, *op. cit.* (note 21), 246/247.
See, furthermore: Aschoff to his mother, 15 August 1916, *ibid.*,
243/244, especially 244.
62 J.H. Dible, *The Lost Years. A Commonplace Book 1914-1919.*
Unpublished war-diary, Imperial War Museum London, signature
90 / 37 / 1, sheets 146,148-152,190-192 (134, 136-140,174-176);

C.L. Oakley, 'James Henry Dible, 29 October 1889 – 1 July 1971', *The Journal of Pathology*, 111 (1973), 65-76, especially 66.

63 P.H. Bahr, 'Clinical and pathological Co-operation', in *JRAMC*, 30 (1918), 525-32.

64 C.C. Booth, 'Clinical Research', in Bynum & Porter, *op. cit.* (note 2), Vol.I, 205-29, especially 221-222; Leishman, 'Organization of the Pathological Service', 17-18, 25-9.

65 *Ibid.*, 16.

66 Keith & Shattock, *op. cit.* (note 44), 574-75.

67 Prüll, *op. cit.* (note 10), 175-76; *idem*, 'Die Leichenöffnung im Spannungsfeld von wissenschaftlicher Medizin und traditioneller Kultur nach 1800'. Paper, presented on 19 March 1994 at the Meeting of the Network 'Geschichte der Epistemologie der Biologischen und Medizinischen Wissenschaften' ('History of Epistemology of the biological and medical Sciences') at Strasbourg; *idem*, 'Der Umgang mit der menschlichen Leiche: Medizinhistorischer Überblick'. Paper, presented at the Congress 'Zum Umgang mit der Leiche in der Medizin' ('Dealing with the Corpse in Medicine') of the 'Akademie für Ethik in der Medizin e.V.' at 8. and 9. July 1994, Heidelberg. Concerning traditional anthropological resistance against autopsy, see the articles in the '*Handwörterbuch des Deutschen Aberglaubens*', ed. by Hanns Bächtold-Stäubli (*Handwörterbuch zur deutschen Volkskunde, Abt.1: Aberglaube*), 10 vols, (Berlin, Leipzig: De Gruyter & Co., 1927-1942). See, above all the articles: P. Geiger, 'Tote (der)', *ibid.*, Vol.VIII (1936/1937), sheets 1019-34; *idem*, "Leiche", *ibid.*, Vol.V (1932/1933), 1024-60; *idem*, 'Leichenschändung', *ibid.*, Vol.V, 1093-94.

68 See – for example – the great number of concerning remarks in the letters of German soldiers: Philipp Witkop (ed.), *Kriegsbriefe gefallener Studenten* (Leipzig, Berlin: Müller, 1918); *idem* (ed.), *Kriegsbriefe deutscher Studenten* (Gotha: Panther, 1916). Furthermore, see: E.M. Kronfeld, *Der Krieg im Aberglauben und Volksglauben. Kulturhistorische Beiträge* (München: Schmidt, 1917); H. Bächtold, *Deutscher Soldatenbrauch und Soldatenglaube* (Strasbourg: Trübner, 1917).

69 *Ibid.*, 16, 26/27.

70 *Ibid.*, 17; P. Fussell, *The Great War and Modern Memory* (London, Oxford, New York: Oxford University Press, 1977), 115, 135, 140.

71 Cf. the letter of the theology student, Gotthold von Rohden, Boiry, Feb. 19, 1915, in Witkop, *op. cit.* (note 68), 40.

72 See, for example: Walther Ambroselli, Im Felde, 19 January 1915, in

ibid., 55-59, especially 58; see the letter of a British soldier, in: D. Winter, *Death's Men. Soldiers of the Great War* (London: Penguin, 1979), 206-207.

73 A. Simpson, *Hot Blood and Cold Steel. Life and Death in the Trenches of the First World War* (London: Donovan, 1993), 107-110; H. Dearden, *Medicine & Duty. A War Diary* (London: Heinemann, 1928), 142-6, especially 142.

74 See, for example: H.S. Souttar, *A Surgeon in Belgium* (London: Arnold, 1915), 179/80.

75 Cf. J. Terraine, *The Smoke and the Fire. Myths and Anti-Myths of War 1861-1945* (London: Sidgwick & Jackson, 1980).

76 Fussell, *op. cit.* (note 70), 116.

77 *Ibid.*, 116-17.

78 Concerning attitudes towards death and dissection in the British Army in the First World War, see furthermore: Joanna Bourke, *Dismembering the Male. Men's Bodies, Britain and the Great War* (London: Reaktion Books, 1996), 210-52. Remarkably enough, concerning the medical treatment of corpses Bourke mentions only resistance against anatomical dissection: *ibid.*, 217-21.

79 C.H. Treadgold, 'Cerebrospinal Meningitis in the Salisbury Main Area during the Early Part of 1916: A Laboratory Study', in: *JRAMC*, 24 (1915), 221-30, especially 229.

80 See, for example: W.R.P. Goodwin, 'The Casualty Clearing Station as a Working Unit in the Field', *JRAMC*, 33 (1919), 42-57, especially 52.

81 Häßner, *op. cit.* (note 14), 309-10.

82 *Ibid.*, 310; G. Ricker, 'Die pathologische Anatomie der frischen mechanischen Kriegsschädigungen des Hirnes und seiner Hüllen', in Aschoff (ed.), *op. cit.* (note 28), 334-83, especially 334.

83 See, for example: *ibid.*, 334.

84 Cooter, *op. cit.* (note 2), 1564.

85 Cf. G.-F. Budde, *Auf dem Weg ins Bürgerleben. Kindheit und Erziehung in deutschen und englischen Bürgerfamilien 1840 – 1914* (*Bürgertum. Beiträge zur europäischen Gesellschaftsgeschichte, Vol.6*) (Göttingen: Vandenhoeck & Ruprecht, 1994), 411-14.

86 Cf. R. Colls, 'Englishness and the Political Culture', R. Colls and Philip Dodd, *Englishness. Politics and Culture 1880-1920* (London, Sydney etc.: Croom Helm, 1986), 29-61; W.H. Greenleaf, *The British Political Tradition, Vol.1: The Rise of Collectivism* (London, New York: Methuen, 1983).

87 There are similarities in the case of German hygiene: W.U. Eckart, '"Der größte Versuch, den die Einbildungskraft ersinnen kann" –

Der Krieg als hygienisch-bakteriologisches Laboratorium und Erfahrungsfeld', in Eckart & Gradmann (eds), *op. cit.* (note 10), 299-319.

88 Foster, *op. cit.* (note 7), 19-51. See also the literature on St. Mary's Hospital and Penicillin, already quoted.

89 Concerning the History of German pathology between the wars, see: C.-R. Prüll, 'Holism and German Pathology (1914-1933)', in C. Lawrence, G. Weisz (eds), *Greater than the Parts: Holism in Biomedicine, 1920-1950* (Oxford: Oxford University Press, in press). About German pathology in the Third Reich, see the rough descriptive study of U. Lampert, *Die Pathologische Anatomie in der Zeit des Nationalsozialismus unter besonderer Beachtung der Rolle einiger bedeutender Fachvertreter an deutschen Universitäten und Hochschulen* (MD Thesis, Leipzig, 1991).

6

The British Medical Officer on the Western Front: The Training of Doctors for War

Ian R. Whitehead

In 1914 the Royal Army Medical Corps (RAMC) was too small to cope with the demands of a protracted war. It needed to increase its supply of Medical Officers (MOs) by recruiting from the ranks of the civilian medical profession. However, the absorption of civilian doctors, into the RAMC, was not without its difficulties. In particular, service in the RAMC involved a modification to the doctors' ethical code, with loyalty to the needs of the State taking precedence over those of the individual. The war also presented medical problems for which neither civilian nor Regular MOs were prepared. With particular reference to the Western Front, this chapter will examine the challenges which the war posed for doctors, and trace the development of RAMC training in response to the demands of war.

Initially, it was not clear that civilian doctors entering the RAMC would require additional training. Unlike the majority of recruits, their military duties were to be closely related to their civil calling. This led to assumptions that the training of MOs would be a relatively easy matter. The supposed advantage which doctors had, is highlighted by one of Warwick Deeping's characters, in his novel, "No Hero This":

> In the infantry we're such utter amateurs. It's easier for you doctors.
> You do know your job.[1]

Writing in July 1917, Colonel T.H. Goodwin considered that medical training was sufficient to instil in MOs the qualities needed to ensure that the sick and wounded received the best possible treatment:

> I have been so impressed by the behaviour of young doctors who
> have gone in without previous training that I think medical training
> alone wonderfully effective for this duty as it teaches self reliance and
> confidence in personal ability, quickness of judgment, and power to
> apply theory to practice in a case of emergency.[2]

Certainly, most doctors were keen to apply their knowledge to war conditions, and to do their utmost for the men. To reach a peak of efficiency, however, doctors required a broader understanding than that given by traditional medical training. They needed to appreciate the differences between civil and military medicine, and to be aware of the mechanics of the military medical organisation. Many doctors had no military experience at all;[3] others had received some training in OTC units or the Reserve Forces; but only a small proportion had seen active service.[4] This lack of experience meant that doctors often arrived at the front unclear about the role that they ought to play. A.A. Martin, in his book *Surgeon In Khaki* describes travelling to France with a group of MOs who were all 'very curious to know the role played by a doctor' in the Army.[5]

The experience of J.M. McLachlan suggests that new MOs were simply left to muddle through. On joining the Seventeenth (Service) Battalion Northumberland Fusiliers, he wrote: 'I'm sort of feeling my way, and am in a slightly fogged condition as to how much I'm supposed actually to do.'[6] One of his duties was to take his men in stretcher drill, and he found that he knew 'jolly little about it'. He also had to lecture to his sanitation and water orderlies, making the uncomfortable discovery that they were better versed in sanitary matters than he was himself.[7] In May 1915, he was stationed at No. 9 Stationary Hospital, Le Havre, in charge of venereal cases, and again admitted to being 'a trifle foggy' as to his duties.[8] Later in the war, it is clear that MOs were still being left to sink or swim. McLachlan (who was by this time MO to the Sixty-fourth Brigade RFA) returned to his unit to find that his relief had known virtually nothing about his duties.[9] And, on another occasion, he had to instruct a newly arrived Medical Officer who had 'made a first class muddle of a sick parade'.[10]

Indeed, many doctors discovered that their civilian experience was poor preparation for military work. Dr. L.W. Batten recalled:

> From October [1914] to March [1915] I had a war-time resident job
> at Barts, busy, responsible fun. It rubbed off a little of my extreme
> prematurity [sic] [he had qualified in September 1914] but did very
> little to fit me for service as a Field Ambulance or Regimental
> Medical Officer which is what I was to become.[11]

The difficulty with fitting doctors for military service was that the urgent need for qualified medical personnel meant that there was often little time for formal training. Consequently, a Medical Officer's training had to rely, to a large extent, on him learning as he went about his duties, adapting his medical skills to meet military requirements. But, it was not only doctors recruited from the civil profession who found themselves inadequately prepared for war. Lieutenant-Colonel G.W. Hughes, a Regular Officer in the RAMC, from 1903 to 1926, remembered nothing in his military training that prepared him for trench warfare. Trench conditions gave rise to difficulties in the evacuation of wounded not previously considered, and diseases and sanitary problems not met with before.[12] In September 1914, Lord Esher informed Kitchener:

> Keogh who organised the RAMC, admitted to me that such a war as this was never thought of. Just as you were called upon to fight through with an army raised to 'reinforce India'; so the RAMC were organised to meet casualties on the South African basis![13]

The RAMC faced a problem not encountered by combatant units. Cavalry, infantry and artillery were organised in peace along the same lines as they were in war. Their daily training concentrated upon their duties in war, and they had no peacetime role to play. However, the RAMC's function in war differed widely from that in peace. Its wartime organisation only sprang into being on mobilisation, and with onerous peacetime responsibilities for dealing with the sick, there was little opportunity to study the changing demands that active service would impose.

As regards surgical practice, the RAMC had to unlearn the lessons of the South African War, where the fighting had been at long range over the clean veldt. In France, the fighting took place at close quarters over land that was highly cultivated; the infection of wounds with this rich soil led to the onset of gas gangrene.[14] In such conditions, early treatment was vital, but at the beginning of the War the RAMC relied on its experience in South Africa, where wounds had been left to heal.

The fact is that both the Regulars and their civilian colleagues had much to learn. Even a consultant of the stature of Sir Wilmot Herringham admitted that he learnt more medicine in his five years with the RAMC than in any previous five years of his life.[15] Some degree of further professional training and guidance was therefore essential for all Medical Officers.

The obvious advantage which Regulars had over the civilian intake was their experience of military procedures. The accounts of temporary commissioned officers demonstrate that they were largely ignorant of the RAMC's ways. Those with Territorial records would have been better placed, but prior to the war concern had been expressed about the effectiveness of Territorial training. In 1913, Major Josiah Oldfield recorded that 'my experience leads me to say that in practice it works out that the Regimental Medical Officer (RMO) has very little training in the duties that will be required of him on mobilisation'.[16] To get the best from civilian doctors some instruction in military procedures was necessary.

In particular, doctors needed to be aware of the differences between military and civilian medicine. Accustomed to clean, well-lit hospitals, with up-to-the-minute facilities and an ample supply of trained assistants, accomplished surgeons had to adjust to working in often cramped, cold and dirty conditions, with only the most basic equipment.[17] Medical Officers also needed to understand that the application of surgical principles varied, depending upon the type of unit to which they were attached. They had to appreciate the differing requirements of work at a Field Ambulance, a Casualty Clearing Station and at the base hospitals. This included being able to discern which cases demanded immediate operative treatment, and which ought to be evacuated to units further in the rear. Even the most able surgeons could not give of their best without an understanding of these differences.[18]

Military requirements also imposed a new set of priorities on doctors. Whereas in civil life the doctor's first duty was to the individual, in the RAMC the needs of the State were paramount. Excessive sympathy and concern ran the risk of desoldierising the men,[19] and wasteful sentimentality was discouraged[20]. In autumn 1915, the Medical Inspector of Drafts with the BEF noted that many inexperienced young doctors were far too ready to find men unfit for service. In his view, Administrative Medical Officers had to impress on doctors the importance of avoiding undue leniency.[21] Medical Officers needed to develop a suspicious attitude towards their patients. J.M. McLachlan noted that:

> The attitude of regarding almost every man who goes sick as a scrimshanker and strafing ad nauseam, isn't acquired in a single day exactly. I think I must be pretty horrible sometimes to the men.[22]

The function of the Army doctor, to maintain the mental and physical well being of the men, so that they might be fit to face death or injury, was bound to give rise to moral dilemmas.[23] Some doctors were clearly uncomfortable with the ethical implications of subordinating the concerns of the individual, in what appeared to be a departure from the Hippocratic tradition. Harold Dearden found difficulty marrying his former understanding of his calling with his military duties, and decided that the best way to cope was not to ask himself any searching questions,[24] and adopt a detached approach. In times of heavy casualties it was difficult to maintain such an attitude. Medical Officers had to discriminate between cases to an unaccustomed extent, often completely ignoring those whose lives could not be saved. These were the harsh realities of war, and no amount of training or experience made it any easier for MOs to accept these limitations on their sense of duty to the sick, wounded and dying. Medical Officers had to put these doubts to the backs of their minds, and make the best of the situation. The problem was not simply one of having to choose between those who might live and the hopeless cases, but of whether to give enemy wounded the same consideration as Allied soldiers. In June 1915, at the opening session of the American Surgical Association, Dr George Armstrong stated that the spirit of antagonism should be far removed from the work of the Army Medical Service.[25] The duty of the doctor in war, as in civil life, was to treat all who came to him in need. Indeed, the evidence from letters and diaries suggests that whatever Medical Officers felt about the enemy cause, they did not allow this to interfere with their treatment of the wounded. Most seem to have treated enemy soldiers ungrudgingly and even those who were less sympathetic did not refuse treatment.[26] Medical training had clearly inculcated in doctors a sense of a higher duty, which neither patriotism, nor even the experience of war, with the loss of comrades to enemy fire, seem able to have undermined. The dominant attitude was summed up by Charles Symonds:

> ...the Prussian ideals I hate and am in favour of continuing the war till we have made sure of crushing them. But individually I don't believe the Hun is really any worse a man than ours is.[27]

In some respects, then, Colonel Goodwin's faith in the sufficiency of medical training was justified. It nurtured in doctors a strong devotion to duty, and a calm, dispassionate approach to their work, that proved of great value in the difficult conditions at the front. But, there were clearly areas in which the doctors required further instruction, if they were to become efficient Medical Officers. James W. Barrett felt that throughout the War not enough had been done to train new Medical Officers:

> ... newly joined medical officers were thrown now into this and then into that position without preparation or adequate training of the kind, and the result ... was a great deal of what is known popularly as 'grouse'.[28]

This state of affairs reflects the urgent demands for Medical Officers, which limited the time available for training, especially during the early months of the war. The benefits of further training were, however, recognised, and steps taken to facilitate this. Prior to the war, there was only one depot for the training of RAMC personnel, situated in Aldershot. But, by the end of 1914 a further seven training centres had been established around the country.

Apart from these centres, the instruction of Medical Officers also took place at military hospitals. The training given here covered medical duties, such as giving inoculations, but there was also an emphasis on military drill and army routine. Complaints from Medical Officers about the amount of drill involved in their training were not unusual. However, Medical Officers' duties did not confine them to purely medical work. They needed to be able to maintain discipline and give effective leadership to the men under their command; skills which drill enabled them to develop. In November 1917, the Under Secretary Of State For War made it clear that there was no question of removing drill from a Medical Officer's training. At the end of 1916, the entire system for training Medical Officers in the U.K. was altered, when the various depots were transferred to Blackpool and concentrated under an administrative headquarters. The change resulted from a need to economise on personnel, by reducing the multiplicity of instruction; and from a desire to achieve greater uniformity in training.[29]

The centre at Blackpool instructed newly enlisted RAMC officers in the various medical and non-medical skills which they would require. Particular emphasis was placed upon preventive medicine. The RAMC School of Hygiene was formed at Blackpool, to meet the urgent need for MOs with a specialised training in preventive work. They were taught the general principles and practice of hygiene, including practical bacteriology and the analysis of food and water. There were also demonstrations of sanitary appliances.[30]

However, the impossibility of adequately preparing every doctor, prior to his embarkation, meant that further training once in the theatres of war, was essential. In spring 1915, Sir Arthur Sloggett issued an order informing all Commanding Officers of medical units that their duties involved taking every opportunity to instruct the MOs under their command; not just in the organisation and function of the unit in which they were currently serving, but of other units to which they might be transferred.[31]

Medical Officers at the front also needed to be made aware of the importance of preventive medicine in keeping an army fit. Slackness in hygiene would severely deplete the strength of an army, undermine its morale, and make its defeat likely. The Boer War had demonstrated to the military authorities the necessity for an efficient sanitary organisation, and progress had been made, prior to 1914, in improving arrangements and teaching RAMC officers the importance of maintaining strict sanitary discipline. An article in the *BMJ* expressed confidence that Medical Officers were now well drilled in the necessary measures for disease prevention, and pointed out the need to ensure that those civilian doctors entering the service received comparable training.[32] Even civilian doctors with a background in preventive medicine needed to learn about the military way of doing things. But, this was not always recognised during the war, and there were instances of civilian Medical Officers of Health, ignorant of sanitary administration in the Army, being placed in authority over men who had made a lifelong study of military hygiene.[33]

As the war progressed, there was an increase in the number of sanitary schools and demonstration areas established in France.[34] In the summer of 1917, a School of Sanitation was established in the Thirteenth Corps. Lectures were given to officers and NCOs on the medical organisation and field sanitation. The intention was to create a better understanding between the combatant and medical branches, and resulted in an improvement of the sanitary situation in the Corps.[35] Throughout France, sanitary schools became 'the rage'[36] in 1917, showing that the Army was making a concerted effort to press home the need for careful attention to hygiene. However, the *Commission On Medical Establishments In France* complained that there was no systematic instruction being given to Medical Officers, and recommended that they be given access to the courses run by the increasing number of sanitary schools.[37] It would appear that some action was taken as a consequence of this recommendation. A number of Medical Officers' papers make refererence to the existence of these schools.

Despite such developments, RAMC training continued to have its critics. In the opinion of Sir Almroth Wright,[38] the Army Medical Service had not taken sufficient action to guide Medical Officers in matters of treatment. He accused the medical service of regarding such questions as outside its responsibility, and being content to leave decisions over 'these professional matters to the arbitrament of the individual Medical Officer, who may sometimes be quite untaught and inexperienced'. The RAMC, in his view, needed to lay down a broad outline of treatment to be adopted.[39] However, his opinions were not shared by other consultants serving with the RAMC. Professor James Swain[40] refuted the idea that matters of treatment were left entirely to the individual Medical Officers, pointing out that various instructions had been issued. At the same time, he felt it inadvisable to lay down too strict a set of recommendations, because 'progress is not made from uniformity'.[41] Sir Berkeley Moynihan[42] firmly agreed with the latter point:

> ... no one ever decided upon the right way of treating wounds. The whole of the progress of surgery has depended upon the different interpretations that different men have given to the different methods of solving the same problem.... It is true of surgery there are many ways of treating the same problem and every one of them is right.[43]

Swain rejected the suggestion that no effort had been made to guide Medical Officers. One means of disseminating information was the publication of memoranda. 1915 saw the publication of a *Memorandum On The Treatment Of Injuries In War*, which summarised the experience amassed in the military hospitals, in France, during the previous ten months, with a view 'to attaining some uniformity in method of treatment based upon definite observation'.[44] Sir Arthur Sloggett felt that this memorandum met Wright's demand that the RAMC set out a broad outline of methods to be adopted[45]. It was the duty of a Deputy Director of Medical Services (DDMS), an Assistant Director of Medical Services (ADMS) and the commanders of medical units to ensure that all Medical Officers serving under them possessed a copy of this memorandum, and that the treatments advocated therein were carried out as closely as possible.[46] A similar publication, issued in 1918, was the *Manual Of Injuries And Diseases Of War*.[47] This set out the role of the various medical units along the line of evacuation, and the recommended treatments to be carried out at each.

Another memorandum was published as a result of work done by the *War Office Committee for the study of Tetanus*; it dealt with the diagnosis and treatment of tetanus, and was constantly updated. In addition, forty Medical Officers, with the necessary experience, were appointed as local inspectors of tetanus, to supervise and advise regarding a disease with which most doctors were unfamiliar.[48]

Taking surgery as an example, we can see that there were various ways in which guidance and further instruction were given. The formation of surgical teams, at the beginning of 1915, was seen by Sir Berkeley Moynihan as a means of preventing junior and inexperienced Medical Officers undertaking serious operations on their own responsibility.[49] Supervision of inexperienced Medical Officers reduced the unnecessary evacuation of patients. Medical Officers were also informed of the latest developments in surgical practice. These included the introduction of blood transfusion and the adoption of the Carrel-Dakin method. Provision was made for MOs to be attached to hospitals and CCSs for practical training in these techniques. The RAMC distributed articles from the medical press, and organised lecture tours of the front, to keep MOs up-to-date. Even so, it became clear that not enough had been done to ensure that MOs serving in forward positions were adequately informed. In particular, they were not receiving adequate instruction in the techniques of blood transfusion. The difficulty of performing transfusions in RAPs and dressing stations was recognised, but there were parts of the line where it was possible, thus saving the lives of men likely to die on the journey back down the line. Consequently, it was decided to form a training centre, attached to a group of CCSs in the Third Army area, where Field Ambulance and Regimental Medical Officers could obtain instruction in the technique.[50]

As Swain pointed out, instructions had been issued to guide Medical Officers as to RAMC procedures or principles of treatment. Moreover, the DGAMS had taken action to ensure that all such instructions were vetted, with a view to securing a high level of uniformity of method and procedure throughout the medical services.[51] At the same time, however, he was anxious not to hamper initiative, and the rigid prescription of medical treatments was avoided. Certain general procedures regarding the recording of symptoms, the treatments adopted and the evacuation of cases, obviously had to be abided by. But, on professional matters, the instructions were intended as guides, leaving Medical Officers some room for manoeuvre.

Such guidance was essential, since many of the conditions encountered during the War were completely new to the doctors. It would, however, have been impossible for the RAMC administration to lay down strict rules regarding prevention and treatment, since in many cases it was equally unfamiliar with the medical conditions which arose. For instance, it was not until 1918 that a link was established between trench fever and the louse,[52] as a result of the work done by the *Committee For The Study Of Trench Fever*, chaired by Major General Sir David Bruce.[53] Only with this discovery could valuable advice be issued to Medical Officers. Gas gangrene, which had never emerged on such a scale in previous campaigns, was a similar case. It was late 1918 before a breakthrough was made in its prevention.[54]

The heavy rains during the winter of 1914-1915 led to terrible conditions in the trenches, and a high incidence of frostbite and trench foot. During November and December 1914 there were 6,378 cases of frostbite amongst British soldiers in France and Belgium; and weekly returns of trench foot cases in the First Army showed an incidence of 3,013 between 27 December 1914 and 28 February 1915.[55] There was, however, no clear idea of how to tackle the problem, as Sir Walter Lawrence indicated to Kitchener in December 1914:

> The pain of this frost-bite seems intense, and no one seems to have any remedy for it. Sir Berkeley Moynihan told me that the best thing was to keep the feet cool, but in every hospital I have seen they swathe the feet in cotton-wool and flannel. No one seems to know how long it will take before these frost-bites can be cured.[56]

As Colonel Arthur Lee noted, there was no effective system of treatment approved by the central authorities. Instead, Medical Officers were left to experiment with various remedies, including putting rum in boots, and wrapping feet in cotton-wool, which often did more harm than good. However, this process of experimentation did enable a recommended programme of treatment to emerge, which was outlined in Army Routine Order 554, issued in January 1915.[57] These recommendations contributed to a reduction in the incidence of trench foot on the Western Front, and helped not only Medical Officers, but all ranks, to better understand the condition.

The use of poison gas was another unexpected development, which called for guidance to be given to Medical Officers. The initial difficulties of protecting the men, however, meant that there was a need for individual initiative and experimentation. Sir John Boyd, who was at Ypres during the first gas attack, was appointed anti-gas officer, Eightieth Brigade, in April 1915. He was given a modicum of instruction, but really knew nothing about the treatment of gas, other than what he termed 'common sense methods'. These included the use of mild cough mixtures, to try and relieve the congestion, but which proved of little use. He was also involved in the development of the first primitive respirators. His job included an educational role. With very little training himself, he had to go around lecturing to units on the precautions to be taken in a gas attack.[58] The RAMC authorities quickly recognised the need to give instruction on gas, and the Director General of the Army Medical Service (DGAMS) issued various memoranda on the subject.[59] Chemical advisers were appointed to the Armies in France, and lectures on gas were arranged.

Gas courses, usually lasting for about five days, were also set up, which, in G D Fairley's words, gave Medical Officers instruction 'in how to deal with Boche vapours and stink pots'.[60]

Shell shock posed another significant challenge to the training of Medical Officers. Understanding about the psychological impact of war was limited. In the early years of the war, it was felt that mental breakdown due to the effects of battle was a new phenomenon; an impression reinforced by the invention of 'shell shock' as a descriptive term. Medically speaking, the term was inaccurate and extremely damaging, as it suggested a causal connection between the effects of a shell explosion and the development of neurotic symptoms which, in the majority of cases, did not exist. In fact, there was no need for a new term, because the symptoms which emerged under the emotional stress of war were virtually identical to those already known in civil life. Once this became apparent, doctors with previous experience of treating psychiatric cases were able to correctly classify the various disorders which comprised emotional shell shock.

Unfortunately few doctors possessed sufficiently in-depth knowledge of psychiatric medicine to make such a definite diagnosis of mental and nervous symptoms. Pre-war, no attempt had been made to give such a grounding to Medical Officers; the course at the Royal Army Medical College had given no consideration to the trauma that war can cause. In an attempt to rectify this deficiency, a training programme was established at Maghull Hospital, which turned out sixty-five Medical Officers, versed in modern psychiatric principles, during the last two years of the war. The remainder of the Army's psychiatric service was recruited from neurological hospitals, mental hospitals and from a group of insufficiently trained volunteers. Amongst these sources of psychiatric personnel, even those with training did not necessarily have experience of dealing with psychosomatic disorders. This inexperience led to the misdiagnosis of many hysterical conditions.[61]

Most doctors lacked the confidence to make firm diagnoses in cases of mental collapse. Reluctant to commit themselves, and wishing to avoid the stigma to the patient of describing his condition as 'mental', the majority of Medical Officers preferred to send cases of this kind down the line, labelled as 'shell shock (wound)'. This led to the unnecessary evacuation to the base of patients suffering from fatigue and mild hysterical disorders, who could have been more effectively treated in a forward hospital; the consequent delay in treatment led to a worsening of these conditions.[62]

The British military authorities were slow to react to the problem of shell shock, and it was not until after the 1916 Somme campaign, where the ferocity of the fighting led to a vast increase in the incidence of psychiatric casualties, that improvements were made in the methods for dealing with such cases. This included better information for Medical Officers on the procedures to be adopted. In February 1917, the Director of Medical Services (DMS) of the First Army distributed instructions for dealing with suspected cases of shell shock and neurasthenia.[63] Later, in June of that year, a General Routine Order (G.R.O.) was issued which laid down the procedure for the classification and disposal of suspected cases.

One of the principal concerns of the instruction was to prevent misuse of the diagnosis. The RMO who first dealt with the case was to beware undue sympathy, and in no circumstances to make a definite diagnosis. The patient was to be transferred to a Special Hospital, marked "Not Yet Diagnosed Nervous" (NYDN), where classification was to take place. From a medical point of view it was clearly important to avoid wrongful diagnosis, but there was concern that financial motives were at work, pushing Medical Officers too far in the other direction, leading to prevention of diagnosis.[64] The fewer cases that were diagnosed the cheaper it would be from the point of view of pensions. Undoubtedly, there were Medical Officers who either from ignorance, or an unsympathetic attitude, refused to class men as NYDN. Moreover, it is clear that the vigour with which Medical Officers were urged to avoid immediate diagnosis was not matched by any attempt to broaden their knowledge of the various mental conditions that comprised shell shock. Conversely, there seems to have been a determined attempt to limit the free-flow of information on shell shock. Even after the Somme experience, the DGAMS felt it inadvisable for articles on the subject to be published in the *BMJ* and the *Journal of the Royal Army Medical Corps.*[65]

The insufficiency of the instructions on shell shock is evident from the difficulties which Medical Officers faced when trying to determine the mental state of men on trial for cowardice or self-inflicted wounding. Without any experience of psychiatry, ordinary Medical Officers were called upon to determine the mental responsibility of men on trial for their lives.[66] In their ignorance, some allowed their distaste for nervous cases to colour their judgment. Others, however, found inexperience in these matters undermining their ability to make confident assertions about an individual's state of mind, especially since, away from the front, it was difficult to assess the strain under which he had been labouring. The Neurologist to the Fourth and Fifth Armies noted that:

it was almost impossible for the medical officer to make a decisive statement that the man had been responsible for his actions when he ran away.[67]

Extensive training in psychiatry would have been impracticable in wartime, except for a few specially selected individuals. Further guidance could, however, have been given to Medical Officers to supplement their limited understanding of mental conditions. That it was not is partly the fault of the military authorities, who reacted slowly to the whole problem of shell shock. But, it was also a reflection of the widespread suspicion and scepticism with which the relatively new science of psychiatry was viewed within the profession. Indeed, MOs generally tended to be more dismissive of psychiatry than many of their combatant colleagues; a fact discernible from the evidence to the War Office's enquiry into shell shock.

Venereal disease was another controversial medical issue on which Medical Officers received insufficient guidance. Some instructions were issued regarding the content of lectures on V.D., and the procedures for the disposal of cases.[68] However, as late as 1918, War Office guide-lines were criticised for 'not really conveying to our doctors any definite instructions of any sort as to what they should do under given circumstances'.[69]

A way of supplementing the knowledge gained from official instructions and orders was through membership of a military medical society. Occasional meetings of Medical Officers began to take place towards the end of 1914, out of recognition of the need for greater interchange of information between hospitals and other medical units. The organisation of these front-line medical societies was actively encouraged by the RAMC authorities. The great value of such societies was the contact they promoted between Medical Officers serving with different RAMC units, and the dissemination of knowledge that grew from this. Discussions covered a wide range of medico-military issues, and often resulted in the publication of papers in the medical press.

The training of Medical Officers was very much a continuous affair, as new information and methods of treatment came to light. The free flow of information which medical societies encouraged was an important part of this process. As mentioned earlier, it was essential that Medical Officers have an understanding of all medical units, not just those at which they were working. In particular, they needed information on the type of treatment given elsewhere, so that patients could receive as rapid and continuous a treatment as possible.

As regards the after treatment of cases, however, the information available to frontline doctors was inadequate, especially in the early months of the War. The belief in the expectant treatment of wounds (based on the South African experience, whereby wounds were left to heal) would not have persisted so long had surgeons at CCSs been aware of the poor recovery rate of cases after evacuation to the Base.[70] H.W. Kaye recorded that greater communication between units was required:

> much of the difficulty in treatment arises from the fact that each set
> of men (Regimental Medical Officers, Field Ambulance, CCS and
> Base Hospital) sees and deals with each patient in the successive
> stages of his way from the Front to the Base, and at different phases
> of his condition. There is thus an inevitable tendency for each stage
> to become a water-tight compartment and for all to criticise (among
> themselves) the men from whom they received the patients; these in
> their turn should be made aware of the nature of these criticisms.[71]

It was the duty of Officers Commanding medical units to ensure that the doctors under their command were familiar with the correct lines of treatment. Kaye, who served with the Forty-third Field Ambulance, in France, found his OC helpful in this regard, as he had spent over nine months at a CCS. He was therefore able to impart information about CCS work, and the observations made there upon the work of the Field Ambulance, which included a suggestion that they had 'erred on the side of doing too much surgically'.[72]

However, insufficient communication between medical units remained a difficulty throughout the war. In 1917, the *Report Of The Commission On Medical Establishments In France* noted that Medical Officers on the Lines of Communication seemed to know little of the medical arrangements at the front, and vice versa.[73] The need for better understanding between Medical Officers was an important lesson of the War, and was not lost on the post-war *Babtie Committee* that looked into the reorganisation of the RAMC:

> In order to achieve the best results in the treatment of wounds, the
> principle of the periodic exchange of Medical Officers (of suitable
> age, physique and qualifications) between General Hospitals and
> Advanced Field Medical Units should be borne in mind.[74]

The employment, as consultants, of eminent civilian surgeons and physicians did help to improve the free flow of information during the war. Part of a consultant's role was to act as a liaison officer, taking news of recent medical developments from area to area.[75] However, there was a problem, in that the consultants themselves were subject to compartmentalism, as a result of the system of deployment. This was a 'concentric' system, whereby the consultant only had jurisdiction over a given area: the consultant at a CCS was not able to supervise the work being done at units in advance or behind of the zone where he was situated.[76] As the *Commission On Medical Establishments* observed, some means of improving consultants' understanding of the problems faced at the various medical units was required. It recommended a method of deployment, known as the radial system, whereby consultants periodically changed places with one another. The advantage of the radial system was that it enabled the consultant to observe the medical arrangements right down the line, see the effects of various treatments and make any necessary improvements. At the same time, he was able to advise Medical Officers, keeping them up-to-date on developments; advice that was infinitely more valuable when based on a wider understanding of the RAMC organisation. The concentric system was not entirely without merit, as it gave the consultant the chance to know his Medical Officers well, and assess their capabilities. Also, because he was travelling less, it enabled him to take a closer interest in the running of the hospitals in his area. But, the radial system was the one which consultants felt enabled them to work most effectively.[77]

Despite the inadequacies of the system, the consultants were able to make a valuable contribution to the diffusion of knowledge, and the regularising of procedures, within their areas. Increasingly, consultants were drawn into the decision-making process. From the time of the Somme, the consultants were brought into counsel and informed of the situation before a battle.[78] The DGAMS regularly summoned the consultants for advice, and issued orders in accordance with their recommendations.[79]

It was the duty of consultants to ensure that Medical Officers were up-to-date on the most efficacious forms of treatment, and aware of the best means of preventing disease. It was essential that consultants keep in touch with developments in medical science, keeping a close watch on the medical press, and passing on relevant information to the Medical Officers in their areas.[80] The distribution of such information helped to stimulate the interest of RAMC Officers in their work, a vital part of the consultants' function. According to Sir Wilmot Herringham:

the most important duty of all was to stimulate an interest in medicine among the officers in charge of medical cases, and to prevent the tendency to careless methods which the circumstances of military work and the deficiency of scientific equipment in the Clearing Stations are apt to produce.[81]

The fact that Medical Officers could not follow up the results of their cases made this task particularly difficult.[82] The consultants were, however, able to stimulate interest by organising conferences, giving lectures and promoting the establishment of medical societies.[83]

Thus, we can trace the process of training, and information gathering, through from the training schools in the United Kingdom; to the demonstration areas and schools at the bases; to the lectures, courses, instructions and medical meetings available to Medical Officers at the front. On the whole, the system provided an adequate grounding for doctors in military medicine, helping them in the transition from civilian work and guiding them on the treatment of unfamiliar conditions. There were defects, in that Medical Officers often became too isolated, and unclear about the work being undertaken elsewhere. Inevitably, because of the extent to which the RAMC grew, and the need to train so many doctors, the arrangements tended to be rather ad hoc. It is therefore not surprising that Medical Officers, even in the later years of the War, were often unsure about the role they were intended to perform.

The necessity for a more systematic programme of instruction for Medical Officers was highlighted by the Commission On Medical Establishments. It recommended that Medical Officers destined for France be sent there immediately upon receiving their commissions. They would then be trained in special frontline schools, and spared the course at Blackpool, which would be reserved for those proceeding to tropical or sub-tropical districts. Such a scheme had a weakness, in that officers initially sent to France might later be despatched to the East, without the benefit of instruction in tropical medicine. However, the Commission felt that this was outweighed by the advantage of having Medical Officers in France completely conversant with their duties and the procedures of the RAMC.[84] In the French Army, the benefits to be gained from some form of frontline education had already been appreciated. During the course of 1915 and 1916, centres of study and instruction were established, and a general scheme adopted, whereby groups of between twenty and forty Medical Officers could be sent for a brief course of instruction, mainly concentrating on the treatment of war wounds.[85] Shortly after the Commission On Medical Establishments concluded its work, a RAMC School of Instruction was formed, in the First

Army, which closely resembled the kind of comprehensive training centre that had been suggested.

In addition to instruction for Medical Officers, there were courses for other ranks of the RAMC; officers and men of the combatant branch; and officers and men of the American and Portuguese armies. Altogether, the school had accommodation for forty RAMC officers and sixty other ranks; ten combatant officers and 130 other ranks.[86] The courses for Medical Officers covered a wide range of medical and military subjects. The value of such a school was soon recognised by Britain's other armies in France, which began steps to establish similar centres in their areas. However, these preparations were disrupted by the German offensive of 1918; only in times of relative quiet could such schools operate.

The war demonstrated that traditional medical training on its own was not sufficient to prepare doctors for military service. Significant differences emerged between the priorities and conditions of civilian and military practice, which required adjustments in a doctor's approach to his work. The principal duty of the Medical Officer was the prevention of wastage. To execute this duty effectively required him to take an interest in matters which few doctors would have been accustomed to regard as within their purview: sanitation; hygiene; and the morale of the men. The problems involved in dealing with a mass of individuals also meant that there was a need for detailed administration. Most doctors were not used to such restrictive rules, and many failed to appreciate the need for them; hence the complaints that were often levelled against the Regular RAMC.

Looking at the development of the system of training for Medical Officers, the picture is similar to that which emerges in other areas of Britain's war experience. Initially unprepared for the numbers of inexperienced doctors with which it had to deal, the system was gradually expanded and adjusted to accommodate the needs of the situation. Given the difficulties involved, especially the fact that time simply did not allow for lengthy training, the system appears to have been fairly successful in turning civilian doctors into efficient Medical Officers. There were some deficiencies (the fact that some doctors appeared to pass through the net; and the danger of isolation), but the formation of schools of instruction, like that in the First Army, would have gone a long way to eliminate these. In the last year of the War, the RAMC was developing an effective training programme, not only for its officers, but for its other ranks and members of the combatant branch.

Notes

1 W. Deeping, *No Hero This* (London: Cassells, 1936), 40.

2 T.H. Goodwin, 'The Army Medical Service', *New York Medical Journal,* cvi (1917), 1. Goodwin was at this time the British liaison officer to the United States Medical Service, in Washington; working to obtain American assistance as regards medical and nursing personnel. See W.G. MacPherson, *Official History of the War – Medical Services – General History,* vol. 1, (London: HMSO, 1923), 147.

3 N. King-Wilson papers, [Liddle Collection, Brotherton Library, University of Leeds (L.C.)] 'Jottings Of An MO' (typescript), 1.

4 In Germany, pre-war conscription ensured that doctors had some military experience, but this did not necessarily mean military medical experience. Colonel H.N. Thompson, who assisted in a German hospital whilst a prisoner, praised the surgical skill of the six doctors with whom he worked, but found their knowledge of administration, sanitation and feeding arrangements to be poor: their pre-war service had been in cavalry, artillery or infantry units, but not in the Medical Corps. See Colonel H.N. Thompson, 'An Account Of My Capture And My Experiences In Germany', *Journal Of The Royal Army Medical Corps,* xxiv (1915), 123.

5 A.A. Martin, *Surgeon In Khaki,* (London: Arnold, 1915), 36-7.

6 J.M. McLachlan papers, [L.C.], letter 321, 3 April 1915.

7 J.M. McLachlan papers, [L.C.], letter 341, 27 April 1915.

8 J.M. McLachlan papers, [L.C.], letter 359, 18 May 1915.

9 J.M. McLachlan papers, [L.C.], letter 699, 14 August 1916.

10 J.M. McLachlan papers, [L.C.], letter 921, 21 August 1917.

11 Dr L.W. Batten papers, [L.C.], letter to son, 18 March 1970, 1.

12 Lieutenant-Colonel G.W. Hughes papers, [Imperial War Museum (I.W.M.)], Autobiographical sketch, 11.

13 PRO 30/57/59, [Public Record Office Kew (P.R.O.)], Kitchener Papers, Letters from Lord Esher to Kitchener: letter 30 September 1914, 3-4.

14 Sir W. Herringham, *Physician In France,* (London: Edward Arnold, 1919), 78-79. Redmond McLaughlin, *The Royal Army Medical Corps,* (London: Leo Cooper, 1972) 35. Owen Richards, 'The Development Of Casualty Clearing Stations', *Guy's Hospital Reports,* LXX (1922), 116.

15 Herringham, *op. cit.* (note 14), 44.

16 Major Josiah Oldfield, 'Regimental And Field Ambulance Training In The Territorial Force', *Journal Of The Royal Army Medical Corps ,*

xxii, (1913), 440.

17 H.M.W. Gray, 'Surgical Treatment Of Wounded Men At Advanced Units', *New York Medical Journal*, cvi (1917), 1013. Herringham, *op. cit.* (note 14), 53.

18 H.M.W. Gray, 'Surgical Treatment Of Wounded Men At Advanced Units', *New York Medical Journal*, cvi (1917), 1013-14.

19 James W. Barrett, *A Vision Of The Possible: What The RAMC Might Become* (London: H.K. Lewis & Co Ltd., 1919), 155-6.

20 L. Gameson papers, [I.W.M.], Typescript, 56.

21 WO 95/52, [P.R.O.], Medical Inspector Of Drafts, Diary, April 1915 – March 1916: 14 October 1915; 17 November 1915; 20 November 1915. Lord Northcliffe wrote that without special training ordinary civilian doctors could not undertake the medical examination of recruits. See Lord Northcliffe, 'The Medical Corps Of The Army', *Journal Of The American Medical Association*, lxviii (1917), 1331.

22 J.M. McLachlan papers, [L.C.], letter 689, 26 July 1916.

23 G.E Berrios & H.L. Freeman, *150 Years Of British Psychiatry, 1841-1991* (London: Gaskell & Royal College Of Physicians, 1991), 246.

24 H. Dearden, *Time And Chance* (London: Heinemann, 1940), 3-4.

25 George E. Armstrong, 'Surgery And War', *Annals Of Surgery*, lxii (1915), 137.

26 It is possible that instances of Medical Officers going out of their way not to treat the enemy did occur, but none have come to light in the course of my research.

27 Charles Symonds papers, [L.C.], extract from letter, 26 April 1917.

28 Barrett, *op. cit.* (note 19), 154-5.

29 MacPherson, *op. cit.* (note 2), 156.

30 An Army School of Sanitation had been established in Leeds, primarily for training American Medical Officers, serving with the British Army, in the details of British field sanitation; it was also used as a demonstration centre for specialist sanitary officers and others. It was, however, a temporary war-time measure, and Blackpool met the need for a more permanent and complete establishment. See W.G. MacPherson, *Official History Of The War – Medical Services, Hygiene Of The War*, vol. 1, (London: H.M.S.O., 1923), 35-61.

31 'Army Medical Procedure', *BMJ*, 1915 (ii), 451.

32 Christopher Childs, 'Prevention Of Typhoid In Our Home Camps', *BMJ*, 1914 (ii), 1087.

33 MacPherson, *op. cit.* (note 30), vol. 1, 63.

34 *Ibid.*, vol. 1, 64.

35 WO 95/903, [P.R.O.], DDMS Thirteenth Corps, Diary: 30 June 1917; 3 August 1917.

36 P.Gosse, *Memoirs Of A Camp Follower: Adventures And Impressions Of A Doctor In The Great War*, (London: Longmans, 1934) 137-8.

37 RAMC 1165, [Contemporary Medical Archives Centre, Wellcome Institute For The History Of Medicine, (C.M.A.C., W.I.H.M.)], Report Of The Commission On Medical Establishments In France, 63.

38 Wright served with the BEF as a Consulting Physician.

39 RAMC 365 [C.M.A.C., W.I.H.M.], Sir A. Bowlby Papers: Memorandum on the Necessity of Creating at the War Office a Medical Intelligence and Investigation Department to get the best possible Treatment for the Wounded, diminish Invaliding, and return the men to the ranks in the shortest possible time, by Colonel Sir A. Wright, 1.

40 Professor James Swain, Consultant Surgeon to the troops serving in the Southern Command, 1914-1919.

41 RAMC 365, [C.M.A.C., W.I.H.M.], Bowlby Papers: Report of the meeting between the DGAMS and Consultants to the Forces held in the Medical Board Room on 15 January 1917, 5.

42 Sir Berkeley Moynihan, Consultant Surgeon to the troops serving in the Northern Command, 1914-1918.

43 RAMC 365, [C.M.A.C., W.I.H.M.], Bowlby Papers: Report of Meeting between DGAMS and Consultants, 11-12.

44 *Memorandum On The Treatment Of Injuries In War*, (London: HMSO, 1915), 1.

45 RAMC 365, [C.M.A.C., W.I.H.M.], Bowlby Papers: letter to Bowlby from Sloggett, 15 January 1917, 3.

46 W.G. MacPherson, *Official History Of The War – Medical Services, Surgery Of The War*, vol. 1 (London: HMSO, 1922), 213-14. WO 95/44, [P.R.O.], DGMS Diary 1915: 1 September 1915.

47 *Manual Of Injuries And Diseases Of War*, (London: HMSO, 1918).

48 MacPherson, *op. cit* (note 46), vol. 1, 151-2.

49 WO 95/44, [P.R.O.], DGAMS, Diary 1915: 27 January 1915. MacPherson, *op. cit.* (note 2), 45.

50 MacPherson, *op. cit* (note 46), vol. 1, 126.

51 WO 95/44, [P.R.O.], DGMS Diary 1915: 16 June 1915.

52 'Transmission Of Trench Fever By The Louse', *BMJ*, 1918 (i), 354. 'The Etiology Of Trench Fever', *BMJ*, 1918 (ii), 120. 'Interim Report Of The War Office Committee For The Study Of Trench Fever', *Journal of the Royal Army Medical Corps*, xxx (1918), 352-3.

53 Commandant of the Royal Army Medical College, 1914-1918.

54 MacPherson, *op. cit.* (note 46), 134-49. McLaughlin, *op. cit.* (note 14), 37.

55 MacPherson, *op. cit.* (note 46), 173.

56 WO 159/17, [P.R.O.], Letters from Sir Walter Lawrence to Lord Kitchener on the medical arrangements in France: letter 31 December 1914, 4.

57 WO 159/16, [P.R.O.], Letters from Colonel Arthur Lee to Lord Kitchener: letter no. 8, 16 January 1915.

58 Sir J. Boyd papers, [L.C.], Recollections, 8.

59 MacPherson, *op. cit.* (note 2), vol. 2, 364.

60 G.D.Fairley papers, [L.C.], Diary: 9 November 1915.

61 E. Miller, *The Neuroses In War*, (London: MacMillan, 1940), 175.

62 W.A. Turner, 'The Bradshaw Lecture On Neuroses And Psychoses Of War', *Journal of the Royal Army Medical Corps*, xxxi (1918), 411. Miller, *op. cit.* (note 61), 140. N. Fenton, *Shell Shock And Its Aftermath*, (St. Louis: Mosby, 1926), 23. A.F. Hurst, *Medical Diseases Of War* (Baltimore: Williams & Welkins, 1944), 163.

63 WO 95/197, [P.R.O.], DMS First Army, Diary: Appendix 14, DMS No. 794/86 Instruction For Dealing With Cases Of Suspected Shell Shock And Neurasthenia, 18 February 1917.

64 Gameson papers, [I.W.M.], Memoirs, 179-180.

65 WO 95/45, [P.R.O.], DGAMS, Diary: 25 November 1916.

66 Gameson papers, [I.W.M.], Memoirs, 163.

67 W. Brown, late Neurologist Fourth and Fifth Armies, France; Wilde Reader in Psychology, University of Oxford. Cited in the Report Of The War Office Committee Of Enquiry Into Shell Shock, (London: HMSO, 1922), 44.

68 WO 293/1, [P.R.O.], War Office Instructions, August- December 1914: Instruction 80, Lectures on Venereal Disease, 6 November 1914. WO 293/2, [P.R.O.], War Office Instructions, January-June: Instruction 127, Venereal Disease, 12 June 1915.

69 WO 32/11404, [P.R.O]., Conference Re V.D. And Its Treatment In The Armed Forces, May 1918, 11.

70 Cuthbert Wallace, *War Surgery Of The Abdomen*, (New York: Blakiston, 1918), 8.

71 RAMC 739, [C.M.A.C., W.I.H.M.], H.W. Kaye papers, Diary, Volume I, 19 September 1915.

72 *Ibid.*

73 RAMC 1165, [C.M.A.C., W.I.H.M.], Report Of The Commission On Medical Establishments, 44.

74 WO 32/11395, [P.R.O.], Report Of The Babtie Committee On The Reorganisation Of The Army Medical Service, 1921-1923, 22.

75 'Consultants With The Armies Abroad', *BMJ*, 1919 (I), 804.

76 George W. Crile, 'Standardization Of The Practice Of Military Surgery – The Clinical Surgeon In Military Service', *Journal of the American Medical Association*, lxix, 291.

77 George H. Makins, 'Introductory', *The British Journal Of Surgery*, vi (1918-19), 11.

78 Herringham, *op. cit.* (note 14), 77.

79 RAMC 365, [C.M.A.C., W.I.H.M.], Bowlby Papers: letter to Bowlby from Sir A. Sloggett, 15 January 1917, 3.

80 'Consultants With The Armies Abroad', *BMJ*, 1919 (i), 804.

81 Herringham, *op. cit.* (note 14), 43.

82 *Ibid.*, 54-5.

83 'Consultants With The Armies Abroad', *BMJ*, 1919 (i), 804. Stephen Paget, *Sir Victor Horsley* (London: Constable, 1919) 302.

84 RAMC 1165, [C.M.A.C., W.I.H.M.], Report Of The Commission On Medical Establishments, 79.

85 'French War Surgery', *BMJ*, 1919 (i), 745.

86 'Recent Developments In RAMC Front Line Education', *BMJ*, 1918 (ii), 141-142.

7

Disease, Discipline and Dissent:
The Indian Army in France and England, 1914-1915

Mark Harrison

During the First World War the ranks of the Indian Army expanded
to over 1.4 million men, swelling what was already the largest
colonial army in the world. Although many of the men who joined
up during the war were non-combatants, and more than half
remained in India, the Indian Army's role in World War I was more
significant than is sometimes claimed.[1] It formed the largest of the
Imperial contingents in both Mesopotamia and East Africa, as well as
serving in France and Flanders, where some 90,000 Indian troops
fought during 1914-15. Thus many thousands of new recruits –
some of whom had been virtually conscripted into the Army or who
had joined up because of adversity at home[2] – found themselves in
some of the most trying conditions ever faced by an army in the field.
The mechanised slaughter of the Western Front, which was entirely
unlike anything sepoys had ever experienced, was enough to test the
mettle of even the best-trained army, let alone one that was poorly
led, poorly equipped and of questionable motivation. Mounting civil
unrest in India in the decade prior to 1914 had raised the possibility
that the Army might be targeted by political agitators. It was feared
that any discontent within its ranks would spread to the population
at home, where it might easily be exploited by nationalist politicians.
Thus, Indian Army commanders and the British government made a
concerted effort to monitor levels of discontent among Indian
soldiers and to ameliorate its causes.

One area in which there was a good deal of disaffection was that
of health and medical care. Medical provisions for Indian soldiers at
the beginning of the war compared very unfavourably with those of
their British counterparts, and even with those enjoyed by colonial
soldiers fighting with the French. Heavy sickness among Indian
troops also sapped their morale and fuelled rumours that Indian lives
were cheap. In the winter of 1914-15 the lack of medical provisions

for sepoys contributed to an acute crisis of morale on the Western Front and created a public scandal which severely embarrassed the British government. This paper assesses the nature and extent of this crisis and the British response – a response which often served to undermine rather than to bolster the moral authority of British rule.

Medicine and authority in British India

Most scholars who have commented on western medicine in British India have agreed that it was, in some sense, a 'tool of empire' but recently our view of 'colonial medicine' has broadened to encompass its 'ideological' role, in the construction of racial differences, for example, and in establishing cultural bridgeheads between rulers and ruled. This 'cultural convergence' has been considered by David Arnold in his book, *Colonizing the Body*, in which he employs Antonio Gramsci's concept of 'cultural hegemony' in order to explain the growing importance of medicine in Indian elite culture from the late nineteenth century. Arnold's conception of hegemony is a dualistic one, embracing both the state's promotion of Western medicine, and its appropriation by sections of the Indian elite, for whom it became a symbol of status, reform and modernity.[3] But the concept of hegemony is a notoriously blunt instrument of historical analysis. Apart from the unresolved question of whether the 'consent' of the masses arises 'spontaneously', or is acquired through more direct intervention on the part of dominant groups, we need to ask whether strategies of control are overt or latent; and, moreover, on which terms the dominant culture is accepted. Might it not be more accurate to speak of 'negotiation' between groups rather than simply their of their domination or subjugation?

In the Indian Army, negotiations over medical intervention centred on the pivotal concepts of honour, duty and dignity. Indian soldiers, I would suggest, came to see the provision of medical care as a duty of the military authorities, as part of an implicit bargain between themselves and the colonial state. But in addition to a sense of reciprocal duties there was also a sense of boundaries and of limits to medical intervention. In order to make sense of this web of customary boundaries and obligations, it is instructive to look again at E.P Thompson's essay on the 'Moral Economy of the Crowd', in which he drew attention to the notions of 'social justice' which informed popular protest in eighteenth-century England. Thompson observed among the 'crowd' a sense of reciprocal obligations and rights – the 'moral economy' – from which arose an uneasy consensus over what were considered legitimate practices in baking, milling, and so forth.[4] Modified versions of the 'moral economy' have since been employed in analyses of peasant protest in South and South East Asia, James C. Scott's, *Moral Economy of the Peasant* being the first and best-known example.[5] There are clearly problems with transposing the concept of the moral economy to a non-European context – not least the appropriateness of Thompson's terminology – and, even more to the military context, since armed forces are not constituted of relations of production and exchange. Yet I would like to preserve at least the notion of a *moral nexus* between the sepoy and the military authorities – a bond which owed its existence to mutual respect of boundaries and to fulfilment of mutually recognised obligations. In the Indian Army these duties were perceived in semi-paternalistic terms, and Indian regiments were conceived, up to a point, as families. But the family metaphor has its limitations, for the web of obligations extended beyond the regiment and army to the King-Emperor himself. Whether or not such bonds were strained or even broken during the First World War is still an open question, and one which will receive further consideration below.

The limits of intervention

Prior to 1914, the Indian soldier (or 'sepoy') had only intermittent contact with Western medicine – far less, certainly, than European troops in India. This relatively *laissez faire* approach was due, in part, to the perception that Indian troops were generally healthier than Europeans (which was true, at least, up to the beginning of the twentieth century) but also to fears that medical intervention might precipitate serious discontent. However, as memories of the Mutiny of 1857 began to fade, Indian soldiers became increasingly the objects of official medical attention. Vaccination against smallpox was made compulsory for new recruits as early as the 1860s, and from the 1890s there were attempts to inoculate sepoys against typhoid and plague although these were never strictly enforced, even during the First World War. Inoculation against typhoid, for example, was considered ritually polluting by many high-caste Hindus, since the bacilli from which the vaccine was made was usually of unknown origin.[6] Other sepoys feared surgical intervention. The American surgeon Harvey Cushing, working as a volunteer in France in 1915, recalled that one Gurkha soldier had refused the amputation of his leg, fearing that he would reincarnated without the limb.[7] In general, though, surgical treatment was welcomed, while measures such as vaccination may have been accepted as a mark of service under the British.[8] Indeed, during the First World War, medicine became a crucial thread in the web of mutual obligations which bound the sepoy to the Raj. Indian troops came to expect adequate provisions to protect them against disease, as well as medical care in the event of their being wounded or falling sick. And, when the military authorities failed in their perceived obligation to provide this care, morale and discipline were severely undermined.

Medicine and morale

Such a situation occurred on the Western Front in the winter of 1914-15. The Indian Army arrived in France wholly unprepared for the rigours of a European winter: Indian stretcher bearers struggled through the snow and mud wearing only the *chappals* (sandals) in which they had arrived from India.[9] Without winter clothing and adequate footwear, thousands of Indian troops fell prey to respiratory illnesses, frostbite, and 'trench foot'. They also suffered severely from infections such as measles to which many had no immunity.[10] Although sickness rates among Indian troops were not much higher than among British soldiers, their experience of illness in France contributed to a feeling that Indian lives were being unnecessarily sacrificed. 'In this sinful country', wrote one Indian patient of his time in France, 'it rains very much and also snows, and many men have been frost-bitten.... All the men will be finished here. In the space of a few months how many have fallen and how many have been wounded.'[11]

During 1915, the authorities became aware that poor health and the dangers of service in France were giving rise to serious discontent. Sir Walter Lawrence, who was appointed Commissioner for the Welfare of Indian Troops in 1914, reported that:

> the conditions of warfare in Flanders were most uncongenial to the Indians. The climate was against them, and the style of warfare was utterly opposed to their ideas and former experiences.... Their suffering from frostbite and the moral and physical shock caused by 'trench back' – when a man is buried and crushed under the falling clay of the trenches – were especially resented by the sepoy. They were bewildered, and had no idea of where they were fighting or whom they were fighting.[12]

In December 1915, Lawrence informed Kitchener that he had noticed 'a considerable falling in vitality', owing to the prevalence of diseases like tuberculosis. There had been a marked increase in the disease among Indian troops, which most MOs attributed to exposure and overcrowding in billets. The Gurkhas, according to

Lawrence, seemed particularly liable to tuberculosis, and those hospitalised with the disease were very depressed. One had even committed suicide.[13] Indeed, morale was at very low ebb throughout 1914 and 1915. Psychiatric casualties and 'melancholia' were common, and certain units (even those composed of the revered Pathans) were deemed unfit for further combat in Europe.[14] According to Lawrence in 1915, the Indian infantry battalions were so dispirited that they were no longer of military value. 'The sepoys', he wrote, 'have been accustomed to look upon their regiment as a family: they have lost the officers whom they knew, and the regiment, which formerly was made up of well-defined and exclusive castes and tribes, is now composed of miscellaneous and dissimilar elements.'[15]

Morale was further undermined by haphazard medical arrangements. Medical provisions for the Indian contingent were based on an organisation designed for frontier warfare in India and were incapable of dealing with the flood of casualties from the Western Front. A shortage of medical personnel necessitated the hasty recruitment in India of menial staff to perform non-technical tasks, while British orderlies and nursing volunteers were employed in more specialised medical duties. But manpower was only one problem among many: the field hospitals brought from India were unsuited to the cold European winter and emergency supplies of bedding and hospital clothing had to be brought in to bring accommodation up to the standard of that enjoyed by British troops.[16] The sanitary conditions inside these hospitals were appalling: basic hygiene was ignored and overcrowding was the rule rather than the exception.[17] In the larger hospitals (located at Boulogne, Hardelot and Montreuil) grave difficulties were experienced in providing Indian patients with an appropriate diet, and burials and cremations were initially conducted without due regard to religious sensibilities. In addition, many of the retired IMS officers recalled to staff the stationary hospitals were out of touch with developments in medicine, and some were patronising in their dealings with patients and subordinate staff.[18]

Plans for the evacuation of sick and wounded Indians were similarly in disarray. The original intention had been to evacuate the sick and wounded via Marseilles to Egypt, and then to India. But this was soon found to be impracticable because of the military situation and arrangements were made for them to be treated in England instead. Hospital accommodation was hastily improvised and provisions were initially no better than those in France. At the end of

November 1914, the only accommodation available for Indian troops in England was two summer hostels at Brockenhurst in Hampshire (grandly titled the 'Lady Hardinge Hospital'), and these were already heavily overcrowded (some wards of the Royal Victoria Military Hospital at Netley had to be used as a temporary measure).[19]

The scandal that erupted over hospitals for Indian troops led, in September 1915, to the appointment of a commission of inquiry under Sir Walter Lawrence. Kitchener, who as Secretary of State for War had appointed the committee, felt a personal responsibility towards the Indian Army, of which he had been commander-in-chief from 1902 to 1909. Paternalistic sentiments were also expressed in various benevolent funds established for sick and wounded Indian Soldiers. The largest of these was the Indian Soldiers' Fund under the chairmanship of John Hewett, which aimed to supplement ambulances and hospitals for Indian troops in France. The fund received donations from the Order of St. John and the Viceroy's Imperial War Fund, and had received upwards of £80,000 by November 1914.[20] Similar funds for Indian troops were established overseas.[21]

However, there were less altruistic reasons for official, if not public, concern for the welfare of Indian troops. Rumours that the British meant to kill off the Indian Expeditionary Force were circulating among demoralised sepoys in France, and the authorities were concerned that these would have 'a very serious depressing effect in India, and a very bad effect on recruiting'.[22] Urgent action was necessary if trust in the British authorities was to be re-established and so a concerted effort was made to expand and improve hospital accommodation in France. According to Sir Walter Lawrence, who inspected the hospitals in 1915, almost all had shown a distinct improvement since his first visit in November. 'When I first saw the hospital in the Jesuit College near Boulogne in the early part of November', he reported, 'I thought it an impossible place. It was transformed by Colonel Wall, IMS, CMG, into a most beautiful and efficient hospital.' Lawrence maintained that Indians were now given preferential treatment in the allocation of buildings. There were also moves to improve the morale of sick and wounded troops by the appointment of YMCA workers from India and the founding of a hospital magazine, which was printed in several Indian languages.[23]

The requirements of caste and religion were another matter which received urgent attention. Many Indian patients refused to eat food that had been touched by British orderlies and special cooks had to be brought in for each religion and caste. In the larger hospitals there were even separate kitchens and slaughter houses.[24] Steps were also taken to quarter convalescent sepoys in more congenial surroundings. Lawrence informed Kitchener in March 1915 that"

> Rouen is not the place for Indians. They speak of it as a ... place of ill luck, whereas Marseilles with the spring approaching already has an effect on their spirits. The atmosphere is Indian – there is sunshine – the supply depot is close at hand, and they cost less to feed than at Rouen; and the authorities have made due arrangements for cremation and Mohammedan burial.[25]

However, the real flagships of imperial benevolence were to be found in England, in the form of the specially-equipped Indian hospitals established at Brighton. The War Office obtained permission to use the town's workhouse (which later became known as the Kitchener Hospital), a school, and the Brighton Pavilion – which, with its oriental domes and 'charming gardens' – was thought especially suitable for Indian patients.[26] The task of converting these buildings into hospitals fell to Colonel P.S. Lelean, RAMC. Lelean, who had some experience of medical work in India, made elaborate rules for the observance of caste and religious differences within the hospital. Caste committees were appointed for each hospital to give advice on dietary and other arrangements and religious occasions such as Ramadan were strictly observed. Special arrangements were also made for funerals, which had been the cause of much discontent in France. Hindus were cremated at a burning *ghat* erected on the Downs at Patcham, just outside Brighton, and a Moslem cemetery was established at Woking. In addition, there were frequent high profile visits by King George V and other members of the Royal family. In short, every attempt was made to give the public in Britain and in India the impression that sepoys wanted for nothing.[27]

The efforts of the British authorities were welcomed by the vast majority of sepoys. Naik Sant Singh of the Garwhal Rifles, a patient at the Kitchener Hospital, wrote in a letter to a comrade: 'I have been in hospital for one month and 22 days... and the Government treated me so kindly that not even my own father and mother could have done more'. 'One gets such service as no one can get in his own house, not even a noble', wrote another Kitchener patient.[28] No accolade seemed too high for the Brighton hospitals: 'Do not worry about me', insisted a wounded sepoy to a friend in Peshawar, 'for I am in paradise. The King came down here last week and shook hands with all the Indians, and asked each one about his wounds and sufferings.'[29]

The considerable pains taken by the British authorities to provide medical care without offence to caste and religion healed the wounds inflicted on Anglo-Indian relations during the first winter in France. Emphasising the paternalistic nature of relations in the Indian Army, one sepoy likened the bedside manner of British medical officers to the 'kindness of fathers to sons'.[30] Improved medical care also reaffirmed the sepoy's loyalty to the King-Emperor: 'The arrangements which the government has made for our people are such as no other King could have made', wrote a Pathan soldier to his uncle in the Punjab.[31] Indeed, as one Sikh patient wrote to a friend in India, 'The wounded soldiers are being treated in England with such great care that my pen fails to describe it. We ought to give our lives for our kind government.'[32]

But the high standard of care available in the flagship hospitals of Brighton raised expectations that could not easily be met elsewhere. Sepoy Ranga Singh, a patient at the Lady Hardinge Hospital, Brockenhurst, complained that: 'There is no fireplace. We are not given milk.... It is very cold. We have to call the nurses "mother" and the European soldiers "Orderly Sahib" – if we do not we are reported. The five Brighton hospitals are good. The others are not good. We are not given soup. We get nothing.'[33] The Barton Court Convalescent Home, lacked organisation according to one Moslem sepoy, and the patients had to cook their own food. 'This place is not equal to Netley', he protested, 'There was everything in plenty. Here no one gets any medicine or anything else and no one asks after us at all'.[34] Despite general improvement, food preparation proved to be a problem in some other hospitals too, especially in the overcrowded stationary hospitals in France. Several complaints were made about the hospital at Boulogne. One sepoy claimed that he and his brother had great trouble in obtaining an appropriate diet. For several days the pair ate nothing in order to preserve their caste.[35] Such protests provide further evidence that medical care had become an important factor in the morale of the Indian Army and that sepoys' expectations had increased substantially whilst serving in Britain and France.

It was not only the lack of medical care which angered sepoys but the conditions under which it was sometimes provided. One of the most frequent complaints, voiced by both patients and Indian staff, was of the harsh disciplinary regime imposed in most of the hospitals in England. The British authorities were concerned that the hospitals would become breeding grounds for indiscipline and dissent: that normally loyal troops would be subjected to political propaganda or otherwise corrupted by the Indian hospital staff. Some of the latter had been hastily recruited just before leaving India from among bazaar coolies in Bombay and were unused to and resentful of military discipline. This group, which performed most of the domestic tasks at the Brighton hospitals, was responsible for the majority of disciplinary offences. During 1915 there were a total of 377 offences under military law committed in at the Brighton hospitals – most were relatively minor in nature, such as breaches of discipline, petty theft, and alcohol related disturbances, and were punished by fines, but 57 were deemed sufficiently serious to warrant imprisonment.[36] The most persistent offenders were returned to India but from those that remained the commanding officer of the Brighton hospitals – Colonel Sir Bruce Seton – was determined to create a disciplined body of men. After subjecting them to six months of RAMC drill, Seton prided himself on having produced a capable body of stretcher bearers and with having reduced the incidence of petty crime to an acceptable minimum.[37]

Similar tactics were tried with the patients – in order to prepare from for a return to military duty – but the effects were less than salutary. Rur Singh of the 15th Sikhs, a patient in Kitchener Hospital, told a friend in Marseilles that 'we are in great discomfort. The sick in all the hospitals are gathered together and paraded. The men cry and moan but no one listens to them'.[38] And there were many similar complaints: 'You probably know that we have parades twice a day', wrote another Sikh to a comrade in a letter suppressed by the military censor, 'We can say nothing. The sick are much worried and harassed'.[39] At the convalescent homes exercise was more vigorous, as Sir Walter Lawrence explained to Kitchener: 'The further the Sepoy gets from his regiment, the more he longs for his native home. As soon as he is fit for light work he should be drilled and have physical exercises, to get back the martial spirit.'[40]

Hospital discipline was deeply resented. Rifleman Ramprashad of the Gurkha Rifles, at the Barton Convalescent Home, told a comrade that 'A new rule has been started which I do not like at all. In the week physical training is held three times. In name it is called a hospital but really it is tyranny.'[41] Indians were not the only troops to undergo PT during convalescence: such procedures were routine in the British Army and do not appear to have given rise to any serious discontent. But in the Indian Army such disciplinary regimes were without precedent, and the sepoy was accustomed to treatment in a regimental hospital, during and after which he would be allowed to recuperate without interference. These measures were seen as unnecessary constraints on the sepoy's liberty and as a blow to his dignity, or *izzat*. Yet Colonel Seton was determined to implement an unusually severe disciplinary code and was encouraged by his early success. 'With the exception of the writers and storekeepers – who are in a chronic state of discontent regarding their military rank and treatment', he reported, 'the personnel has given extraordinarily little trouble'.[42]

Seton's remarks were not unfounded. Storekeepers at the Kitchener complained of being in an 'evil plight' and that the officers treated them badly.[43] But discontent was not confined only to the storekeepers. The sub-assistant surgeons – who were essentially hospital assistants and orderlies – were equally disaffected. They had long campaigned for improvements in pay and conditions of service but had made little headway in the years before 1914.[44] Like the storekeepers, many complaints concerned harsh treatment by the IMS officers in charge of Indian hospitals. Others questioned the professional competence of the old-India hands who had been brought out of retirement during the war. Sub-assistant surgeon J.N. Godbole claimed that 'good treatment is only to be seen where British and not Anglo-Indian officers are in charge. As soon as the latter have control confusion reigns.... As a result of such treatment men in the hospital prefer to go to the front. Such are the methods of our Anglo-Indian officials.'[45]

For the most part, the protests of subordinate hospital staff were muted. Their grievances were long-standing and were not in themselves sufficient to trigger serious unrest. But, when compounded by other grievances, the situation became explosive. Such a mixture occurred in Brighton in the spring of 1915, when Colonel Seton imposed a police cordon around the Indian hospitals to prevent patients and staff from visiting the town. This step had been taken partly to prevent unruly elements among the staff from gaining access to intoxicating liquor, but also to avoid any scandal that might arise from liaisons between Indians and British women. The latter had clearly taken a shine to the Indians. 'Brighton is covered with girls who make a lot of the natives', wrote a British orderly to his wife in India, 'They are seen to arm in arm with ward servants and are very fond of coloured people'.[46] Some Indians were shocked by the advances made by British women. 'The women have no modesty', wrote Surjan Singh, a patient in the Kitchener hospital', 'but walk with the men who please them most'.[47] But others had fewer reservations. 'I am very happy in this place', wrote another Sikh patient, 'There are lots of women to be had. They write letters to us to come to their house and have food with them, and that we can get a woman. I am very much confused in mind'.[48]

British officials were concerned that sexual relationships with

British women would diminish the *izzat* of the Raj. Indeed, letters referring to the availability of European women were often suppressed by the military censor.[49] For the same reasons, female nurses were never employed in the Kitchener Hospital, although a few were engaged at some of the other Indian hospitals at the start of the war.[50] Similarly, all personnel were kept in the hospital area: the only exceptions being convalescent Indian officers and warrant officers, who were provided with passes with restricted hours.[51] But the confinement of nearly 600 Indians within the hospital area was, as Seton acknowledged, 'no easy matter'. The walls were supplemented by barbed-wire palings and a police guard consisting of convalescents was placed around the perimeter.[52] Not surprisingly, these restrictions gave rise to a great deal of discontent, among both patients and staff. 'They do not let us out to the bazaars', protested a patient at Kitchener Hospital to a comrade in the 40th Pathans, 'They do not let the French or English girls talk to us, nor do they let us talk to them. The English have now become very bad. They have become dogs. Our Indian soldiers are very much oppressed, but they can do nothing .... There is abundance of everything but there is no *izzat*.'[53] Other patients complained increasingly of being depressed and miserable, and of being punished even for very minor breaches of hospital regulations such as eating the pears which grew in the hospital garden.[54]

As was so often the case in British India, rebellion was heralded by rumour, including one which claimed that medical officers had deliberately inflicted pain on Indian patients. 'Here there is a great tyranny on the part of the doctor', wrote a patient at Kitchener Hospital, 'Anyone whose hand is wounded or who has a pain in his back [i.e. suspected of malingering] is branded with a hot iron. No one is allowed outside ... altogether the treatment is harsh.'[55] Another patient at Brighton claimed that a doctor had pulled him off his bed and poured cold water over him as a punishment, causing him to lose face before his comrades.[56] The Indian staff, too, began to consider handing in their resignation *en masse* as soon as they returned to India.[57] But protest was not always deferred. The most serious incident to occur in the English hospitals was the attempted murder of Colonel Seton by a sub-assistant surgeon from one of the Bournemouth hospitals, in protest against the confinement of his comrades in the hospital compound. He had walked into Seton's office armed with a revolver but had missed his target. The man in question was sentenced to seven years' 'rigorous imprisonment': a comparatively light sentence which may have reflected the authorities' concern not to provoke further unrest.[58] Unsurprisingly, the incident was never mentioned in Lawrence's official report to the War Office, for this would have irreparably damaged the high reputation the hospital enjoyed. The same was true of suicide attempts on the part of some of the patients. However, Lawrence never failed to inform Kitchener personally when such incidents occurred.[59]

The attack on Seton was unusual in that it may have been overtly nationalistic in motivation. There was disproportionate number of political agitators among the aggrieved sub-assistant surgeons from which Seton's would-be assassin was drawn and India Office secret servicemen had been posted to many of the hospital and convalescent camps in France. As Lawrence informed Kitchener in March 1915, 'The staff of the Hospitals, both in Britain and France, have very black sheep in the matter of sedition. These are very carefully watched. We have had to get rid of two in England, and there is one man now under close observation in France'.[60] Political agitators had also infiltrated the Indian Bearer Corps raised by M.K. Gandhi from amongst Indian students in Britain. Two members of the Corps had been removed from France by the end of March, and one who was caught persuading Indian patients against returning to the firing line had been suspended.[61] Indian visitors to medical establishments in Europe were also suspect and were kept under close surveillance. In April 1915 staff at the Marseilles Convalescent Depot were surprised by the sudden visit of the Raja of Kapurathala, who insisted on a tour of the camp during which he asked many questions about the diet provided for the Sikhs. The answers to his questions were satisfactory, according to Lawrence, but had he been allowed to go around the camp unescorted his questions might have led to trouble.[62] There were fears that Sikh units had been infiltrated by Ghadrites: revolutionaries based mainly in the USA among Sikh immigrants. On the outbreak of war, many had returned to their homeland and, with German encouragement, had instigated an uprising against the British.[63] Letters from Indian soldiers, which passed through the hands of the official censor, also reveal that Sikh militants had attempted to contact soldiers in France.[64]

Such agitation fed upon the grievances of hospital staff and patients – particularly restrictions on their liberty – but also upon the resentment caused by the of the return of wounded sepoys to the firing line: a policy without precedent in the Indian Army.[65] This directive came about because very few sepoys were prepared to return voluntarily to their units. 'There is a form of trades unionism in

India', wrote Lawrence to Kitchener, 'and any man who volunteers to go back will be regarded as a black-leg by his comrades'.[66] 'Only men who are wholly useless are sent back to India' one sepoy told his family,[67] and many unfit men were employed on fatigue duty, giving rise to 'many complaints'.[68] Some men encouraged their friends and relatives back in India not to enlist: 'I say emphatically that no one should enter military service', wrote Krishen Singh, a ward orderly at the Kitchener Hospital to his brother.[69] Another Sikh gave similar advice to his family, but stressed his continuing loyalty to Britain.[70]

Some sepoys accepted their lot fatalistically: 'No one has any hope of survival', wrote a patient at Kitchener hospital, 'For back to the Punjab will go only those who have lost a leg or arm or an eye. It is as God pleases.'[71] But many were prepared to avail themselves of any opportunity to escape the firing line. A few Indian troops deserted and encouraged others to do the same,[72] although most seem to have thought desertion shameful and inimical to military honour.[73] More commonly, sepoys, like their comrades in the British Army, took refuge in their own bodies. 'Malingering' (the attempt to feign illness or to make the most of one's wounds) and self-inflicted wounds were common. Malingering was part and parcel of life in the Indian Army prior to the war and some men took to feigning illness as a means of gaining an early discharge with pension.[74] And, as in most armies, malingering was a time-honoured ritual which established the bounds of military authority, and which tested the mettle of new officers and NCOs. But during the Great War malingering took on epidemic proportions and troubled the authorities more than is generally acknowledged. Lawrence had apparently come across 'many cases of malingering' during his tour of Indian hospitals in France,[75] and Sadar Singh, a patient at the Brockenhurst Hospital, claimed that 'hundreds of thousands' of sepoys in France had resorted to such measures.[76]

Many sepoys regarded malingering as dishonourable but there were at least as many who exhorted their comrades to 'swing the lead'. 'If you can, do not remain fit for duty', urged a Pathan soldier in India to his brother in France, 'Go "sick" and do not return to the battle again. God will then help you'.[77] 'You should tell the doctor that you got ill through carrying ammunition boxes from the support trenches to the firing line', wrote another Pathan who had been invalided back to India, 'That will probably get you a pension, and if so it will be an excellent thing'.[78] Another inmate of the Kitchener explained to a comrade: 'There are many subterfuges for a man, and you should endeavour in every manner to protect your life, there are a hundred things you can say... [that you are] weak, [have a] pain in the chest, or asthma'.[79] There were numerous other examples of men feigning such complaints as deafness, venereal disease and 'trench back'.[80] 'Shell-shock' was particularly favoured because of the apparent ease with which genuine cases could be aped. 'In the case of the Mahsuds', reported Colonel Seton, 'it was difficult at times to separate the true signs of organic disease from the functional and the feigned. The first of them had undoubted hysterical fits in addition to his mental disturbance, the other men of the 129th Baluchis in the ward copied these with more or less accuracy'.[81]

Judging by the letters of Indian sepoys, self-inflicted wounds were less common than attempts to fake illness. Nevertheless, the incidence of suspected SIWs was still considerable, and there is no reason to suspect that they were less common than in the British Army, in which special hospitals were established to cope with the large number of such cases. Soon after the arrival of the Indian Corps in France in September 1914, medical officers noticed that many sepoys were wounded in the left hand: the most usual site of the self-inflicted wound. One study showed that over 1049 (57 per cent) of the wounded Indian soldiers admitted to hospital by November 1914 had been so injured.[82] However, some officers were determined to quash what they regarded as a vicious rumour which impugned the honour of the Indian Army. Colonel Sir Bruce Seton conducted a study of his own, based on 1000 wounded soldiers admitted to the Kitchener Hospital. The wounds chosen for study were those regarded as most likely to be self-inflicted: wounds of the hand, of the arm and forearm, and simple wounds of the leg and foot. Seton claimed to find no evidence of any self-inflicted wound at the Kitchener and explained away the seemingly high incidence of such wounds in the Indian Army as mere chance. (A similarly high proportion of hand wounds had been observed in some distinguished British regiments, whom no one would dare accuse of self-infliction.)[83]

Conclusion

The true incidence of self-inflicted wounds is impossible to gauge. In all probability it was exaggerated by those who had a low opinion of the martial qualities of Indian troops and underestimated by those who leapt to defend the Indian Army. But it seems clear that the lines of evacuation served as safety valves releasing the war-weary from the front and, had this flow been arrested altogether, it is likely that more serious unrest would have occurred. It is, perhaps, significant that there were only six mutinies in the Indian Army during the First World War: a record no worse than that of the British Army and considerably better than that of the French. That more serious outbreaks of unrest did not occur was also due to the ameliorative action of the authorities combined with close surveillance of Indian troops. Sensitivity to the needs of sepoys was politically essential, for the British government and the Government of India could not afford to alienate the moderate nationalists and the more traditional elements that were the bulwark of British power in India. Equally, they could not afford to offend public opinion in Britain, where the welfare of Indian troops had become a *cause célèbre*. Ultimately the government was able to turn an unwelcome burden into a propaganda coup and the Kitchener Hospital and other such institutions became flagships of imperial benevolence, of considerable use in promoting the myth of imperial unity.

Medical care was also a constituent of what might be termed the moral nexus of the Indian Army. Sepoys had grown accustomed to a degree of medical care in the event of their falling sick or wounded, and during the war these expectations markedly increased. Where good medical provisions existed they served to reaffirm the bonds that existed between the sepoy, his officers, and the King-Emperor. But where such expectations were not fulfilled there was considerable resentment and disillusionment; especially when poor medical care was accompanied by a lack of respect for caste and religion. Even the most opulent medical provisions counted for little when the sepoy was deprived of his liberty and honour, as events at the Kitchener Hospital so amply demonstrate. Restrictions of personal liberty, harsh discipline, and the condescending manner of some British staff, were the final straw as far as many sepoys and hospital assistants were concerned. Small wonder then, that hospitals were among the principal foci of political agitation and unrest.

Yet overtly nationalistic or revolutionary dissent was rare in the Indian Army, and in the case of the hospitals was confined mostly to hospital staff who had long nursed grievances about their status and conditions of service. This is not so say, however, that this dissent was not 'political' in the sense of having a specific pattern or purpose. Rather, grievances were articulated in the more traditional idiom of duty, honour, and customary rights: conceptions of social justice which were essentially the same as those which constituted the moral universe the Indian peasant. The shortcomings of medical care in the Indian Army did not reveal any fundamental or irreconcilable contradiction between British and Indian interests. Indeed, many sepoys continued to profess loyalty to Britain despite their disillusionment with the war. But the conditions attached to medical care, and the loss of many customary 'rights', served to undermine the moral legitimacy of British rule to the extent that both recruitment and morale were materially effected.

Notes

1 Correlli Barnett, *The Collapse of British Power* (Stroud: Alan Sutton, 1993), 79.

2 Sumit Sarkar, *Modern India 1885-1947* (Delhi: Oxford University Press, 1983), 169.

3 David Arnold, *Colonizing the Body: State Medicine and Epidemic Disease in Nineteenth-Century India* (Berkeley: University of California Press, 1993), 241-6.

4 E.P. Thompson, 'The Moral Economy of the English Crowd in the Eighteenth Century' and 'The Moral Economy Reviewed', in his *Customs in* Common (Harmondsworth: Penguin, 1991), 185-351.

5 James C. Scott, *The Moral Economy of the Indian Peasant: Rebellion and Subsistence in Southeast Asia* (New Haven: Yale University Press, 1976). For a critical introduction to peasant protest in British India see David Hardiman (ed.), *Peasant Resistance in India 1858-1914* (Oxford: Oxford University Press, 1992).

6 Evidence of Surgeon-General William Babtie, Procs. Mesopotamia Commission, qq.7480 & 7586, CAB 19/4, PRO.

7 Harvey Cushing, *From a Surgeon's Journal 1915-1918* (London: Constable, 1936), entry of 4 May, RAMC 971, CMAC.

8 Arnold, *op. cit.* (note 3), 95.

9 A. Ghosh (ed.), *History of the Armed Forces Medical Services* (Hyderabad: Orient Longman, 1988), 106.

10 War diaries of Lt.-Col. Beveridge, ADMS Sanitation; 23 & 29 October 1914, RAMC 543, CMAC.

11 Censor of Indian Mails: extracts from letters to and from Indian members of the Expeditionary Force. Letter no.3, 16 January 1915; wounded sepoy in Brighton Hospital to a relative in Kumaon, Censor of Indian Mails (hereafter CIM), L/MIL/5/825/vol.1, IOR.

12 Lawrence to Kitchener, 27 December 1915, WO 32/5110, PRO.

13 Lawrence to Kitchener, 14 December 1915, WO 32/5110, PRO.

14 Colonel Sir Bruce Seton, 'A Report on the Kitchener Indian Hospital, Brighton', pp. 34-5, L/MIL/1/5, IOR; Lawrence to Kitchener, 27 December 1915, WO 32/5110, PRO.

15 Lawrence to Kitchener, 15 June 1915, WO 32/5110, PRO.

16 Papers of Sir Anthony Bowlby, diary, 3 November 1914, RAMC

2008/7, CMAC; War diary of Sir Arthur Sloggett, DGMS France, 6 August 1915, WO 95/44, PRO; War diary of DGMS France, 6 January 1916, WO 95/45, PRO; W.G. MacPherson, *The Medical Services on the Western Front, and During the Operation in France and Belgium in 1914 and 1915* (London: HMSO, 1923), 123-30.

17   War diaries of Lt.-Col. Beveridge, ADMS Sanitation, 27 October & 10 November 1914, RAMC 543, CMAC.

18   Ghosh, *op. cit.* (note 9), 106.

19   Report by Sir Walter Lawrence on 'Arrangements made for sick and wounded in France', 1, WO 32/5110, PRO.

20   *Lancet*, 14 November 1914.

21   *Egyptian Gazette*, 16 January 1915.

22   Lawrence to Kitchener, 15 June 1915, WO 32/5110, PRO.

23   Lawrence, 'Arrangements', 4-5, WO 32/5110, PRO.

24   *Behind the Lines* (the unofficial magazine of No.10 Stationary Hospital), October-November 1916, RAMC 1601, CMAC.

25   Lawrence to Kitchener, 3 March 1915, WO 32/5110, PRO.

26   Lawrence, 'Arrangements', *ibid.*

27   'His Majesty's Approval of the Emergency Provision for Indian Troops Sick and Wounded at Brighton', Lelean Papers, RAMC 565, CMAC; 'Report on the Kitchener Indian Hospital', p.10, L/MIL/1/5, IOR.

28   Cited in Lawrence, 'Arrangements', WO 32/5110, PRO.

29   Letter 20, 30 January 1915, CIM, L/MIL/5/825/vol.1.

30   Letter 33, 27 March 1915, *ibid.*

31   Letter 6, 10 April 1915, CIM, L/MIL/5/825/vol.2, IOR.

32   Letter 17, 15 February 1915, CIM, L/MIL/5/825/vol.1, IOR.

33   Letter 19, 8 January 1916, CIM, L/MIL/5/826/vol.1, IOR.

34   Letter 36, 6 March 1915, CIM, L/MIL/5/825/vol.1, IOR.

35   Letter 10, 5 June 1915 & letter 40, 29 May 1915, CIM, L/MIL/5/825/vol.3, IOR.

36   'Report on the Kitchener Indian Hospital', pp.5-6, L/MIL/1/5, IOR.

37   *Ibid.*, 7.

38   Letter 8, 11 September 1915, CIM, L/MIL/5/825/vol.5, IOR.

39   Letter 32, 25 September 1915, CIM, L/MIL/5/vol.6, IOR.

40   Lawrence to Kitchener, 5 August 1915, WO 32/5110, PRO.

41   Letter 56, 25 September 1915, CIM, L/MIL/5/825/vol.6., IOR.

42   'Report on the Kitchener Indian Hospital', p.7, L/MIL/1/5, IOR.

43   Letter 24, 23 October 1915, CIM, L/MIL/825/vol.6, IOR.

44   Mark Harrison, *Public Health in British India: Anglo-Indian Preventive Medicine 1859-1914* (Cambridge: Cambridge University

Press, 1994), 12-13.

45 Letter 22, 27 March 1915, CIM, L/MIL/5/825/vol.1, IOR.

46 Letter 19, 4 February 1915, CIM, L/MIL/5/825/vol.1, IOR.

47 Letter 81, 26 June 1915, CIM, L/MIL/825/vol.3, IOR.

48 Letter 33, 28 August 1915, CIM, L/MIL/825/vol.3, IOR.

49 For example, (censored) letter 29, Umed Singh Bist (Gurkha Rifles) to a friend in the Punjab, 13 November: 'If you want any French women there are plenty here and they are very good looking', CIM, L/MIL/5/825/vol.6, IOR.

50 'Report on Kitchener Indian Hospital', 5, L/MIL/1/5, IOR; Nicholas Thornton, 'A Passage to Brighton', *Nursing Times*, 87, 44, 30 October 1991, 44-6.

51 'Report on the Kitchener Indian Hospital', p.7, L/MIL/1/5, IOR.

52 *Ibid.*, 7-8.

53 Letter 22, 12 June 1915, CIM, L/MIL/5/825/vol.3, IOR.

54 Letter 1, 19 June 1915, CIM, L/MIL/5/825/vol.3; letters 8 & 50, 11 September 1915, CIM, IOR L/MIL/5/825/vol.5; letter 2, 2 October 1915, CIM L/MIL/5/825/vol.6., IOR.

55 Letter 21, 12 June 1915, CIM, L/MIL/5/825/vol.3, IOR.

56 Letter 2, 27 November 1915, CIM, L/MIL/5/825/vol.5, IOR.

57 Letter 60, 11 September 1915, CIM, L/MIL/5/825/vol.5, IOR.

58 'Report on the Kitchener Indian Hospital', p.7, L/MIL/1/5, IOR.

59 Lawrence to Kitchener, 14 December 1915, WO 32/5110, PRO.

60 Lawrence to Kitchener, 10 March 1915, *ibid.*

61 Lawrence to Kitchener, 22 March 1915, *ibid.*

62 Lawrence to Kitchener, 30 April 1915, *ibid.*

63 David Omissi, *The Sepoy and the Raj: The Indian Army 1860-1940* (London: Macmillan, 1994), 137.

64 Letter 26, 30 January 1915, CIM, L/MIL/5/825/vol.1, IOR.

65 Omissi, *op. cit.* (note 62), 118.

66 Lawrence to Kitchener, 15 June 1915, WO 32/5110, PRO.

67 Letter 5, 19 June 1915, CIM, L/MIL/5/825/vol.3, IOR.

68 Letter 52, 19 June 1915, *ibid.*

69 Letter 7, 5 June 1915, *ibid.*

70 Letter 1, 4 February 1915, CIM, L/MIL/5/825/vol.1, IOR.

71 Letter 4, 16 January 1915, *ibid.*

72 Letter 5, 15 February 1915 & letter 33, 27 March 1915, *ibid.* There were 92 soldiers suspected of deserting from the Indian Expeditionary Force in France, L/MIL/17/5/2043, IOR.

73 For example, letter 12, 10 April 1915, CIM, L/MIL/5/825/vol.2, IOR.

74 Omissi, *op. cit.* (note 63), 118-19.

75 Lawrence to Kitchener, 10 March 1915, WO 32/5110, PRO.
76 Sadar Singh to friend in the Punjab, CIM, L/MIL/5/825/vol.3, IOR.
77 Pathan sepoy to friend in Punjab, L/MIL/5/825/vol.1, IOR.
78 Rahman, 57th Rifles to friend in France, CIM, L/MIL/5/825/vol.2, IOR.
79 Naik Main Ram to sepoy friend in India, CIM, L/MIL/5/825/vol.3, IOR.
80 Sikh soldiers at Kitchener Indian Hospital to comrade in France, CIM, L/MIL/5/825/vol.1; Khair Mohammed Khan, 129th Baluchis (invalided to India) to Jamadar Zarif Khan, with the same Regt. in France, CIM, L/MIL/5/825/vol.2; Sadar Singh, Lady Hardinge Hospital Brockenhurst, to relative in the Punjab, CIM, L/MIL/5/825/vol.3, IOR.
81 'Report on Kitchener Indian Hospital', 35, L/MIL/1/5, IOR.
82 Omissi, *op. cit.* (note 63), 119.
83 Colonel Sir Bruce Seton, 'An Analysis of 1,000 Wounds and Injuries received in Action, with special reference to the Theory of the Prevalence of Self-Infliction', L/MIL/17/5/2402.

8

'War always brings it on':
War, STDs, the military, and the civilian population in Britain, 1850-1950

Lesley A. Hall

'War breeds vice and venereal', claimed Brigadier-General F. D. Crozier in 1930.[1] This association has the status of an accepted truism, but does the connection, in fact, exist? Certainly, it has been noticeable that, in England, public anxiety about sexually transmitted diseases has tended very largely to emerge either in times of war or in the context of military fitness. This paper looks at the particular manifestations of such anxieties during a hundred-year period in which both war and society in general changed radically, from the revelations about the parlous state of health in the army generated by the Crimean War, to the Second World War and the advent of what seemed, at the time, the miracle cure of penicillin for these age-old complaints.

The topic of venereal disease in the fighting forces of the Crown, and how to prevent it, did not suddenly surface in the middle of the nineteenth century. Ballhatchet, in *Race, Sex, and Class under the Raj*, depicts anxieties about the venereal transactions between British soldiers and native women in India dating back to the eighteenth century. He delineates the persistent ambivalence that hovered around sexual indulgence by soldiers: was resort to prostitutes a concomitant of manliness, or was it likely to 'rapidly and certainly [sap] the principle, the courage, the animal power and the life' of the European troops? Controversy raged over the appropriate measures to deal with the problem: statistics as to the efficacy of a lock hospital system varied widely in different areas of the subcontinent and thus could be used to argue a plausible case either for or against such a measure. 'Decent' native prostitutes who lived in regimental bazaars and submitted to medical examination, were differentiated by authority from the 'disorderly' prostitutes who did not.[2]

Back in the mother country, the subject of venereal disease treatment or prevention was ignored in public health anxieties about the general population, even at a time of growing concern with these matters. The voluntary hospitals which were founded in great numbers from the mid-eighteenth century usually refused patients suffering from these ailments, specialist lock hospitals had difficulty in obtaining financial support, friendly societies refused sickness benefit to venereal sufferers. Such evidence as there is about how poor law administration dealt with venereal disease among the section of the population which fell within its remit suggests a combination of the punitive and the neglectful – punitive to individual cases which came to attention, and neglectful of the wider implications.[3] The upper classes, of course, could obtain treatment from private practitioners, but as the Royal Commission on Venereal Diseases pointed out as late as 1916, given the almost complete silence on public discussion of these diseases, even the better-off were frequently 'misguided by advertisement or misleading recommendations' to seek remedies from quacks in no way qualified to deal with the disease.[4]

The Victorian army was seen as a realm of its own distinct from the civil realm, having its own concerns over venereal diseases as a military problem, distinct from civil health anxieties. This emphasis on the military perspective in venereal disease control, the relative neglect of it as a more general problem within the population at large, may have some connection with the fact that in the nineteenth century, subsequent to the Napoleonic Wars, for the British public war was something that took place on foreign soil, often very distant foreign soil. Following the fall of Napoleon, Britain was not even involved in wars with contiguous European nations. War was out there a long way away and the people who fought it were not part of normal society. It seems plausible, in the light of this, to suggest that anxieties around venereal diseases had a good deal to do with a perception that these were diseases generated at the interface between the extremely clearly demarcated domains of the military and civilian life: i.e. they were particularly threatening because they partook of a liminal quality. As anthropologists tell us, the liminal is an area or state often perceived to be full of risk and danger, a perilous 'no man's land', the space between clearly defined categories where instead of being safely separated they mingle in a potentially explosive way.[5]

The Contagious Diseases Acts of the 1860s were passed in the aftermath of the Crimean War and the revelations resulting from that conflict about the poor state of health and hygiene that existed in the Army. The figures of hospitalization of other ranks for venereal diseases in 1860 ran at 394 per thousand, a figure which equalled the sum total of figures for tuberculosis, respiratory infection, and fevers, which were the most obvious concomitants of overcrowded, insanitary and badly ventilated barracks. Furthermore, this figure was several times greater than that for the Navy, and compared very unfavourably with the venereal disease rates reported for the armies of other European nations.[6] The CD Acts, which were aimed at reducing this practically epidemic rate of venereal infection, affected an apparently well-defined group of women in specific garrison and port towns, the prostitute population to whom the soldiers resorted. They were to be treated with a severity more appropriate to martial law than to civil legislation, by being subjected to compulsory physical examination if suspected of being diseased, and incarcerated in Lock Hospitals if they were.

Soldiers were themselves a stigmatized group. The British Army in the nineteenth century was not a conscript force, its ranks were made up of (largely working-class) men who had 'taken the Queen's shilling', committing them to extensive periods of service – indeed, prior to 1847, for life – which might take them to all parts of the Empire. They were subject to brutal discipline, and forced to live in conditions that were squalid even when they were not as appalling as those which became notorious during the Crimean conflict. Only a handful, a mere 6%, of men were permitted to marry 'on the strength', and their wives were looked at askance – 'their quarrels and complaints, their... want of care and cleanliness... their habits of dissipation'[7] – and little provision was made for married quarters even for this handful of licensed couples.

Among the lower classes themselves there was a persistent tradition that 'enlistment [is] the last step on the downward career of a young man', and the use of the army at home in aid of the civil power in activities such as strike breaking and evicting tenants in Ireland, was not likely to endear it as a career choice.[8] Problems were often caused among local populations by the billeting of troops in inns and private households prior to the increasing erection, from the 1850s, of proper barracks for home-based troops: though Myna Trustram has suggested that the housing of soldiers in regimented barracks led to a growing divide between them and civilian society, as the masses of hangers-on and camp-followers formerly associated with troops were excluded.[9] This may in fact suggest that the boundary between the military and civil populations was becoming more rather than less definite and thus more perilous to transgress.

There was a pervasive notion that the army was 'the dustbin of the nation', providing a lifestyle 'fit only for paupers and hardened criminals'. In 1869 an article in *The Contemporary Review* advanced the argument that every reckless, wild, debauched young fellow, the refuse of the beershop, the sweepings of the gaol, every one who is too idle to work, too stupid to hold his place among his fellows, who had come into unwelcome contact with the law, or generally involved his fortunes in some desperate calamity, is considered, by general consent to have a distinct vocation to defend his country.[10]

In 1880 a senior military officer wrote in *Colburn's United Services Magazine* of the widespread conviction that the soldier's life is one of unbridled debauchery and black-guardism; that to 'go for a soldier' is to take a final plunge into the lowest depths of degradation. Soldiers were treated as pariahs: excluded from parks and places of public amusement, and prevented from travelling second-class on public transport.[11] These attitudes, which persisted well into the twentieth century, are depicted in various texts, for example the works of Kipling, who, himself sympathetic to the common soldier, dramatized popular attitudes in poems such as 'Tommy':

> I went into a public 'ouse to get a pint of beer,
> The publican 'e up and sez, 'we serve no redcoats here'...
> I went into a theatre as sober as could be,
> They gave a drunk civilian room, but 'adn't none for me.[12]

There was a strong class dimension involved in these attitudes towards the army: it was not perceived as a suitable middle-class career in the mid-nineteenth century – the officers were drawn from the upper classes and the ranks from the lower echelons of the working classes, and moreover an element often perceived as riffraff and semi-criminal; not the respectable and self-improving poor but the barely literate. There was scarcely any possibility of making the transition from the ranks to the officers' mess. The Army itself was thus composed of two almost impermeable groups (in spite of the occasional 'gentleman-ranker', or NCO who received a commission), both of which had strong and longstanding associations with low morals and debauchery (aristocratic vice, lower-class immorality). It was not a 'respectable' career, and the diseases suffered by soldiers were not the diseases of the respectable.[13]

The serving soldier was marked off from the general population. The other ranks were, it might be conceded, brave boys prepared both to kill and to die for the protection of their country and its civilian population, but they were set aside as a group which did not fit in to the normal social patterns of marriage and family and settled residence. They were discouraged from marrying and from perpetuating themselves and they could be moved about to the ends of the earth at the will of their superiors. As a group, therefore, they had many of the complex characteristics of the marginal and dangerous as described in Mary Douglas's *Purity and Danger*, 'left out in the patterning of society... placeless'.[14]

Myna Trustram has made a powerful case for the familial nature of the army as an institution, and the strong element of paternalism in its prevailing ideology.[15] It could be argued that the regimental family was felt to replace the familial relationships of civil life, or to act as a substitute for them. However, within this model the other ranks were perpetual children or at least adolescents. This has powerful resonances with the position and status of adolescent boys in the societies described by Douglas in which boys, on reaching the age of puberty, undergo a period of initiation as a *rite de passage* between childhood and manhood. As she describes them, initiation ceremonies were themselves often described as dangerous and potentially lethal to the participants (as a soldier's life could literally be). Between their ritual dying to their childish lives, and their rebirth as fully adult men integrated into the social structure, these boys were outcast, without a place within society. Sometimes they actually had to leave physically and go far away. If they remained nearby, any contacts between them and the full members of society were perceived as anti-social, and violence and lawlessness might even be expected of those undergoing initiation.[16] Soldiers were withdrawn from society, but they were not reintegrated into it at the end of an initiatory rite of manhood as adolescents were. They were set apart from normal social life for a particular purpose, and therefore when they were not in the battle-field or its vicinity, performing that purpose, they were dangerously out of place with a powerful potential to disrupt social norms. Their powers, which exercised in the right place were benign and protective, became ambiguous and even malign taken out of that location.

The Contagious Diseases Acts, in their way, seem to have been attempting to create an equivalent cadre of women to supply the sexual needs of these men regarded as outcasts from decent society: almost, one might suggest, a *cordon sanitaire* protecting society at large from the potential dangers they threatened. As Skelley has pointed out in his important study of *The Victorian Army at Home*, the attitudes towards soldiers cited above extended to those members of the civilian population who associated with them for either professional or personal reasons.[17] The women affected by the CD Acts were presumed, like soldiers, to be volunteers, but subject, through practising their trade in a garrison or naval town, to militaristic rigours of discipline. This militarization of the prostitute was almost explicit in the Indian context, where proposals were made for the enforced examination of prostitutes residing within regimental cantonments, and their expulsion if found to be diseased.[18] While attempts to define and segregate prostitutes as an unclean group have a long history, in this particular case it may be suggested that the particular group of 'dirty women' identified by the CD Acts was particularly 'dirty' because they consorted with soldiers, who were themselves a stigmatized group and thus contaminated their associates.

Mark Harrison has asked the pertinent question 'Why were the military authorities so determined to maintain a system of regulated prostitution?'. The evidence for the effects of the CD Acts on the VD rate in the army was extremely ambiguous, and the Continental system upon which the Acts were modelled was not a particularly shining example of the benefits of regulated prostitution. Harrison rightly suggests that regulating sexual activity of the troops in this way formed part of a more generalized anxiety about policing the contact between the military and civilian domains, shared by both sides. The idea prevalent among officers that interaction with civilians 'exposed soldiers to inappropriate habits and values' may well have had ramifications which extended well beyond disciplinary concerns about intemperance and disorder.[19] During the 1850s and 60s the Peace Society put forward arguments that 'the purifying influences of domestic life' ran counter to the requirement of the military authorities that the soldier should be 'a useable instrument for killing', something which was inimical to any ties which 'tend[ed] to render him more of a man and less of a machine'.[20] Thus the civilian domain was also positioned as something that was dangerous to the soldier's continued capacity to operate effectively as a fighting machine.

The campaign against the CD Acts suggests that some, however, did not assume this widely accepted absolute hiatus between the civil and the military. In the same way that the proponents of the repeal of the Acts were arguing for the common humanity of the prostitute, they were arguing for the humanity of the soldier. In 1870 Harriet Martineau claimed that the reason why the common soldier tended to sink into 'gross animalism' was clearly demonstrated by the revelations made in the sanitary reports on the army at home and in India of the pervasive assumption that the ranker's 'animalism is a necessity which must be provided for.'[21] The repealers believed that the soldier should no longer be treated as the slave of his lowest animal instincts.

210

The clear-cut distinction which the Victorians had nonetheless largely succeeded in maintaining between military and civil spheres became considerably more blurred during the First World War, which apart from anything else was taking place much nearer home, just across the Channel. There had been persisting concerns around venereal diseases as a problem to do with military fitness, in India and as a significant element in the anxieties around national physical deterioration which followed the Boer War. Significantly, the earliest experiments with Salvarsan, Paul Ehrlich's 'magic bullet' against syphilis, were conducted by Colonel L. W. Harrison in the military hospital in Rochester Row. However, in 1913 the extent of sexually transmitted disease as a problem within the general population was finally recognised by the setting up of a Royal Commission on Venereal Diseases, to investigate their prevalence and the existing provisions for treatment, and to make recommendations for both preventive and curative measures.

It was therefore in this context of the emergence of a hitherto absent public concern with the entire subject that quite early in the war it was recognized that a particularly delicate problem was posed by venereal disease, which became even more sensitive when conscription came into force. Instead of the notion of the soldier as someone who was not encouraged to breed, there was a whole new picture of the eugenically desirable 'flower of manhood' setting off into the dangers of war. Contemporary commentators (and much subsequent historiography) tended to define the problem as having to do with the sudden proliferation of 'amateur prostitutes' suffering from 'khaki fever' who were, it was alleged, positively besieging soldiers with offers of gratuitous amorous favours. The professional prostitute took on a new guise, perceived less as a dangerous anarchic force than as a sensible tradeswoman who 'knew how to take care of herself' unlike these 'amateurs'. However, it is possible to take a somewhat different perspective in looking at the new versions of policing the old civil/military divide which arose during the Great War.

The facilities for early diagnosis and treatment were significantly better developed in the military in 1914 than they were in civil life, as the Royal Commission on Venereal Diseases discovered. This system however was placed under considerable stress by the outbreak of war, although the Official War History claimed that the rates of infection 'compare[d] favourably with the rates for the three previous peace years 1911-1913'.[22] Absolutely larger numbers of men however, were involved, and they were not professional soldiers but volunteers and conscripts who would – if they survived the war –

return to normal civil life. They were not a distinctive group set off from the general population in the same way. The issue of VD control thus became important not merely because of the enormous wastage of man-power it caused during this period of national emergency, but because these diseases 'incurred the likelihood of permanent damage to the individual, infection to others, and an heritage which might stain an innocent life'[23] – as already mentioned, the men who marched away during the war of 1914 to 18 were envisaged as prime breeding stock. F. D. Crozier writing of his experiences as *A Brass Hat in No Man's Land* noted that 'many of the boys were new to the big drums', and the ranks were filled by an entirely different group of men: 'some of the finest middle- and lower-middle-class stock in the Kingdom'.[24]

Crozier presents an evocative picture of life as it was for the Regular Army, by its nature and traditions alien from the kind of life the young men joining the colours in 1914 and later had been living and would have expected. There was a considerable culture clash, quite distinct from the general abnormality of times in which the uncertainties of the situation led to the feeling 'why not have a fling and enjoy the pleasures of sexual intercourse while the chance was there?' Crozier considered that it was not only the 'absence from home' but the 'inculcation of barbaric habits in our manhood' as these young men were thrown into an alien way of life with standards often completely contrary to those they had been brought up in, which contributed to 'The abnormal life, the shattered nerves' leading to sexual promiscuity.[25]

It was recognized that sexually transmitted diseases posed particular problems for medical officers. With other infectious diseases the task was to prevent infection from reaching the personnel or spreading among them. In the case of STDs, the causes were known, and the risk was individually undertaken in spite of awareness that it existed.[26] Means of reducing the prevalence of these diseases among the troops varied, and their success was similarly varied. Exhortations to sexual continence, most famously Lord Kitchener's address to the British Expeditionary Force, were sometimes employed. Particularly in France reliance was placed on the traditional medically-inspected regulated prostitutes. Not all the Medical Corps considered this the most effective course of action, at a period when advanced medical opinion favoured the medical approach rather than social control.

According to the official History of the War 'during war the sexual instinct is stimulated in both sexes, and gratification of the

impulse is more easily obtained.... there is a tendency towards
slackening of moral principles'.[27] This, like Crozier's comment that
'prostitutes and loose women always follow the big drum', with the
result that 'war breeds vice and venereal', was scarcely the timeless
truth we sometimes think.[28] This perception that 'social conditions
operated strongly during the war in favour of a high venereal rate'[29]
was perhaps largely about this particular war, when the traditionally
perilous zone of interaction between the military man and the
women who associated with him was vastly extended. It is perhaps
pertinent that this was the first war in which women took a
significant official – as opposed to the traditional, irregular, camp-
follower – part, as nurses, ambulance drivers, doctors, and in a variety
of auxiliary roles in the new women's forces.

Some authorities accepted that the prostitute was a necessary
concomitant of combat. However expedients such as licensed brothels
were put into practice behind the front lines in areas dominated by the
military, and in foreign countries. Furthermore, it was discovered that
'Over 60 per cent of the infections resulted from intercourse with
women who were not prostitutes in the ordinary sense of the word'.[30]
The 'promiscuity' of women who could not be legitimately be
described as prostitutes, or at least not 'professionals', undermined
arguments for controlling venereal disease by regulating prostitution,
and created enormous anxiety by its transgression of normal peacetime standards differentiating respectable from unrespectable women.
Men's preference for women who at least appeared to be not of the
prostitute class was even attributed to the campaign against venereal
disease with its emphasis on the dangers of consorting with
prostitutes. R. A. Lyster of the National Society for the Prevention of
Venereal Disease claimed the fear being drummed up around sex with
prostitutes was a misguided approach to venereal disease control. He
argued that 'it frightens people from the professional... and drives
them to the non-professional'. Lyster was of the opinion that 'The
average soldier... was convinced that if he had sexual relations with a
woman who was not a professional prostitute, he was safe, and no
amount of argument would convince him otherwise.'[31]

What actually constituted the most effective medical preventive
approach to venereal diseases in the fighting forces remained
contentious. Early treatment of the potentially infected was one
recommendation: this involved ablution areas where treatment could
be given as soon as possible after exposure: Crozier noted as an effect
of the disruptions of war that 'young men find themselves in this
strange queue, who would, in times of peace, have hesitated to line

up outside a music hall'.[32] The American and Dominions model of the issue of prophylactic packs was much cited and it was argued that the means of self-disinfection should be supplied (it was almost always the provision of chemical means of protection, not condoms, which was under discussion in these debates). There was a perceptible, though far from absolute, shift of emphasis away from the provision of a special group of women to cater for the needs of a particular group of men, to means whereby contamination could either be washed away, or a barrier set up against it at the critical moment. While this accorded with medical developments, it may also have had to do with the aforementioned issue of the composition of the British Army fighting the First World War: it was a less specific and distinct group of men. The men who were contracting VD from women who were not 'real' prostitutes were in the majority of cases men who were not 'real' – full-time, professional – soldiers. However, the change in approach may also relate to changes in the nature of warfare and the type of soldier it demanded, capable of taking on more personal responsibility in a more 'scientific' age, as Mark Harrison as argued.[33]

By the time of the Second World War, the distinction between the Army out there fighting the war and the civilian population well behind the lines had thoroughly broken down. In the age of war in the air the population in general were in as much or more danger than troops at the front, were involved in fire-watching and air-raid patrol, queued for rations, were subject to direction into employment as deemed necessary for the conduct of the war. Anxieties over the effect of venereal diseases on manpower focussed on potential erosion of the workforce in the factories as well as the fighting forces in the field. Among the forces, in spite of the existing mechanisms for dealing with VD, this was, once again, 'the most difficult of all diseases to control'. Theoretically information was disseminated to all servicemen about risks and provisions for treatment but many 'denied ever having had a lecture on the subject'. Measures of prevention and treatment were introduced: condoms issued, educational films shown, lectures given and poster campaigns initiated. In 1943 regulation 33B under the Defence (General) Regulations provided for notification of carriers: in theory this was not the traditional measure overtly discriminating against women, but nonetheless it bore more punitively upon women. It was not until 1944 that the new wonder-drug penicillin was used to treat syphilis, which could be done effectively in the field with a course of treatment lasting days rather than the years which Salvarsan therapy had necessitated: however there was considerable resistance to allocating this scarce resource to the treatment of VD.[34] The advent of antibiotics had a major impact (at least for a few decades before resistant strains developed and new diseases emerged) on attitudes towards sexually-transmitted diseases.

In spite of the various measures taken, by 1942 venereal diseases had risen at an appalling rate from an all time low just before the outbreak of war, even though syphilis had been effectively treatable by the arsenical drug Salvarsan since 1910, and gonorrhoea had recently (1937) proved amenable to the first antibiotics, the sulphonamides. The Ministry of Health therefore launched a campaign to raise public awareness of these diseases, and to alert the public to the facilities for treatment. Although the campaign had been intended to be hard-hitting and forthright a certain degree of censorship of the advertisement copy was exercised by the press. The initial accessible demotic language of the copy, employing vernacular usages like 'pox' and 'clap', was replaced by more technical terms acceptable to squeamish sensibilities. This euphemism was criticized as seriously vitiating the impact of the campaign, by addressing the problem in a way less likely to communicate meaningfully to the population it was intended to reach.[35]

In 1942 Mass Observation was commissioned by the Government to investigate the efficacy of its educational campaign around venereal disease. MO had been established in 1937 with the aim of producing what was described as 'an anthropology of ourselves'. A nationwide panel of observers drawn from among the general population took on the task of reporting upon their own everyday lives and all that went on around them, by both 'field study' of 'actual behaviour under normal living conditions' and more subjective reportage from what were described as 'voluntary, candid informants in all works of life'. Unlike opinion pollsters or market researchers, they were to look and listen, as well as, or instead of, asking.[36] In its 1942/43 venereal disease survey MO's method was to approach individuals in the street and ask them a set schedule of questions, beginning by ascertaining whether they had actually seen the Ministry's advertisements. Male observers were to approach men, and female, women, and find out what they felt about the press campaign, whether they felt they were getting too much or not enough information about VD, if there was anything special they wanted to know, what their views were about the dissemination of this information, were there any words they felt should not be used, and their own views on prevention. Indirect comments not specifically related to these questions were also to be recorded, as were refusals to respond, and assessment of the degree of embarrassment. The Observers were struck by 'the great willingness, and often active desire' of the public to know more about the subject and have it brought into the open.[37]

The reports by the observers of their interviews are extremely fascinating and a number of interesting reiterated themes occurred among the returns. In spite of the press campaign which had explicitly stated that various superstitions about the way the diseases could be caught were not true, and that it was not possible to identify sufferers, these were recurrent motifs in the replies.

The educational campaign had emphasized that prostitutes were not the only or even the main source of the diseases, but the idea that they were was obviously still very prevalent. (All the ascriptions of class and age to respondents seem to be rather approximate and based on the interviewer's assessment, but have been included here to give some indication of social and age range). According to a middle-class man between 50 and 60:

> you must tackle the source of it – the woman with the germs. Why were the troops free from venereal disease in the last war? Because women had to have a doctor's certificate once a week. Exactly what I say – a medical examination of prostitutes.

(The elison from the woman with the germs to women to prostitutes is itself interesting, as is the assumption that last time, in the First War, the solution to the problem had been got right: this was a persistent if somewhat misguided belief.) A 45-year-old middle-class man advocated 'rigorous inspection of that class of individual through whom the infection is contracted' and a lower middle class male of 40 thought that 'all members of the "oldest profession" should have to submit to compulsory examination at least every month'. Opinions were not necessarily consistent: a middle-class woman of 55 said 'Prostitutes should be examined, or stopped': but then went on 'It's not necessarily prostitutes. They often have to take more care of themselves'. This reflects the pervasive but not necessarily accurate idea that professionals knew how to take care of themselves, as one 35-year-old admitted prostitute remarked (several times in slightly different words) 'I am a prostitute but a woman of the world. That is why I know how to protect myself against the disease.' However, she added that 'But if ever anything goes wrong and I do get the disease, well then I shall put my head in the gas oven. No treatment for me then, the gas-oven and that will be the end.'[38]

suggesting that even if she did know how to take care of herself she did not have very much idea of the curative possibilities available if she did become infected.

Other respondents, though they located the diseases in specific bodies, did not necessarily see these as those of professional prostitutes. In some cases the bodies were gender free, or at least of both sexes: a 20-year-old lower-middle-class woman blamed 'bad people and bad women'. For a 21-year-old middle-class male, those to blame were the ones in 'West End night clubs' of unspecified gender.[39] Soldiers were also victims of blame: a 35-year-old middle-class woman thought 'of course it's the soldiers and the ATS'; and a lower-middle-class woman of 45 said 'of course, they say its the troops' (which does suggest a little scepticism about this view). [40]

Usually the dangerous bodies were very definitely those of women. One working-class man of 67 suggested 'Keep away from women' as the remedy for the disease, but most respondents specified particular groups of women as the danger: a male of 50, middle-class, thought that 'any woman who's had four men is bound to either have it or be a carrier'; a 55-year-old middle-class male put the problem down to

> young girls roaming about not caring for their sense of decency and honour what can you expect. If you sit in a train or bus there they are it would seem sat in such a position as to be suggestive.

'Girls of fifteen picking up soldiers' were the cause, thought a 30-year-old lower-middle-class woman, and a 55-year-old middle-class woman considered that 'These little cheap loose-living girls – they should be dealt with'. However one 30-year-old working-class woman asked 'Why should I know. I would never run into it':[41] which is perhaps just another way of saying that the disease did not inhabit bodies like the respondent's. Young girls, either as dangers or in danger themselves, recurred: several working- or lower-middle-class women said things like 'The girls should use pessaries to protect themselves' (aged 40); 'Quite young people know already more than we do. Lots of hot baths with Dettol douching' (35); 'Girls should look after themselves' (25); 'due to the lack of privacy nowadays, it is impossible for young girls to use the syringe'(45).[42]

Sometimes the stigmatized bodies were specifically those of foreigners: a 55-year-old lower-middle-class male said 'Increased has it? must be the foreigners here', while a 30-year-old middle-class woman remarked 'it's all these blinking foreigners'.[43] Two women, 25 and 30, working-class and lower-middle, said in almost exactly the same words

217

'It's all those foreign soldiers'. Sometimes particular nationalities were mentioned: a middle-class woman of 45 said 'Well I haven't read much about it but I've a friend a Doctor at St Mary Abbots she's doing VD she says its the Americans'.[44] The Mass Observers themselves remarked that 'It is a great pity that so much blame should be put on American and various allied members of the services'.[45]

The converse idea to its location in specified bodies, was that the disease was somehow both horrible and all pervasive and could be contracted by means other than sexual contact, a viewpoint often voiced. A considerable group of women, their ages ranging from 20 to 73, mostly from the lower social groups, expressed anxieties around this, and emphasized the general benefits of 'Great cleanliness', 'always have a good wash', because 'Cleanness keeps a lot of things away'. Lavatory seats and their dangers figured prominently: 'People should not use any lavatory seat'; 'women have to be very particular about using public conveniences'; 'one has got to be very careful when using public lavatories'; 'one has got to be careful in strange lavatories'; 'be careful about using lavatories, about touching banisters, when boarding buses'; 'Never to sit on any lavatory except the one in your own home'. Ideally, 'Every woman should keep herself clean, scrub herself, not to sit on any lavatory seat'.[46]

In spite of this idea that the disease was somehow miasmatically present and capable of striking anywhere, attitudes towards those actually infected were frequently punitive, stressing not merely compulsory treatment but severe punishments. A man of 56, middle-class, thought there was 'no way other than sterilisation... Compulsory – heavy punishment for anybody failing to comply'; working-class males of 40 suggested 'Male complaint notifiable under a severe penalty'; 'making it a punishable offence for not reporting' One man of 45, middle-class, went so far as to recommend 'making promiscuous intercourse a punishable offence' and another, of somewhat lower social status said 'The best thing to do would be to burn the "dirty bastards" who are walking about with it and won't be treated'.[47]

Several, mostly from the lower social groups, saw some form of segregation as the solution: a 30-year-old male said 'they shouldn't be allowed to contaminate anybody else. Let them live their own lives in misery'; two women of 40 suggested 'People suffering from the disease should be isolated from the general public' and 'trying to catch the guilty one and shutting him up away from people who are clean'; and a working-class woman of 30 thought that there ought to be 'An order forbidding people having the disease to mix with other people.' The model here was presumably derived from existing public health measures for infectious diseases with which the respondents might already have come into contact: one woman of 25 suggested that 'One should isolate everybody who has got it' but also argued that 'One should have a "toxoid" for it, the same thing as they have for diphtheria'. A woman of 50, of a somewhat higher social group, similarly suggested 'I suppose it would be good to have children inoculated against it, I had all my children inoculated against small-pox'.[48]

Others, however, took the view that if prostitution were properly contained the problem would be eradicated, with a traditional, if somewhat misguided belief, that such things were better ordered on the Continent. Men in their forties, mostly of the lower social echelons, spoke of 'having proper places for the purpose of this "pastime" where every precaution and constant examination should be given'; 'Recognis[ing] brothels by properly licensing them when proper medical examination there should be enforced'; 'Firstly by instructing the people as above, and secondly by regulating the places where intercourse takes place and making medical inspection compulsory there'; though one did explicitly suggest 'licensing this business where people could go if they must, where proper examination of *both* parties should take place'. A lower-middle-class woman of 45 similarly suggested 'Controlled houses as they have on the continent, but men to be examined too beforehand'.[49]

However, set against views which located VD in specific, and usually 'other', bodies, were those who advocated general medical examination of everyone. A middle-class-woman of 51 thought it would be: a very good idea if State made everybody have a medical examination every so often. Say every five years. Many things would be found out which should be attended to, and are not. An 18-year-old working-class youth considered 'the only way to prevent it is examine everyone in the country" similarly a lower-middle-class male, 25, remarked 'I think the only way to stop it is to have medical examination every year for everybody, and especially before marriage'; a lower-middle-class man and woman, both 45, thought 'Compulsory medical examination periodically'; 'Only one remedy – be examined every so often by a doctor. Compulsorily'. A middle-class man of 50 stated 'I think it's absolutely essential that every man woman and child in the country should have test', and a man of 45 and somewhat lower social class recommended 'Compulsory medical Inspection and Instruction in all districts according to age'.[50]

It should be emphasized, however, that there were, in fact, many respondents who did not believe that it was possible to control the diseases by compulsion, and that the way forward was rather through education and perhaps scientific medical advances. Some recommended prophylactic packets: two men, both 45 and lower-middle-class suggested 'the issue of a prophylactic packet to all the services as now issued to the US Navy'; 'Issue of a preventative – free to troops and on sale to all at Chemists'.[51] Many wanted a campaign of information, sometimes with such specifications as 'the full facts of the danger of this scourge, and not being namby-pamby about it' (lower-middle-class male, 50); 'By the authorities telling us in plain language about it and not being windy of the subject' (45-year-old working-class male).[52] However, a middle-class woman of 25 pointed out 'we're getting so many instructions about so many things I don't know if people would notice.... There's so many nagging advertisements about this and that already'.[53]

Yet others were concerned that by passing regulations such as 33B 'they will persecute prostitutes by it' whereas the first necessity was to 'eradicate fear surrounding matter' (male, 50, middle-class), and similarly a middle-class male of 40 considered that 'Compulsion may drive it underground. Let people be frank'. An 'old soldier' of 60 said 'Listen, mate.... the only way to prevent it is let people stop treating sex as shameful and secret', a view concurred with by a lower middle class 20 year old: 'The whole trouble is fear and shame. If you can get rid of them, it would be easy.' This attitude was shared by an upper middle class man of 55: 'of course if you drive it underground it's no good. The main thing is to encourage people to go for treatment. If you make it repressive people will simply hide it.'[54] This was possibly related to the perception of one lower-middle-class man of 55: 'I'm against compulsion – it's too much like the Gestapo'.[55]

Individuals' attitudes to a specific group of diseases could be related to a number of more general concerns which the war was likely, if not to have created, to have exacerbated. Some people saw the disease as harboured in specific, identifiable bodies – a definable enemy – and it is perhaps not to be wondered at that 'foreigners' were seen as particularly likely to be its agents, though at least one respondent a 45-year-old, lower-middle-class woman recounted that 'My husband used to go to Covent Garden – they've a place there [a VD Hospital] he said you'd be surprised the nice looking fellows going there', suggesting that the venereally diseased looked like anyone else – -unsuspected fifth columnists, as it were – but she did add 'where did they get it? – Dirty Women!'.[56] Others, in the midst of a war in which the Home Front was in as much danger as the fighting forces, saw it as all-pervasive, and likely to strike anyone at random, if precautions were not taken (a frame of mind perhaps analogous to air raid precautions – being careful about the blackout, and taking refuge in shelters). The ideas of compulsory examination and/or punitive measures can be related to wider issues of the militarization and regulation of society in a nation at war. The ideas about public education and advances in scientific medicine can also, of course, be related to contemporary discourses: the variety of contradictory discourses which abounded, and were sometimes expressed in the course of one interview by a single individual, can readily be discerned.

These statements of the early 1940s suggested that it could be possible to link the attitudes to venereal disease which emerged from the usual conspiracy of silence when it became a matter of military significance, to wider attitudes around war, the military, and the civilian population. There were demonstrable changes in the specific character of this connection over the hundred years from 1850 to 1950. Although many attitudes clearly persisted throughout this time, there do seem to have been alterations in the nature of war, while the relationship between the army and the civil population also changed. What certainly did persist was an enduring link in people's minds between war, soldiers, 'vice and venereal' as associated disruptions of the natural order.

To conclude, a couple of final quotations from respondents to Mass Observation, which are thought-provoking – in rather different directions – about the transgression of normal sexual and gender relations caused by war, and perceptions of the way this generates sexual disease: Working-class man of 65: 'War always brings it on. And now that women are in the forces, it makes it worse'; 54-year-old male, lower-middle-class: 'You... get all these waves of venereal disease when wars come, and men are segregated away from women. One of the chief ways to prevent venereal disease is to prevent wars'.[57]

Notes

1 Brig-Gen F. D. Crozier, *A Brass Hat in No-Man's Land: A Personal Record of the European War* (London: Jonathan Cape, 1930), 67.

2 K. Ballhatchett, *Race, Sex, and Class under the Raj: Imperial Attitudes and Policies and their Critics, 1793-1905* (London: Weidenfield and Nicolson, 1980), 10-39.

3 L. A. Hall, '"The Cinderella of Medicine": Sexually Transmitted Diseases in Great Britain in the Nineteenth and Twentieth Centuries', *Genitourinary Medicine*, lxix (1993), 314-9.

4 Royal Commission on Venereal Diseases: Final Report Cd 8189, 1916, §133, §188.

5 M. Douglas, *Purity and Danger: An Analysis of the Concepts of Purity and Taboo* (London: Ark 1984- first published 1966), 96-7.

6 A. R. Skelley, *The Victorian Army at Home: The Recruitment and Terms and Conditions of the British Regular, 1859-1899* (London: Croom Helm, 1977), 25.

7 M. Trustram, *Women of the Regiment: Marriage and the Victorian Army* (Cambridge: Cambridge University Press, 1984), 39: citing *United Services Gazette*, 1854.

8 Skelley, *op. cit.* (note 6), 243-4.

9 Trustram, *op. cit.* (note 7), 12-4

10 Skelley, *op. cit.* (note 6), 245.

11 *Ibid.*, 247.

12 R. Kipling, *'Tommy', Barrack-Room Ballads*, 1892.

13 Skelley, *op. cit.* (note 6), 204.

14 Douglas, *op. cit.* (note 5), 96.

15 Trustram, *op. cit.* (note 7), 23.

16 Douglas, *op. cit.* (note 5), 95-7.

17 Skelley, *op. cit.* (note 6), 247.

18 Ballhatchett, *op. cit.* (note 2), 10-39.

19 M. Harrison, 'The British Army and the Problem of Venereal Disease in France and Egypt during the First World War', Medical History, xxxix (1995), 133-58.

20 *The Herald of Peace*, cited in Trustram, *op. cit.* (note 7), 135.

21 Cited *ibid.*, 131.

22 W.G. MacPherson (ed.), *History of the Great War Based on Official Documents: Medical Services: Diseases of the War Volume II* (London: HMSO, 1923), 119.

23 *Ibid.*, 74.

24 Crozier, *op. cit.* (note 1), 143.

25 *Ibid.*, 67.

26 MacPherson, *op. cit.* (note 22), 72.
27 *Ibid*, 78.
28 Crozier, *op. cit.* (note 1), 64.
29 MacPherson, *op. cit.* (note 22), 121.
30 *Ibid*, 121.
31 Evidence of Dr R A Lyster, 15 Dec 1919, to Committee of Enquiry into Sexual Morality 1918-19. Association for Moral and Social Hygiene archives, Box 49 in the Fawcett Library at London Guildhall University.
32 Crozier, *op. cit.* (note 1), 143.
33 Harrison, *op. cit.* (note 19).
34 Hall, *op. cit.* (note 3).
35 R. Porter and L. Hall, *The Facts of Life: The Creation of Sexual Knowledge in Britain, 1650-1950* (New Haven: Yale University Press, 1995), 241-2.
36 T. Harrisson, *Britain Revisited* (London: Victor Gollancz Ltd, 1961), 15-22.
37 Tom Harrisson-Mass Observation Archive at the University of Sussex: MO A9, 'Sex Surveys', Box 1, VD Survey, file A.
38 MO A9 1/E Nov-Dec 1942, 1/D Nov-Dec 1942, 1/B Dec 1942 London.
39 MO A9 1/B, 1/E.
40 MO A9 1/B
41 MO A9 1/B Dec 1942 London; 1/E Nov-Dec 1942, 1/G Feb-Mar 1943; 1/C Nov-Dec 1942 London.
42 MO A9 1/C Nov-Dec 1942 London, 1/B Dec 1942 London.
43 MO A9 1/B Dec 1942 London ('Indirect').
44 MO A9 1/B Dec 1942 London ('Indirect').
45 MO A9 1/A.
46 MO A9 1/B Dec 1942 London.
47 MO A9 1/E Nov-Dec 1942, 1/D Nov-Dec 1942, 1/G Feb-Mar 1943.
48 MO A9 1/E Nov-Dec 1942, 1/B Nov-Dec 1942.
49 MO A9 1/D Nov-Dec 1942, 1/B Nov-Dec 1942.
50 MO A9 1/D Nov-Dec 1942, 1/E Nov-Dec 1942, 1/B Nov-Dec 1942.
51 MO A9 1/D Nov-Dec 1942.
52 MO A9 1/D Nov-Dec 1942.
53 MO A9 1/C Nov-Dec 1942.
54 MO A9 1/E Nov-Dec 1942.
55 MO A9 1/B London Survey
56 MO A9 1/B.
57 MO A9 1/E Nov-Dec 1942, 1/B Nov-Dec 1942.

9

Sex and the Citizen Soldier:
Health, Morals and Discipline in the British Army
during the Second World War

Mark Harrison

Measures to control sexually transmitted diseases (STDs) have traditionally focused on women far more than on men. The common principle underlying the Contagious Diseases Acts introduced in Britain during the nineteenth century, and legislation enacted in Britain and other nations during the two world wars, was that women were the main source of infection. These measures also rested on very different conceptions of male and female sexual conduct. Although men might be permitted a temporary lapse from virtue, a woman who had contracted 'venereal disease', as it was then generally known, was tainted for life.[1] The 'double standard' inherent in legislation to control STDs has rightly attracted a good deal of attention but, in seeking to reveal and account for this injustice, attempts to regulate male sexual behaviour in relation to venereal disease have been generally overlooked.[2] As I have argued elsewhere, such measures were most apparent in the armed forces, where venereal disease was one of the most important causes of ineffectiveness among troops. Attempts to regulate the sexual behaviour of British soldiers were also linked to ideals of masculinity which emphasised the virtues of chivalry, physical fitness and moral purity. During the Victorian period 'muscular Christianity' espoused by individuals such as Gen. Gordon and Henry Havelock, and the Stoical, neo-Spartan ethos present in some of the public schools, began to show itself in appeals for sexual abstinence and in the provision of 'wholesome' recreations for troops.[3]

Such high-mindedness sat uneasily with the Army's traditional tolerance towards sexual promiscuity and prostitution, although it was widely accepted by the late nineteenth century that rational control over body and mind would prepare young men for the conduct expected of them on the battlefield.[4] These attitudes were still in evidence at the beginning of the First World War, and military virtue was identified with sexual restraint far more than in the French or German armies; such concerns being a product of the British Army's closer involvement – both as actor and subject – with movements for moral reform. An influential elite, counting among its members the Secretary of State for War, Lord Kitchener, and the Commander-in-Chief of the British Army in France, Sir Douglas (later Earl) Haig, sought positively to discourage sexual promiscuity. As a result, measures to control venereal disease (VD) were punitive in nature and, where local circumstances permitted, as in Egypt, vigorous measures were taken to outlaw prostitution and associated vices.[5] Although sections of the army were tolerant of prostitution, attitudes towards the sexual behaviour of troops were far from *laissez faire*, as is usually claimed.[6]

Focusing mainly on the British Army in the Mediterranean theatre of operations, this paper considers the extent to which such attitudes had changed by 1945. The conventional view is that the Second World War brought a liberalisation of sexual behaviour, as well as greater frankness in the discussion of related problems such as venereal disease. There is a good deal of truth in this, but it is a view which stands in need of qualification. Although the war was, for many, a time of unprecedented sexual freedom, influential sections of British society sought to reassert control over the body in the name of health, democracy and good citizenship.[7] These attempts at sexual control centred, once again, on venereal disease; a major source of anxiety in wartime because of its implications for military effectiveness and racial vigour. The armed forces and prostitutes – traditionally seen as the main sources of venereal infection – were the targets of a health campaign which portrayed promiscuity and its attendant evils as an offence against the state.

The approach to VD control in the British Army both shaped and reflected a new conception of citizenship that had been emerging prior to the war, but which now took on an added dimension as a result of the conflict against the Axis powers. The typical British male was portrayed as free and self-directed, but his freedom (including his sexual freedom) was bounded by a sense of responsibility, moderation and 'good form'. In these respects, he was supposedly different from the men of Axis countries, who were represented variously as cruel, promiscuous and undisciplined. But this new vision of the British serviceman was crucially compromised as both his self-discipline and capacity for education were called into question by increasing rates of VD in foreign theatres.

The British government's decision to embark on a campaign of public education about VD was a direct response to the huge increase in the disease in the UK at the beginning of the Second World War. In 1941 the incidence of VD among servicemen and male civilians increased by 113%, and among women by 63%. In addition to the likely consequences for national efficiency, these figures seemed to indicate a national moral decline, going hand-in-hand with a rise in the number of births occurring outside of wedlock. The government's decision to increase the number of treatment centres for VD, and to introduce compulsory treatment for women suspected of having the disease (Regulation 33B), were reminiscent of its response during the Great War. But the frankness of anti-VD propaganda marked an important break with the past. In 1942 the Ministry of Health launched a campaign to make the facts about VD and its treatment more widely known, and for the first time in Britain the subject was deemed fit for a radio broadcast.[8] As the new Central Council for Health Education (successor to the British Social Hygiene Council) put it, 'hush-hush' was being banished'; the causes, effects and treatment of VD were to be discussed far more openly than before.[9]

'Total War' acted as midwife to a new culture of citizenship that had been developing since the late nineteenth century, and which had acquired new meaning following the enfranchisement of men and women over the age of 21 by the Representation of the People Acts of 1918 and 1928. The concept of 'citizenship', as introduced into British political vocabulary by the Liberal philosopher T.H. Green, entailed a reciprocal relationship between the individual and the state; the former owing duties and responsibilities in return for the rights and privileges conferred by membership of British society. One of the most important of these duties, as expressed in numerous books and articles from the end of the nineteenth century, was the responsibility of the citizen to bear arms, and to keep himself fit for military duty.[10] Ideas of citizenship also found expression in writings on welfare and social insurance: benefits were given in return for individual contributions and in relation to the individual's willingness and capacity to serve the state. The notion of citizenship, therefore, gradually acquired a social as well as a political dimension.[11]

This interest in citizenship, education and health was part of the more general trend in public health identified by David Armstrong in his study of medical knowledge in twentieth-century Britain; namely, the shift in focus from the 'environment' to the 'individual'. According to Armstrong, the 'old' public health, typified by nineteenth-century sanitarianism, treated the body as an object and sought to control its relationship with the environment; the 'new' public health, by contrast, was concerned with the minutiae of social life, with the individual and his or her social relations.[12] As both Armstrong and Abram De Swaan have observed,[13] the 'new' public health was a product of the belief that individuals were bound together in a web of 'mutual dependency' nurtured by the state.[14] Venereal disease, in particular, was no longer used to forbid certain sexual relationships but became a mechanism through which to observe them'; instead of condemning 'illicit' relationships, sexual hygiene organisations aimed to promote 'social progress' and family life.

It would be misleading to draw too strong a contrast between the 'old' and the 'new' public health, since nineteenth century conceptions of public health were by no means exclusively environmental; just as 'environmental' controls continued to be an important feature of the 'new' public health. However, the change in emphasis captured by the new buzz-words 'social hygiene' and 'sexual hygiene' is undeniable and can be discerned in other spheres of state involvement. The rhetoric of 'citizenship', or at least of civic duty, began even to effect a change in the traditionally elitist British Army, and during the Second World War, an Army Bureau of Current Affairs was created by the Adj.-Gen. Sir Ronald Adam. Adam believed that it was the soldier's right – but also his responsibility – in a modern democracy to reason why.[15] These two features – *rights* and *responsibilities* – were integral to the notion of citizenship as it developed in Britain during the war – among soldiers and civilians.[16] However, this emphasis on education owed as much to the changing nature of modern warfare – which demanded increasing technical expertise – as it did to the promotion of citizenship in any highly developed sense. As Maj.-Gen. Sir Ernest Cowell, Chief Surgeon with the Allied Forces in Italy put it in 1944, 'The modern soldier is not a body; he is a highly trained specialist, a man taught to think for himself.'[17]

The idea that VD could be fought effectively through a combination of education and propaganda stemmed from the belief that is was primarily a problem of attitude and motivation. Lt.-Col. Robert Lees, Consulting Venereologist for British Middle East Forces, considered that

> control of V.D. is a matter of discipline and "morale" much more than of medical measures. Self-discipline comes first, with pride in being fit to fight, and fit to serve. Secondly comes unit discipline which depends on the C.O., officers and senior N.C.Os. It is my

impression that the units with the highest reputation as crack fighting men and famous for good discipline have a low rate of V.D. and base units have a high V.D. rate.[18]

There was, it seemed, a need to provide soldiers with wholesome forms of recreation, and to dispel the ignorance which still surrounded venereal diseases. But propaganda had to be of the right kind. According to Lees, that which aimed to frighten the soldier by describing in graphic detail the symptoms of gonorrhoea or syphilis was likely to fail, since modern forms of treatment had robbed VD of much of its horror. He suggested that 'the impairment of military efficiency of the soldier, and his duty to his unit, the army and the country by keeping "fighting fit" should be the basis of the appeal'.[19] In a report to Ernest Cowell in December 1943, Lees pointed out that 'It should be clearly understood by every man that it is a disgraceful act to endanger his health while on active service, by consorting with any loose women. A high code of personal morality must be followed and all must be taught that complete abstinence from sexual intercourse is not detrimental to health or vigour. Association with public prostitutes is "conduct unbecoming an Officer and a Gentleman".'[20] Thus, while the emphasis may have changed considerably since the Great War, the Army continued to regard venereal disease as a moral as well as a medical problem, although there were clearly different views on the matter. In a letter to the *British Medical Journal* in August 1941, Col. P.F. Chapman, a retired colonel of the Indian Medical Service, denounced appeals to chastity as 'worse than useless', advocating in its stead chemical prophylaxis and frank discussion of the problem: 'Men are surprisingly shy about these matters', he claimed.[21] But his comments soon met with an indignant response from a serving officer of the Royal Army Medical Corps (RAMC) who stressed that chastity was still 'strongly encouraged' in the Army; troops received lectures on 'maintaining a high moral standard and on abstention from illicit sexual relations'.[22]

Related issues, such as masturbation, proved equally controversial. The practice had previously been denounced on moral and medical grounds but was now being reconsidered in the light of the enforced separation of soldiers from their wives and sweethearts. While not actually encouraging the practice, some medical men argued that masturbation ought not to be discouraged since it offered troops a means of sexual gratification free from the risks associated with prostitution. The 'Any Questions?' column of the *British*

Medical Journal posed the question 'Would it be true and right to tell a man aged 20 in the forces that masturbation was a lesser evil than fornication?', to which an anonymous expert responded in the affirmative. The ethical decision was, he insisted, a matter for the individual concerned, while, medically speaking, occasional masturbation could be practised without danger to health or virility, with the proviso that 'it should be resorted to only when it becomes essential to obtain relief for a sexual tension which has become unbearable'. 'If masturbation is used in this way and not merely for pleasure', he counselled, 'it will be unlikely to become a preferable substitute for normal intercourse in the future.'[23] But concern over VD in the armed forces was not sufficient to raise the taboo surrounding the practise. Dr J. Luxford Meagher informed the journal that he had read the column 'with feelings of disgust' and warned of the danger of habit formation. 'It is precisely those who are weak of will to which it appeals....', he claimed: 'Surely an act universally condemned throughout the ages cannot suddenly, owing to any "trend of opinion", become permissible. The remedy for all natural urges is strenuous resistance, reinforced by prayer, also sublimation of those urges ... by athletic and intellectual interests'.[24] The same reactionary impulses constrained the discussion of homosexuality in the armed forces. A man whose friend's son had been demoted within the Officer Training Corps, and sentenced to 90 days in military prison for homosexual acts with young boys, bemoaned the lack of medical advice available to such individuals. In the absence of any military authority prepared to discuss the subject he had written to the National Society for the Prevention of Venereal Disease (NSPVD) who had unsuccessfully pursued the matter on his behalf. He praised the Society for 'openly fighting the hush-hush ... and destructive tactics normally applied in cases such as this'.[25]

These discussions took place against the backdrop of more general concerns about venereal disease and sexual behaviour in wartime. The NSPVD (successor to the National Council for the Combating of Venereal Disease), and related 'progressive' or Left-leaning organisations like the Progressive League and the National Social Hygiene League, were engaged throughout the war in a battle against what they perceived as 'obscurantism'; an unholy alliance between Church and State which kept people in the dark regarding sexual matters. Their principal opponent was the Archbishop of Canterbury, the Most Rev. W. Temple, who was appointed to the presidency of the Central Council for Health Education in 1942 in an attempt to assuage religious opinion. The Archbishop had angered the Society and many army MOs by his opposition to Regulation 33B and chemical prophylaxis against venereal disease. At a meeting on VD staged in London in 1943 by the Central Council for Health Education, Temple spoke out against the distribution of prophylactics to troops on the grounds that it would be an inducement to fornication. Army education, he insisted, should stress the sacredness of sex and the possibility of chastity.[26]

For most advocates of prevention, however, the 'moral' or religious approach to VD control was *not* incompatible with the 'medical' or 'secular', although many 'progressives' viewed the moralising of the Church as unworldly and restrictive.[27] Organisations like the Progressive League and the Communist Party of Great Britain went so far as to accuse the government of giving way to religious opinion and of failing to make chemical prophylaxis readily available to civilians.[28] Nor were such suspicions confined to the Left: *Reynolds News*, a low-brow London newspaper, carried a story alleging a 'behind the scenes fight at the Ministry of Health'; one section stressing the need for 'clean living', the other for greater frankness about VD. The former, it lamented, had won.[29] These suspicions appear to be borne out by the fact that the Ministry of Health actively discouraged local authorities – many of which were subscribers to the NSPVD – from disseminating information on chemical prophylaxis.[30]

Yet the debate over VD prevention cannot be characterised simply as one between 'moralists' and 'pragmatists', since the meaning of 'morality' itself had undergone a change. Morality in sexual matters was now construed not so much in religious terms, but in terms of civic responsibility. Posters exhorted soldiers to 'Guard against VD. Keep straight – keep sober. You owe it to yourself, your comrades, your efficiency',[31] while army health educators sought to dispel the apparently common belief that good health was contingent upon sexual activity. Cowell noted in a memorandum on health in December 1943 that 'Continence is a duty to oneself, to one's family and one's comrades. A man can keep fit without a woman'.[32] Or, as the British forces newspaper in North Africa, the *Union Jack*, put it in July 1942, 'As for the moral aspect, well, we leave it to you, but remember the women folk waiting at home – will you be able to face them with a clear conscience on your return?'.[33] The soldier was also made aware of his responsibility to future generations. A Central Council for Health Education leaflet distributed to soldiers in North Africa described VD as 'a great black snowball which, unless we check it, will go rolling down the years of peace and reconstruction.... The problem is one which the community as a whole must face seriously and resolutely because it affects the whole nation and the future of our race'.[34] The possible effects of syphilis and soft chancre on soldiers' wives and children were underscored by such films as 'Sex Hygiene', which were shown to all Allied servicemen in overseas theatres.

It is necessary, however, to make distinctions between attempts at health *education* and health *propaganda*; while the former appealed to reason, the latter sought to elicit a more emotional response. Appeals to chivalry, pride of self and patriotism all fell into the category of 'propaganda'; propaganda which distinguished the character of the British soldier from what Cowell referred to as the 'wanton promiscuity' of the Germans and Italians.[35] But lack of moral discipline was not the only feature which allegedly set British and Allied troops apart from the Axis forces. Japanese soldiers, though widely regarded as paragons of military efficiency, were perceived as brutal and sexually deviant; an image which fed on reports of rape and other atrocities during the Japanese invasion of Nanking and countries occupied after 1941. A report on the psychology of the Japanese soldier by Maj. John Kelnar of the RAMC, for example, made much of the sado-masochistic tendencies of the Japanese, which he saw as arising from the deep conformity and subordination which allegedly pervaded Japanese society. According to Kelnar, the Japanese character was the antithesis of the independent-minded Briton: 'The basic mechanism of the sado-masochistic character of the Japanese is his tendency to give up his independence and individuality, and to acquire the strength which he needs as a compensation for his sense of individual insignificance and powerlessness in the society in which he lives.'[36] This report, intended for the War Office in London, was one of many so called 'national character' studies which informed wartime propaganda in Britain and the United States.[37]

It is questionable how far British servicemen thought of themselves as morally or psychologically superior to their Axis counterparts, but propaganda which instilled a sense of duty to comrades and country was invaluable, according to the venereologist Lt.-Col. Lees. In his opinion, it reached 'the man to whom reason does not appeal – the rather stupid sensual fellow who indulges most of his appetites and who is the type most commonly infected'.[38] Lees was referring mainly to the rank and file, whose education and upbringing had not instilled the virtues of self-discipline and sexual restraint expected of the officer class. A medical report on the Italian campaign declared that other ranks were far more likely to contract

VD than officers because of 'their more limited resources for sublimation through social and intellectual interests'.[39] It was alleged that other ranks were more likely to include persons with an 'inadequate personality', as the psychiatric jargon of the day described them. A study conducted by the RAMC officers Maj. E. Wittowker and Capt. J. Cowan in 1942 found that VD patients were far more likely than other categories to include persons with a history of instability or indiscipline. Contrasting 200 VD patients with a control group of 86 impetigo patients, they found that some 59 per cent of VD patients were classified as 'immature personality types' as against only 19 per cent of impetigo patients. Some 54 per cent of VD patients were classed as discontented with army life, a s against only 29 per cent of impetigo patients. The classification was made on the basis of a questionnaire and simple psychiatric interview. A supposedly typical VD case was 'Corporal A.B.', aged 28, and labelled an 'unaggressive dependent' personality. He was described as 'A self-centred, selfish individual whose role in life is to make money and to have personal comforts. Has never been able to hold his own. Married two-and-a-half years and got on well with his wife who mothered him a good deal'.[40] The study is interesting chiefly for two reasons. First, it draws a picture of the typical VD patient as a selfish mother's boy, who shirks his responsibility to comrades and country in his desperate search for comfort. He is, in many respects, the antithesis of the model British citizen, lacking both independence and self-control. Secondly, virtually every case discussed in the report is drawn from the other ranks, giving the impression that such behaviour was class-based. Thus, despite echoing the rhetoric of citizenship, psychiatry may have served to confirm latent stereotypes of a dependent working class.

Most health educators realised that appeals to sexual abstinence would make little impact on the immature and self-centred. So, in the event of their urges being too strong to control, Maj.-Gen. Ernest Cowell urged soldiers to use a condom or prophylactic packet, both of which were provided from the very beginning of the war.[41] He also warned them to report sick at once if symptoms appear: failure to do so was a crime under military law, and those reporting sick with VD faced the loss of wartime proficiency pay. Those engaged as tradesmen or acting NCOs also lost their rank and position.[42] Measures against VD were, therefore, never entirely free from penal stigma. But the sanctions against contracting these diseases were far less severe than during the First World War, when all pay was stopped during the period of hospitalisation and leave cancelled for up to

Incidence of VD amongst British troops in India (per 1,000 troops)

Type of VD	1939	1940	1941	1942	1943	1944	1945
syphilis	8.5	12.7	12.6	9.5	8.2	9.4	11.7
gonorrhoea	32.4	30.9	33.8	27.1	26.3	31.6	25.6
other VD	10.3	14.5	18.1	33	29.4	31	42.5
Total	51.2	58.1	64.5	70.2	63.9	72	79.8

Incidence of VD amongst British troops in the Middle Eastern Force (per 1,000 troops)

Type of VD	1939	1940	1941	1942	1943	1944	1945
gonorrhoea	30.2	22.4	16	8.5	-	4.3	7.2
syphilis	2.5	4.13	4.3	2.4	-	3	5.4
other VD	6.26	7.6	19.7	14.7	-	8.4	11.8
Total	39	34.2	40	25.6	15.9	15.7	24.4

Incidence of VD amongst British troops in Italy (per 1,000 troops)

Type of VD	1944	1945
gonorrhoea	25.9	50.3
syphilis	3.7	7.1
chancroid	9.7	8.9
lympho-granular	0.1	-
other VD	11.3	4.9
Total	50.6	71.2

Incidence of VD amongst British troops in North West Europe (per 1,000 troops)

Type of VD	1944		1945			
	1st quart.	2nd quart.	1st quart.	2nd quart.	3rd quart.	4th quart.
gonorrhoea	1.2	7.6	9.18	6.1	11.2	10.5
syphilis	0.8	1.4	2.2	1.6	7.1	11.2
soft chancre	-	-	0.2	0.1	0.1	0.3
other VD	0.1	0.7	2.2	3.8	3.8	3.7
Total	2.1	9.8	13.8	9.9	22.3	25.7

Incidence of VD amongst British troops in the United Kingdom (per 1,000 troops)

Type of VD	1940	1941	1942	1943	1944	1945
gonorrhoea	6.4	8.8	11.3	8	5.1	8.9
syphilis	0.9	1.4	2.5	2.9	2.4	3.2
soft chancre	-	0.1	-	-	-	-
other VD	0.1	0.2	0.2	0.3	1.2	1
Total	7.4	10.5	13.9	11.3	8.7	13.1

Source: W. Franklin Mellor (ed.), *Medical History of the Second World War. Casualties and Medical Statistics* (London: HMSO, 1972), 119, 192, 264, 282, 334.

twelve months.[43] This more tolerant attitude reflected the observation, made during the First World War, that punishment tended to produce concealment and was therefore counter-productive.[44]

The combination of discipline and health propaganda met with little success. In the Middle East there was some improvement as admissions from VD fell from almost 40 per 1,000 troops per year in 1941 to 15.7 in 1944, rising somewhat in 1945. In Italy, however, the rise in VD seemed inexorable, climbing from the already high figure of 50.6 per 1,000 in 1944 to just over 71 in 1945. The war years also brought an uneven increase in VD in India from 51.2 per 1000 before the start of the war to almost 80 per 1,000 by its close. VD rates in northern Europe were lower than most other overseas theatres and, until after victory in Europe, did not differ significantly from those in the UK.

In 1941, before the introduction of penicillin to treat gonorrhoea (which comprised around 80 per cent of cases), infection with this disease usually entailed absence from duty averaging around 25 days in some theatres.[45] During 1943, as the use of penicillin replaced treatment with sulphonamide drugs,[46] the average number of days spent absent from duty for each gonorrhoea patient declined to just a few days, the course of treatment lasting only 24 hours. Before the advent of penicillin, soldiers who had contracted syphilis might be absent from duty for between 40 and 50 days – a very substantial period of time.[47] With the introduction of penicillin this average declined to four or five days, but it was found that syphilitics were 50 per cent more likely to contract 'jaundice' or 'infective hepatitis', as it was then known. It was thought that soldiers may have been infected with the latter from an intra-muscular injection of the drug, although this conclusion was purely speculative.[48]

The persistence of VD among the British Army overseas was attributed to a combination of sexual opportunity and lack of alternative recreations; other factors specific to certain theatres also played their part. The 1945 edition of *Field Service Hygiene Notes* for India listed the factors thus:

1. Distance from home and the diminished feeling of shame at having contracted VD.
2. The long duration of the Indian tour. Few men consorted with prostitutes during their first year in India but became habitual users after 3-4 years.
3. The lack of social amenities.

4. Lack of (respectable) European female company.
5. The availability of facilities for cheap sexual activities.
6. Climatic conditions: it was generally agreed that the 'sex glands' of persons in a hot climate were more active than in a temperate or cold climate, increasing the strain on the 'sex-starved soldier.'
7. The effect of war: the ever present prospect of active service, with the chance of death in action, tended to induce the attitude of 'getting as much out of life as possible'.[49]

Though the rank and file were thought specially liable to succumb to such temptations, it was generally acknowledged that the moral discipline of the officer class could also be eroded during a long tour overseas. One MO in Italy reported that 'The newcomer to any formation which has been serving overseas for a considerable length of time observes a subtle peculiarity of psychology which is difficult to define, but which is reflected in the case of officers in a narrowing of intellectual activity and in the type of conversation and humour which finds favour.'[50]

But in which circumstances, precisely, was VD usually contracted. Overseas, it was generally acknowledged that most infections were contracted at brothels and from so-called 'amateur prostitutes operating on the streets of cities such as Cairo or Bombay. In Britain, however, the situation was more complex. A survey of 200 VD patients showed that the majority (76 per cent) allegedly contracted VD from sexual partners 'picked up' at public houses, cinemas, and so forth, by soldiers on leave. Some 22 percent of these were married women whose husbands were away, over 4 per cent were 'service girls', and 1 per cent were men. Only six per cent of patients claimed to have been infected by a prostitute.[51] Well over half those interviewed (some 68.5 per cent) owned up to not using a condom, the majority because they had regarded it as unnecessary. In other words, that their partner had 'looked respectable'.[52]

These figures provide some insight into the behaviour of soldiers but one suspects that some may have concealed the true circumstances of the infection; being unwilling to own up to visiting a prostitute for example. It is therefore useful to consider the unmediated statements of soldiers themselves; what do their memoirs and recollections tell us about the impact of army health education and propaganda on sexual behaviour? Certainly, not all were rampantly or thoughtlessly promiscuous. Private Frank Kelly, for example, was only occasionally tempted by the numerous sexual opportunities open to him in occupied Germany at the end of the war. 'I am a lazy blighter with girls', he claimed, 'but it wasn't possible to keep out of bed with some of them. It's not going to bed with them I mind, but bed and sleep go together with men. Sometimes they would get angry. Rosemary [his sweetheart] was all right most of the time, but now and then would get a romantic mood, and I had to do something about it.'[53] George MacDonald Fraser tells a similar story in his best-selling account of the war in India and Burma, *Quartered Safe Out Here*. He noted that his section, which had been deprived of female company for months in the jungles of Burma, did not run amok when permitted leave in Calcutta: 'They eyed what talent there was in the bars of Chowringhee, danced with abandon at the service clubs, and chatted up the Wrens, Waafs, ATS, and nurses, and that was about it.' Considering why they had been so restrained, MacDonald-Fraser explained that they were a more 'inhibited, pious and timid generation' who felt that illicit sex was immoral. He also noted the effect of medical advice against promiscuity: 'it may have been that the risk of infection was the great restrainer ... clap was reputed to be excruciatingly painful; syphilis, which was rumoured to be incurable, was regarded much as AIDS is today.' He recalled that 'the Army propagandised unceasingly, with lectures, short-arm inspections, and terrifyingly explicit films'; one poster showed a statuesque blonde surrounded by leering Japanese, with the caption 'Is this the face that loved a thousand Nips?'[54]

VD rates testify to the fact many British soldiers were less timid than MacDonald Fraser suggests. However, it does seem likely that fear of venereal infection – of both its medical and social consequences – may have reinforced any natural reserve among soldiers, while prompting the more sexually adventurous to take precautions. Letters from service-men and women to organisations such as the NSPVD, requesting further information on prophylaxis, indicate that venereal infection was a risk not accepted lightly. In the first years of the war, the Society claimed it had received 'many thousands' of such requests and, although the number of letters in its archive suggest this may have been an exaggeration, letters from service people were fairly common. One young man from Renfrewshire, Scotland, wrote 'As I expect to be called up for military service in the near future, I should be grateful if you would inform me of the best prophylactic measures against venereal disease'.[55] Another, from Bethnal Green London, asked for information on the grounds that, 'I am about to join the army and I may possibly find myself in the category of those many men who find palliative relief from the strains of war in occasional promiscuity'.[56]

Such letters suggest that there was widespread acceptance that military service – or, at least, wartime conditions – tended to encourage promiscuity in the normally chaste or monogamous. Indeed, there may have been some truth in the criticisms made of the Society by Church leaders that its 'realism' actually encouraged such beliefs. Letters from serving soldiers confirm that military service, particularly sedentary duties centred around base camps and the like, presented tremendous sexual opportunities. As one military correspondent to the NSPVD explained, writing of his station in India, 'The heat is great here and the temptation enormous'.[57] The need for guidance on prophylaxis was also acknowledged by servicewomen,[58] who generally suffered far lower infection rates than their male colleagues.[59]

However, it should be emphasised that the majority of service people who expressed an interest in chemical prophylaxis to the NSPVD were members of the medical services, who would have been more familiar with the practice than most. Some of these were medical officers who joined the NSPVD in order to obtain its educational materials.[60] But most correspondents were rank and file members of the medical services, eager to improve their knowledge of VD, for both professional and personal reasons. Quite a lot of interest seems to have been aroused by an article on 'scientific prevention' which appeared in the journal *New Statesman and Society* in November 1940. It was this article which induced Pte. O.P. Hollander to inquire about a technical problem of some urgency: 'Have been to the chemist and got myself a mixture containing 33% calomel cream and 2.5% Protargol. Is this correct? How is it to be applied and within how long of infection? What probability of its being *ineffective* [original emphasis] is there; and, above all, while granting me immunity, can it leave me in a condition liable to infect others?'[61]

But the high rates of venereal infection which existed in certain theatres indicate that few British soldiers were as well informed. Throughout the war, the NSPVD continued to receive complaints from soldiers that they had not received any information regarding prophylaxis; not because the Army disagreed with the practice, but simply because medical officers were overwhelmed with other tasks. In 1943 John Finlayson, Organisational Secretary and Lecturer of the National Social Hygiene League, told Herbert Jones of the NSPVD that 'It is certainly untrue to say that Medical Officers lecture to all units, many men tell me that they have not had a lecture at all and they have been in the army three years'. He also claimed that: 'In many units there are no facilities whatever for the men to keep themselves free from Venereal Diseases should they take risks. No condoms are provided even at a price, or douche departments. I am very often able to give the Commanding Officers ... the address of condom manufacturers and they readily avail themselves of the chance to purchase and supply their men at about 3d each.'[62]

An even greater obstacle to VD prevention was posed by the Army's policy of regulated prostitution. In garrison states such as India red-light districts in ports and military stations were frequented regularly by soldiers, even though regimental brothels had been (officially) closed for years.[63] Recalling his arrival in Bombay in 1942, one British soldier recalled that: 'In the evening four of us ... mounted a ghari and instructed the driver ... to show us the sights. A look of comprehension dawned on his unprepossessing countenance and he made straight for what proved to be the brothel quarter (Grant Road).'[64] The same soldier noted that the only real entertainments available to troops stationed at Bareilly were 'undesirable female company and three bottles of indifferent beer a month.'[65] Brothels were equally numerous in Egypt, Greece, Italy and Palestine, although technically illegal in the latter. In Sudan and Eritrea there were no brothels but plenty of so-called 'amateurs', who plied their trade in streets and bazaars.[66] These 'amateurs' were said to be the product of a society which possessed no moral or religious bar to sexual intercourse outside of marriage.[67] In countries such as Italy, the abundance of prostitutes was attributed largely to the poverty and economic dislocation caused by the war. But, whatever the reason, it was generally recognised that prostitution was a complex social and economic problem not capable of immediate solution, and that the only effective means of controlling the situation was to bring prostitution under medical and military control.[68]

British policy in most overseas theatres was initially to contain the problem by establishing regulated brothels where prostitutes were inspected for venereal disease. This procedure was standard in the armies of most nations, including those of Germany and the United States.[69] This was a continuation of practices established during the 19th century, and which had received a new lease of life during the First World War in France and Egypt, until the brothels were closed under pressure of public opinion.[70] Inspection was usually carried out by military MOs but in some areas, such as Eritrea, the Army resurrected the Italian system of inspection by a municipal doctor. The consultant venereologist in Eritrea, Capt. Bell RAMC, paid surprise visits to test the effectiveness of the system and to investigate all instances where military personnel alleged to have been infected.[71]

The inspection of brothels was accompanied by a crack down on unregulated and 'amateur' prostitution. In Egypt, reported Robert Lees, 'The civil and military police are constantly vigilant and active against street walkers and other clandestine prostitutes. During the first quarter of 1941 the Cairo police arrested 732 such women, and on medical examination 175 (23.9%) were found to suffer from venereal disease'.[72]

In Egypt, and in other countries where British troops were stationed, many of these arrests were made on the basis of information supplied by soldiers who had contracted VD. VD patients among the Expeditionary Force sent to France in 1940 were supplied with a form which requested information that would enable military policemen to identify 'diseased prostitutes'. They were required to furnish details of the date of exposure, the first occurrence of symptoms, the location of the woman's house or brothel, and her name, nationality and appearance.[73] The system remained in place wherever the British Army was permitted to operate it.

The contradiction between this system of officially-tolerated prostitution and exhortations to sexual abstinence in army hygiene propaganda became increasingly apparent. Although some MOs favoured the continuation of regulated prostitution, the majority, including most senior officers and venereologists, denounced the practice for undermining their efforts. The existence of medically-inspected brothels created a false sense of security: the Deputy Director of Hygiene (DDH) for the Middle East noted in January 1942 that 'the idea is extremely prevalent that ... the brothels are safe, and it is considered that far larger numbers of men are consequently visiting these places than would otherwise associate with loose women'. He claimed that over 45,000 men were visiting the Cairo brothels every month.[74] Surveys of those admitted to hospital with VD also revealed that very few soldiers had bothered to wear condoms or perform chemical prophylaxis after intercourse.[75] The Consulting Venereologist, Lt.-Col. Lees, reported in 1943 that only 1 soldier in 20 who acquired VD had carried out any form of personal disinfection.[76] Attendance at brothels also raised the spectre of infection with deadly diseases such as typhus, which had broken out amongst the civilian population on several occasions. The DDH reported that 'The state of these brothels, although much has been done to improve them, is still sordid, degrading, and insanitary in the extreme, and in close proximity to forbidden areas, the conditions of which are indescribably filthy'. Further, the effects of brothels on the 'mental hygiene, discipline and morale' of a 'young, raw, civilian army' were such as to corrode military authority.[77]

But these concerns were not shared by all British officers and there were some combatant officers who continued to view promiscuity as inevitable, or even as essential to the maintenance of morale. To such men regulated brothels were the lesser of two evils. The opposing views of medical and (some) combatant officers are clearly discernible in the debate over regulated prostitution in Cairo. At the beginning of 1942, the DDH pressed for the closure of licensed houses on the grounds mentioned above, and because they would provoke a an outcry 'of the first magnitude' in Britain and the Dominions should their existence become known.[78] Medical opinion at this stage was virtually unanimous that brothels in Cairo and Alexandria should be placed out of bounds to British troops, and that alternative recreational facilities should be provided. But the Deputy Adj.-Gen. was firmly opposed to this and doubted whether such moves would reduce the incidence of VD, despite the allegedly beneficial effects of an experimental closure of brothels in the Canal Zone.[79] The case made by the DDH was further weakened in March 1942 when, at a conference on VD, several MOs previously committed to the closure of brothels, including the DDMS, had sided with the Deputy Adjutant.[80] The DDH suspected that some pressure had been exerted upon them, and wrote in 'the strongest possible terms' to the Deputy Adjutant's superior.[81]

By the late summer, however, the tide was beginning to turn in favour of medical opinion. The political storm of which the DDH had warned had erupted in Britain and 'numerous charges had been made in speeches, in the Press and by letter against the Army by dignitaries of the Church, morality societies and others of encouraging the soldier in fornication.'[82] Some combatant officers had also begun to share his concerns. At the beginning of August the DDH received a copy of a letter from the commander of Cairo Area to all zone and unit commanders declaring that the Berka – a military brothel – would shortly be placed out of bounds.[83] Although the commander faced considerable resistance from other officers, he stood firm in his decision to close the brothels. The DDH recorded in December 1942 that

> It is gratifying to record that the Commander ... thinks that the closing of the Berka has removed a grave blot on British prestige in Egypt; that the behaviour of the troops has improved to a very material extent since the closure; that, even if a slight increase in V.D. did occur as a result, it is quite offset by other advantages....[84]

241

These comments are significant because they illustrate the perceived importance of preserving the image of British purity and 'good form'; a trait of character which set the British – and other Allied troops – apart from the allegedly promiscuous Germans and Italians. The statement made by the DDH appears to show that such considerations may even have outweighed anxieties caused by manpower wastage from VD. After all, treatment with penicillin (from late 1942) drastically cut the recovery time of those hospitalised with most forms of these diseases. The need to maintain an air of moral superiority was especially important in those countries under Allied military government and, particularly, in Egypt where anti-British sentiment had increased during 1942.[85] In mainland Italy, during the first few months after the invasions of September 1943, it was impossible to impose any restrictions on access to prostitutes though, by December, MOs were proposing that brothels be placed out of bounds, and that steps be taken to prevent soliciting. Maj.-Gen. Cowell was convinced, on the basis of his North African experience, and the rising incidence of VD among Allied troops in Italy, that propaganda would be ineffective so long as the army tacitly endorsed prostitution. In December he reported that 'The V.D. rate now seriously threatens to limit the effectiveness of Armies and Formations. In some instances the V.D. rate is equal to the malaria rate, larger than the hepatitis rate and is the chief cause of sickness.'[86] In some units of the British Army the VD rate was a high as one in ten of the total strength.[87]

Pleas to control prostitution were received sympathetically by the Allied Military Government in Italy, which quickly issued instructions to control soliciting and to commence the medical examination of prostitutes in brothels. Treatment centres for civilians were also established and women infected with VD were compelled to attend.[88] Yet the measures fell short of those desired by Cowell and his consultant venereologist Lees, who had just been sent to Italy from North Africa. Again, they urged that brothels be placed out of bounds to troops, not only because of the heavy wastage from VD, but because 'An Army, especially one occupying a country, is judged by the conduct of its troops, both on duty and off duty, and we noted with regret very lax discipline evidenced by careless drinking and insulting attitudes to apparently respectable civilian women, who obviously resented any approaches made.' As in Egypt, Lees recommended that closure of brothels be accompanied by an intensification of propaganda, improved welfare and recreational facilities, and the employment of the Women's Auxiliary Service in all bases. He argued that the 'presence of women from the home counties, with their high standards, will improve the conduct of the troops'. In view of the seriousness of the VD situation in Italy, which exceeded that in North Africa, these recommendations were accepted before long by the British Army Council and by US forces, and soon became Allied policy.[89] Similar measures were taken in North-West Europe, though it seemed that many soldiers still managed to attend brothels despite agreement between the Allies that they be placed out of bounds.[90] 'Amateur' prostitution was also common and measures to contain it were frustrated by tensions between military and civilian administrations. Military officers often alleged that the latter were corrupt and inefficient, and that police and other civilian officials took bribes from pimps and prostitutes to prevent their arrest.[91] It was also believed that women infected with VD had evaded diagnosis and treatment with the connivance of civilian doctors, rendering routine examination of prostitutes ineffective. Efforts therefore came to concentrate on the Allied Provost Staff and the arrest of pimps and prostitutes.[92]

Conclusion

The methods used in Allied-occupied countries towards the end of the war show that the control of venereal disease in the British Army was guided by far more than the need to prevent wastage of manpower. Sexually transmitted diseases were a serious military problem in Italy, but less so in the Middle East, India and North West Europe. But in all these theatres the *political* and *disciplinary* implications of venereal disease were grave, for its associations with vice and intemperance blackened the reputation of British and other Allied forces overseas. Such considerations were vitally important in view of the often awkward relationship that existed between Allied forces and civilian administrations, and also in terms of the challenge which VD and rampant promiscuity dealt to images of Britishness, as expressed in wartime propaganda. Although this propaganda seems to have had little impact on the behaviour of British troops, it tells us a great deal about the ways in which national identity and citizenship were represented during the war. It also reveals a decided shift away from a religious discourse surrounding sexually transmitted diseases to one which was predominantly secular. But this is not to say that those on the 'progressive' wing of the anti-VD campaign had fully succeeded in ridding these diseases of their stigma. Although fewer people regarded illicit intercourse as an offence against God, to have risked infection with VD was to have failed in one's duty as a soldier, spouse, parent, and, above all, as a British citizen.

Notes

1   Edward J. Bristow, *Vice and Vigilance: Purity Movements in Britain Since 1700* (Dublin: Gill & Macmillan, 1979); Judith R. Walkowitz, *Prostitution and Victorian Society: Women, Class and the State* (Cambridge: Cambridge University Press, 1980); Richard Davenport-Hines, *Sex, Death and Punishment: Attitudes to Sex and Sexuality in Britain Since the Renaissance* (London: Collins, 1990); Mary Spongberg, 'The sick rose: constructing the body of the prostitute in nineteenth century medical discourse', Ph.D. thesis, University of Sydney, 1993.

2   An important exception is Lesley Hall, *Hidden Anxieties: Male Sexuality, 1900-1950* (Cambridge: Polity, 1991), 32-39.

3   See Olive Anderson, 'The growth of Christian militarism in mid-Victorian Britain', *English Historical Review*, 1971, 86, 46-72; Stephen Koss, 'Wesleyanism and empire', *Historical Journal*, 1975, 18, 105-18; Alan R. Skelley, *The Victorian Army at Home: The Recruitment and Terms and Conditions of the British Regular, 1859-1899* (London: Croom Helm, 1977); Bruce Haley, *The Healthy Body and Victorian Culture* (Cambridge, Mass.: Harvard University Press, 1978); J.A. Mangan, *Athleticism in the Victorian and Edwardian Public School: The Emergence and Consolidation of an Educational Ideology* (Cambridge: Cambridge University Press, 1981); J.A. Mangan & J. Walvin (eds), *Manliness and Morality: Middle-Class Masculinity in Britain and America, 1880-1940* (Manchester University Press, 1987); Frank Mort, *Dangerous Sexualities: Medico-Moral Politics in England Since 1830* (London & New York: Routledge & Kegan Paul, 1983); Norman Vance, *The Sinews of Spirit: The Ideal of Christian Manliness in Victorian Literature and Religious Thought* (Cambridge: Cambridge University Press, 1985); Allen Warren, 'Citizens of the empire: Baden-Powell, scouts and guides and an imperial idea, 1900-40', in J.M. MacKenzie (ed.), *Imperialism and Popular Culture* (Manchester: Manchester University Press, 1986), 233-56.

4   Frank Mort, *Dangerous Sexualities: Medico-Moral Politics in England Since 1830* (London: Routledge & Kegan Paul, 1987), pp.75-6. By the turn of the century, however, there was considerable anxiety over whether these masculine virtues were being undermined by the cultural and physical environment of modern cities, see George L. Mosse, 'Masculinity and the decadence', in R. Porter & M. Teich (eds), *Sexual Knowledge, Sexual Science. The History of Attitudes to Sexuality* (Cambridge: Cambridge University Press, 1994), 251-266.

5 Mark Harrison, 'The British Army and the problem of venereal disease in France and Egypt during the First World War', *Medical History* (1995), 39, 133-58.

6 Edward H. Beardsley, 'Allied against sin: American and British responses to venereal disease in World War I', *Medical History* (1976), 20, 189-202; Suzann Buckley, 'The failure to resolve the problem of venereal disease among the British troops in Britain during World War I', in Brian Bond & Ian Roy (eds), *War and Society: A Yearbook of Military History*, vol.ii (London: Croom Helm, 1977), pp.65-85; Bridget A. Towers, 'Health education policy 1916-1926: venereal disease and the prophylaxis dilemma', *Medical History* (1980), 24, 70-87.

7 In other words, sexuality was still controlled, but through new (and predominantly medical) modalities of power. This is a qualified re-statement of the argument presented in Michel Foucault's *The History of Sexuality: An Introduction*, vol.1 (New York: Vintage Books, 1978). However, as has been suggested elsewhere, Foucault probably went too far in denying that any meaningful liberalisation of sexual behaviour had taken place in the second half of the twentieth century. See Roy Porter & Lesley Hall, *The Facts of life: The Creation of Sexual Knowledge in Britain, 1650-1950* (New Haven and London: Yale University Press, 1995).

8 Angus Calder, *The People's War: Britain 1939-1945* (London: Pimlico, 1992; first edition, Jonathan Cape, 1969), 313.

9 Ministry of Health and Central Council for Health Education leaflet, 'A Great Black Snowball'.

10 See for example James Cantlie, *Physical Efficiency: A Review of the Deleterious Effects of Town Life upon the Population of Britain, with suggestions for their Amendment* (London & New York: G.P. Puttnam & Sons, 1906); Charles Porter, 'Citizenship and health questions in wartime', *Journal of State Medicine*, 25 (1917), 276-82.

11 On citizenship and welfare in Britain see Jose Harris, 'Enterprise and welfare states: a comparative perspective', *Transactions of the Royal Historical Society*, 5th ser. 40 (1991), 175-95; *idem*, 'Society and state in twentieth-century Britain', in F.M.L. Thompson (ed.), *The Cambridge Social History of Britain, 1750-1950*, vol. 3; Geoffrey Finlayson, *Citizen, State and Social Welfare in Britain, 1830-1990* (Oxford: Clarendon Press, 1994).

12 David Armstrong, *The Political Anatomy of the Body: Medical Knowledge in Britain in the Twentieth Century* (Cambridge: Cambridge University Press, 1993), 10-13.

13 Abram de Swaan, *In Care of the State: Health Care, Education and*

Welfare in Europe and the USA in the Modern Era (Cambridge: Polity Press, 1988).

14 On the history of the 'social', see Patrick Joyce, 'The end of social history?', *Social History*, 1995, 20, 70-91.

15 Calder, *op. cit.* (note 8), 251.

16 See T.H. Marshall, *Citizenship* (Cambridge: Cambridge University Press, 1950).

17 Papers of Sir Ernest Cowell, RAMC 466/36, memo on health to combatants, 16 December 1943, CMAC.

18 Lt.-Col. Robert Lees, memo on prevention of VD, 14 April 1942, WO 222/1302, PRO.

19 Lees, Report for January.-March 1941, 6, WO 222/1302, PRO.

20 Lees to Cowell, Recommendations for the prevention of VD amongst Allied Forces in the CMF, December 1943, RAMC 466/36, Cowell papers, CMAC.

21 Col. P.F. Chapman to editor, *British Medical Journal* (hereafter: *BMJ*), 1940, 3 August 1940, 169.

22 Lt.-Col. T.E. Osmond, RAMC, to editor, *BMJ*, 1940, 236.

23 'Any Questions?', *BMJ*, 1944, 1 January, 31.

24 Dr J. Luxford Meagher to editor, *BMJ*, 1940, 2 September, 328.

25 J.H. Brannagh to Secretary NSPVD, 24 January 1940, SA/PVD/6, CMAC.

26 The Most Rev. W. Temple, 'The Church's Approach', *Proceedings of the Central Council for Health Education Conference on Health Education and the Venereal Diseases, 26 February, 1943* (London: CCHE, 1943), 9-10.

27 Discussion point by Dr Maitland Radford, MOH St. Pancras, *ibid.*, 19.

28 'We demand prophylaxis', *PLAN*, 11, 2, 1944, 1. Secretary to J.B.S. Haldane, University of London Dept. of Biometry, to NSPVD, 28 November 1942, re. article on VD by Haldane in the *Daily Worker*, SA/PVD, CMAC.

29 *Reynolds News*, 27 February 1944, 2.

30 H.R. Hartwell, on behalf of Minister of Health, to Town Clerk, Bournemouth, 31 July 1944 and A. Lindsay Clegg, Town Clerk of Bournemouth, to Ministry of Health, 15 August 1944, SA/PVD/11, CMAC.

31 Copy of poster in RAMC 1542, CMAC.

32 Cowell, memo on health to combatants, 16 December 1943, RAMC 466/36, CMAC.

33 'Health hints for soldiers', *Union Jack*, 5 July 1942.

34 Ministry of Health and Central Council for Health Education

leaflet, 'A Great Black Snowball'.

35 Cowell, 'Report on the health of the army in North Africa', 7,
    RAMC 466/38, CMAC.

36 Maj. John Kelnar, 'Report to the War Office on the psychological
    effect of upbringing and education on Japanese morale', RAMC
    1900/18/19, CMAC.

37 See John W. Dower, *War Without Mercy: Race and Power in the
    Pacific War* (New York: Pantheon Books, 1986).

38 Lees, 'Methods of prevention of venereal disease', 14 April 1942,
    WO 222/1302, PRO.

39 Medical report on the Italian campaign, RAMC 1849, CMAC.

40 Maj. E. Wittowker & Capt. J. Cowan (with the assistance of Lt.
    D.C.T. Sullivan), 'Some aspects of the V.D. problem in the British
    Army', GC/135/B.1, MacKeith Papers, CMAC.

41 Monthly report of Deputy Director of Hygiene, France, September
    1939, 2, WO 177/1, PRO.

42 Cowell, 'Health memorandum', 16 December 1943, RAMC
    466/36, CMAC.

43 Harrison, *op. cit.* (note 5), 139.

44 See L.W. Harrison's comment on E.T. Burke, 'Venereal disease: its
    prevention and treatment on active service', *Bulletin of War Medicine*,
    1, September 1940, 41.

45 These figures relate to gonorrhoea. See 'Medical Quarterly Report',
    No.1, V.D. Treatment Centre, Oct. 1941-March 1942, Middle East
    Force, p. 3, WO 222/1334, PRO.

46 Brig. Robert Lees, Report of the Consulting Venereologist, July-Sept.
    1944, 2, WO 222/1300, PRO & 'Report on Penicillin in VD',
    BMJ, 25 March 1944, 428.

47 Wittkower & Cowan, *op. cit.* (note 40), 1 & *BMJ*, 25 March 1944,
    429.

48 Brig. Robert Lees, Report of the Consulting Venereologist, first
    quarter of 1943, 2, WO 222/1300, PRO.

49 *Field Service Notes – India, 1945* (Calcutta: Government of India
    Press, 1945), 418-20.

50 'Medical report on the Italian campaign', 149, RAMC 1849, CMAC.

51 Wittkower & Cowan, *op. cit.* (note 40), 2.

52 *Ibid.*, 9.

53 Frank Kelly, *Private Kelly* (London: Evans Bros., 1954), 47-8.

54 George MacDonald-Fraser, *Quartered Safe Out Here: A Recollection of
    the War in Burma* (London: Harvill 1993), 182.

55 Hector MacKenzie to Secretary NSPVD, 28 November 1940,
    SA/PVD/6, CMAC.

56 A. Deaner, Bethnal Green, London to Secretary, NSPVD, 6 December 1940, SA/PVD/6, CMAC.

57 L.A.C. Dodwell, 87 R & R Party, RAF, India, 18 August 1944, SA/PVD/11, CMAC.

58 Sgt. J.C. Hall, D Company, 1st Batt., Gold Coast Regiment, R.W.A.F.F., Accra, Gold Coast Colony to Secretary NSPVD, 15 January 1940.

59 Editorial, *BMJ*, 1941, 9 August, 208.

60 Maj. Crawford Campbell, RAMC, to Secretary NSPVD, 22 October 1940, SA/PVD/6, CMAC.

61 Pte. O.P. Hollander, 2 Company, NCC, 219 FA, Chatteris, Cambs., 25 November 1940, SA/PVD/6, CMAC.

62 John Finlayson to Herbert Jones, 18 January 1943, SA/PVD/9, CMAC.

63 Government of India, *op. cit.* (note 49), 420. On regulated prostitution in British India see Kenneth Ballhatchet, *Race, Sex and Class under the Raj: Imperial Attitudes and Policies and Their Critics* (London: Weidenfeld & Nicolson, 1980); David Arnold, *Colonising the Body: State Medicine and Epidemic Disease in Nineteenth-Century India* (Berkeley: University of California Press, 1993), 83-7; Mark Harrison, *Public Health in British India: Anglo-Indian Preventive Medicine, 1859-1914* (Cambridge: Cambridge University Press, 1994); Philippa Levine, 'Venereal disease, prostitution, and the politics of empire: the case of British India', *Journal of the History of Sexuality*, 4 (1994), 579-602.

64 *The History of the Fourteenth General Hospital R.A.M.C. 1939-1945* (Birmingham: The Birmingham Printers, c.1946), 19.

65 *Ibid.*, 24.

66 Lees, 'Report of Consulting Venereologist', 28 April 1941, 5, WO 222/1302, PRO.

67 Lees, 'Report on visit to Eritrea', 15 November 1941, 6, WO 222/1302, PRO.

68 Lees, 'Report on methods of prevention of venereal disease', 14 April 1942, 1, WO 222/1302, PRO.

69 See Franz Seidler, *Prostitution, Homosexualität, Selbstverstümmelung. Problem der deutschen Sanitätsführung 1939-1945* (Neckargemünd: Kurt Vowinkel, 1977); Christa Paul, *Zwangs Prostitution: Staatlich Errichte Bordelle im Nationalsozialismus* (Berlin: Hertrich, 1994); T.H. Sternberg *et al*, 'Venereal Diseases', in L.D. Heaton, *Medical Department U.S. Army. Preventive Medicine in World War II, Volume V: Communicable Disease* (Washington DC: Office of the Surgeon General Department of the Army, 1960), 260-8.

70 Harrison, *op. cit.* (note 5), 149-156.

71 Lees, 'Report on visit to Eritrea', 6, WO 222/1302, PRO.

72 Lees, 'Report of Consulting Venereologist', 28 April 1941, 5, WO 222/1302, PRO.

73 Medical administrative instructions, No.12, 23 November 1939, WO 177/1, PRO.

74 DDH MEF, 'Notice for DMS', 19 January 1942, RAMC 2048/1, CMAC.

75 Report of Brig. Robert Lees, Consulting Venereologist CMF, 13 April 1945, WO 222/1300, PRO.

76 Consulting Venereologist – Summary of Policy and Action, Sept. 1939-31 August 1943, WO 222/12, PRO.

77 DDH MEF, 'Notice for DMS', 19 January 1942, RAMC 2048/1, CMAC.

78 DDH MEF, War Diary, 19 January 1942, RAMC 2048/1, CMAC.

79 DDH MEF, War Diary, 13 February and 16 February 1942, RAMC 2048/1, CMAC.

80 DDH MEF, War Diary, 19 March 1942, RAMC 2048/1, CMAC.

81 DDH MEF, War Diary, 20 March 1942, RAMC 2048/1, CMAC.

82 Consulting Venereologist, 'Summary of policy and action, September 1939-31 August 1943, 9.

83 DDH MEF, War Diary, 4 August 1942, RAMC 2048/1, CMAC.

84 DDH MEF, War Diary, 1 December 1942, RAMC 2048/1, CMAC.

85 P.J. Vatikiotis, *The History of Modern Egypt: From Muhammed Ali to Mubarak* (London: Weidenfeld & Nicolson, 1991), 352-354.

86 Cowell, War Diary, 10 December 1942 and recommendations on VD, 6 December 1942, RAMC 466/36, CMAC.

87 Cowell, Medical circular, 11 December 1942, RAMC 466/36, CMAC.

88 Cowell, Medical arrangements Allied Force Command, RAMC 466/36, CMAC.

89 Lees, Recommendations for the prevention of VD amongst Allied Forces in the CMF, 1, 3.

90 Report from Medical Division, Rear HQ, 21 Army Group to Director of Hygiene, 27 September 1944, RAMC 761/3/52, CMAC.

91 C.R.S. Harris, *Allied Administration of Italy 1943-1945* (London: HMSO, 1957), 427-8.

92 Lees, Report on venereal disease for the first quarter of 1945', 13 April 1915, WO 222/1300, PRO.

10

The Repression of War Trauma
in American Psychiatry after WWII

Hans Pols

Let me start with a literary anecdote from another war and another country, to illustrate some of the relations between war, trauma, and language that are the topic of this paper.[1] The notorious writer Louis-Ferdinand Céline, in his *Journey to the End of the Night*, narrates his experiences as a French soldier during World War I.[2] The main character of the novel, Bardamu (bearing some, but mostly a deceptive resemblance to Céline) was duped into army service by following a parade through Paris soon after the outbreak of the Great War, happy to be honoured by streets full of 'civilians and their wives cheering us as we passed, and throwing flowers at us.' Soon after he arrived at the front-line, his enthusiasm waned; Bardamu was desperately finding ways to get wounded or be taken prisoner (by either side, for whatever reason) in order to get out. The continuous threat to be killed by German soldiers or the French military police – 'The only uncertain thing in the whole business was what uniform one's executioner would wear' – had completely undermined his morale. So had the continuous abuse by his superiors, the poor quality of the food and lack of sleep and shelter, and his utter disbelief in the higher purposes of the war had completely undermined his morale. He envied the deadly sick horses of his troupe, all with large open wounds on their back, raw and running with pus, because they were not required to approve of the war or to believe in it. He loathed to be cannon fodder in service of some patriotic ideals he did not subscribe to and, in addition, to be ebullient about his condition at the same time. The horses suffered but were free. 'Enthusiasm', however, 'was our dirty prerogative, reserved for us!'[3]

After being wounded, Bardamu returned to Paris, where he encountered the complicity of the medical establishment to the war effort. The first few weeks, he appeared to be in good spirits. However, it did not take very long before increasingly intense memories of the war started to plague him. Obsessive thoughts kept intruding whatever he did to find distraction. One evening, he suddenly stood up in a chic restaurant, screaming 'Run, all of you! Get out! They are going to fire!' He was taken to a hospital 'especially organized to receive cases like myself, whose patriotic ideals had either been slightly shaken or else entirely warped.' The doctors were kind when questioning the patients, while 'in the most charming way in the world dangled our death warrants in front of our noses.' There were only three ways out of the hospital: the front line, the firing squad, or the insane asylum. Fortunately, Bardamu was placed in the last. The asylum (the Bicêtre) was led by an energetic psychiatrist who derived many new insights from his treatment of shell shock. According to him, the war acted 'as wonderful revealer of the human spirit.... We have broken into the innermost precincts of Man's mind, painfully, it is true, but as far as science is concerned, providentially, decisively.' This psychiatrist had developed a new psychotherapeutic regime in order to restore patriotism 'by electrical treatment of the body and strenuous doses of the ethics of patriotism for the soul, by absolute injections of revitalizing morale.' Bardamu nodded with feigned enthusiasm and in a whim of melancholy realized that he was 'twenty years old and already had nothing but the past.'[4]

In order to please their physicians and visitors – and in order to delay their return to the front lines – the patients of the Bicêtre started to imitate one particular patient who had received honourable attention for praising the Fatherland during an epileptic attack. In a short time, the clinic became known as a center of intense patriotic fervor. Several well-known high-society visitors came to visit the clinic, while the patients attempted to out-do each other in singing the praises of the glorious war. Bardamu, eager to please an attractive actress, provided 'so many and such vivid and highly colored details, that from the moment he started she never took her eyes off me.' In order to keep the attention of visitors, the patients fabricated increasingly fantastic heroic war stories; they all vied with each other to see who could invent even more sublime records of the war in which they themselves played fabulously heroic parts. These stories were only a thinly veiled cover-up for their real emotions: 'We were living a tremendous saga in the skin of fantastic characters, deep down we ourselves derisively trembled in every corner of our heart and soul.' The actress asked Bardamu permission to have his experiences memorialized as poetry by a sickly poet-friend of hers. On one of those many official events celebrating the honour of the

252

Fatherland and the sacrifices young men had made rushing to her defense, the poem was recited. Bardamu was appalled that this sickly poet had 'monstrously enlarged upon my fantasies with the help of fine-sounding rhymes and tremendous adjectives which rolled out solemnly in the vast, admiring silence.'[5] At this moment, the contrast between the virile heroism of France's soldiers and the dejected state of the mentally wounded patients sent to the insane asylum came out particularly strongly. After the applause, another soldier claimed credit for the heroic deeds related in the poem, depriving Bardamu from his moment in the limelight. Bardamu did not even achieve praise for the heroic travails he concocted. Not long after, he is discharged as incurable.

Two issues make Bardamu's involvement with the war a particularly horrendous experience: first, the loathed the continuous threat to his life, and, second, he detested the denial of this threat in the official rhetoric of the glorious nature of the war. Bardamu could not be very enthusiastic about being butchered for whatever reason; not even for the honour of the Fatherland. The grand narratives around honour, the Fatherland, heroic sacrifice, and reinvigorated masculinity sounded hollow to him; they had no relation whatsoever to his own war experiences. Nevertheless, this rhetoric was continuously forced upon him by the military, by physicians, and by civilians; providing the only way to gain attention (from physicians and actresses), recognition, and some form of respect and self-esteem. The only way, ironically, to prolong his stay in the hospital and avoid being sent back to the front was to partake in that self-same vocabulary he despised so much. 'The whole thing', he said, 'was pure theater; you had to play your part.'[6] One feature of these grand narratives of masculine vigor, the Fatherland, and honourable sacrifice is the impossibility of expressing trauma, pain, and suffering in their vocabulary. In a sense, these grand narratives denied the trauma and suffering related to the war effort and thereby to justified the war and its cost in human lives, injury, and pain. Bardamu's discontent and opposition to the war; his continuous sense of dread could not find expression in this language – he could only fall silent and become sick.

In this paper, I concentrate on reactions to the trauma of World War II by American soldiers, psychiatrists, and American society at large. I argue that while American psychiatrists who were stationed close to the front-lines explained the incidence of war neuroses by referring to the extraordinary stresses of battle, their colleagues after the war came to emphasize the pernicious predisposing influence of family life on the vulnerability of America's men to mental breakdown. The first explanation referred to the circumstances in which soldiers succumbed to war neuroses as causative factors in its onset. The second explanation considers these circumstances only incidental to the nature of mental breakdown and instead insists on analyzing the early childhood experiences of soldiers debilitated by war neuroses. It is my central contention that a public recognition of the existence and the nature of trauma – completely absent in Bardamu's case – is necessary before individual traumatized soldiers can start to make sense of their war experiences and work them through.[7] In this sense, trauma is never an individual experience but dependent on public means for its articulation. This paper is an attempt of recent historical scholarship to relate individual and collective memory, in particular of war, by focusing on trauma as a dislocation in time.[8] In this paper, I will describe how psychiatric theory during the war provided the means to express and work through traumatic battle experiences while after the war this opportunity was lost as a consequence of changes in the ideas of psychiatrists.

The grand narratives embraced by the home front and the army to make sense of the war made it impossible for soldiers and veterans to express their experiences of suffering, loss, and trauma. In this way, there was a collision between events experienced by soldiers and the language available to describe them. During the war there was a brief period of time when psychiatrists related war trauma to actual battle experiences to be re-lived and abreacted in psychotherapy. However, when the war was over psychoanalytically oriented psychiatrists displaced the trauma of individual soldiers onto a drama of a threat to the nation's masculinity – stirringly embodied in the traumatized, crippled, or mutilated veteran. American psychiatrists displaced this threat in particular on the American mother. Psychoanalysis rose in unprecedented popularity in American culture after World War II by initially acknowledging and treating war trauma and subsequently repressing and displacing this concern with a grand narrative about the threat mothers posed to the masculinity of the nation. This was the particular American displacement of the traumas of warfare that impeded the national 'working-through' of trauma as we witnessed in Bardamu's case.

War

The war constituted a breakthrough both for psychiatrists' professional self-confidence as well as for the esteem in which the public held the profession. The war accelerated trends that transformed psychiatry from a profession based in mental hospitals, relying on somatic treatment methods to an eclectic approach characterized by psychotherapy, out-patient treatment, and prevention.[9] During the war, new psychotherapeutic approaches were developed to meet the unprecedented challenge posed by mentally crippled soldiers. These approaches displayed an interesting range of influences from ego-psychology, psychoanalysis, and the older social-adjustment psychiatry. The purportedly high success rates of these new approaches enormously increased the confidence of psychiatrists in their ability to treat the neuroses of daily life as well as those of the battlefield. Second, during and after the war, these psychotherapeutic methods became available to an unprecedented group of practitioners. During the war, they were disseminated on a wide scale to army physicians. At the close of the war, general practitioners displayed a strong interest in psychotherapy as well – not only because of the great number of veterans with vague complaints they found in their offices. Third, the war experience influenced a generation of post-war research into psychosomatic disorders and the influence of stress on well-being. In the fourth place, the war experience fueled an unprecedented high public regard for psychiatry and a corresponding popularization of psychiatric knowledge. After the war, American psychiatrists addressed the problems of war and peace in the conviction that conflict on an international scale was closely related to war and peace in the home, where frustration bred aggression and faulty parenting styles fostered authoritarian personalities.[10] During the post-war years, the public consumed psychological advice to an unprecedented degree, as presented in child-rearing manuals (Dr. Spock), radio programs, lectures, child-study groups, and pamphlets.[11] The immediate post-war years were the heyday of American psychiatry. As a specialty, the discipline grew enormously. As a cultural force, psychiatric and psychological insights became part of popular culture to an extent as they had never been before.

When the American army became involved in the hostilities of World War II, psychiatrists had no role in it except for screening out mentally unfit conscripts.[12] Despite the extensive experience in treating 'shell-shock' during the first World War, the psychiatric profession was not prepared to treat this condition a mere twenty years later. In an act of professional amnesia, practitioners completely ignored the lessons of World War I in treating shell-shock. The endless and violent battles of World War II resulted in great numbers of injuries and disabilities. Many of these were so-called neuropsychiatric casualties; during the 1943 Tunisian campaign, they made up 20 to 34 percent of all patients. Sufferers from war neuroses were as baffling as they were irritating to army physicians, since they seemed not to be particularly amenable to treatment. The manifestation of war neuroses varied in different persons, depending on their background and personal history. In addition, their expression at a particular moment also depended on the etiology, the current distance to the battle zone, the nature of the military occupation, and war conditions in general. War neuroses did not constitute a stable or clearly identifiable clinical entity with characteristic and invariable symptoms. Moreover, symptoms tended to mimic those of organic disease. After some battles, a significant number of the soldiers broke down and suffered from severe and debilitating anxiety attacks, tremors, stuttering, and amnesia. Most of them were no longer able to perform the most basic functions.[13]

In his well-known article about shell-shock during World War I, Martin Stone analyzed the relation between morale, war conditions, and shell-shock.[14] War neuroses during the first World War characteristically took the form of conversion hysteria. Understood as hysteria, the shell-shocked soldier's body could be interpreted as protesting the war-time demand to function as a de-skilled cog in a mechanized killing machine. By displaying a hysterical paralysis, the soldier ultimately defied the extensive training, 'drill', as the inculcation of blind obedience. Conditions during World War II were different in many aspects. The purpose and justification of war were not particularly compelling to many soldiers. In addition, this global war proved to be much less predictable – fatal attacks could be undertaken at any time and by any means by an invisible enemy. With the absence of a strong ideology and with the invisibility of the enemy, group cohesion and the bonds with one's friends proved to be the most important factor for maintaining morale. For many soldiers, their 'buddies' were the only reason they could persevere.[15] Breakdown incidence appeared to depend mostly on the conditions of combat, internal group cohesion, and the quality of military leadership.[16]

Only in 1943 did the army enlist psychiatrists in an attempt to stem the flood of psychiatric casualties. Roy G. Grinker and John P. Spiegel, two psychoanalysts who had been interested in psychosomatic medicine before the war, wrote a widely used manual for medical officers on the treatment of war neuroses.[17] Since an adequate theory detailing aetiology and treatment was still lacking, the manual consisted of a compilation of illustrative case histories, such as the one of a twenty-year-old platoon sergeant, who could protect himself from severe shell-fire only by flinging two dead bodies over himself:

He lay there for a long time, trembling and terror-stricken, until finally an artillery shell exploded very close by and blew the two bodies off the patient, ripping off his shirt at the same time. The two dead soldiers had actually saved his life. His mind at that point went blank. He wandered about, and was picked up by some men from his company.... When he entered one of the forward hospitals he had acute anxiety, persistent tremor, great restlessness, loss of appetite, and insomnia with battle dreams.[18]

This soldier was confronted in the most horrendous manner with death, the senselessness of the war he had not chosen to fight in, probably a strong sense of survival guilt, and the definite dissolution of his community – it was the death of his fellow soldiers and the mutilation of their corpses that saved his life. These case histories morbidly illustrate the nature of trauma as resisting and even destroying language; the inability of the suffering soldier to express what had happened to him. These traumatized soldiers disrupted psychiatric knowledge at the time as well: In order to elucidate the nature of war neurosis, Grinker and Spiegel had to stay very close to the actual experience of the mentally wounded soldier. Abstractions and generalizations seemed utterly out of place – trauma could actually best be narrated by relating the actual circumstances under which it came into being. Re-experiencing these actual conditions in a therapeutic setting provided a key to treatment. Grinker and Spiegel relied on basic psychoanalytic notions by arguing that, under severe battle conditions, even the strongest and most mature soldiers could regress to the condition of a helpless child: 'The ego reacts with the anxiety and helplessness of a child and abandons the scene altogether (stupor), or refuses to listen to it (deafness), or to talk about it (mutism), or to know anything about it (amnesia).'[19]

In a sense, war trauma constituted a dislocation of time: it provided a temporal delay in experience that carried the individual soldier beyond the shock of the first moment; a shock of such magnitude that it could not be fully experienced at the time. In this sense, the individual removed himself from a situation that was too ominous to handle. In another sense, because the event was not assimilated or experienced fully at the time it occurred, it could only be experienced belatedly, in repetition, in the form of repeated nightmares, memory flashes, and intrusive hallucinations. The event repeatedly possessed the individual suffering from war trauma – not as memory of events that occurred in the past but as currently present. This paradoxical nature of trauma is summarized as follows by Cathy Caruth: 'Trauma is repeated suffering of the event, but it is also continual leaving of its site.'[20] In a sense, the story re-experienced in a night-mare or a flash-back is a story that literally *has no place*, neither in the past, in which it was not fully experienced, nor in the present, where its images and re-enactment is not fully understood. These characteristics: a delay in experience, the repetitive nature and the directness of its memory, and the lack of response to traditional treatment methods constitute the resistance of trauma to full theoretical understanding. In a way, only the particular stories, and their repetition, provided an insight into the nature of the particular trauma an individual soldier was suffering from.

War neuroses disrupted psychiatrists' theoretical understanding of mental breakdown; which they had thus far related to predispositions, be they genetic, neurological, or Oedipal in nature. During the war, this perspective was temporarily replaced by an environmental outlook. For Grinker and Spiegel, soldiers succumbing to war neuroses were neither cowards nor weaklings. Quite the contrary, their reaction appeared to be entirely normal given the horrendous front-line conditions. They stated that 'it would seem to be a more rational question to aks why the soldier does *not* succumb to anxiety, rather than why he does.'[21] Army psychiatrists were not treating abnormal conditions in pathological individuals, but pathological conditions in perfectly healthy and previously well-adjusted individuals who had been exposed to an extraordinarily horrid situation. This perspective, emphasizing environmental stress as a cause of mental breakdown, justified psychiatric intervention at the front lines. Psychiatrists were not treating cowards but heroes.

The treatment offered by Grinker and Spiegel incorporated both the demands of morale and the feeling of comradery by offering a repetition of the initial experience in a protective environment.[22] In his theater of operations, the psychiatrist induced a narcosis with a Pentothal injection. This stimulated a regression to an almost pre-natal situation in which a libidinal transference to a protective, reliable – but firm – father-figure could be established easily. After reaching a state of twilight sleep, the patient was symbolically returned to the battle-field which had maimed his mind so severely. While the psychiatrist fulfilled the regressed soldier's need for protection and dependence, the soldier's ego was nurtured and encouraged to re-experience his anxiety – or, one could argue, the soldier could fully experience his trauma for the first time. This cathartic experience was not debilitating; instead through his libidinally over-determined identification with the psychiatrist the soldier 'absorb[ed] further strength'.[23] Using these maternal metaphors, psychiatrists portrayed themselves as strong, spiritual fathers who could nurture mentally wounded soldiers back to health and vigor, enabling the soldier's ego to take control over the situation. Already before the war, psychiatrists had cast doubt on the ability of raising children without their supervision; mothers could only avoid mentally maiming their children by closely following the advice and professionals and, preferably, have their growing children closely monitored by them. This sibling rivalry between 'natural mothers' and 'spiritual fathers', psychiatrists at times unwittingly portrayed themselves as masculine mothers or properly mothering fathers, in a blending of gender roles.

Losing one's closest friends or buddies proved to be a particularly traumatizing event during World War II. In order not to exacerbate the consequences of mental breakdown, army psychiatrists repeatedly emphasized the importance of keeping the mentally wounded soldier close to his unit by providing treatment close to the front lines. Removing a traumatized soldier often strengthened his feelings of isolation and solidified his symptoms; keeping him close to his buddies kept at least a semblance of a community of support present. Most soldiers felt already dissociated from the home front, where nobody seemed to have an inkling of what was going on during battle. Removing them from their buddies, their only source of communal and emotional support would be traumatizing in itself. Restoring their mental health also healed the ties with the prime reference group of fellow soldiers – however, it did not take away the continuous sense of danger.

In the reports of army psychiatrists, success rates of treatment exceeded anything ever achieved in civilian life. Grinker and Spiegel portrayed the power of psychiatry in almost Messianic terms: 'The stuporous become alert, the mute can talk, the deaf can hear, the paralyzed can move, and the terror-stricken psychotics become well-organized individuals.'[24] Curing mentally wounded soldiers resulted in the restoration of military authority over the efficient and fighting solider. The psychiatrist's authority over their patients structured the psychotherapeutic process in a most efficient way, blending the military authority of their army position with the ideal of a nurturing father derived from their professional ideals. The psychiatrist as nurturing father restored both the fighting unit of the army and the libidinal bonds between buddies. The traumatizing experience of the soldier was validated, recognized, and shared by individuals who knew about its nature. The isolation of the mentally suffering soldier was overcome. What army psychiatrists did not realize was their persistently ambiguous position: their stated interest was in healing mentally wounded soldiers but, in doing so, they dangled death warrants in front of their patients' noses. A healed soldier would return to his fighting unit, risking death and mutilation once more. Military psychiatrists often emphasized the importance of their military position in effecting therapeutic cures. Psychiatrists and physicians could not question the higher purposes of the war; instead, they reinforced these purposes with all the professional means they had at their disposal. The fact that their military position placed them in a rather ambivalent position with regard to their patients was not explicitly discussed by army psychiatrists during the war. Their new environmental theories and their successful therapeutic intervention made them ease the pressing manpower shortages in the American army.

Front-line psychiatrists emphasized time and again that they were treating *normal* soldiers suffering from *extraordinary* stresses. Their activities within the military enabled them to extend the domain of psychiatric intervention implicitly as the treatment of essentially normal individuals suffering a temporary lapse in war neurosis. Referring to the extraordinary stresses of war removed the stigma from psychiatric war casualties and justified psychiatric intervention on the battle field. The therapeutic techniques developed by Grinker and Spiegel and information about the basic techniques of psychotherapy was provided to all army physicians by William Menninger in a technical bulletin.[25] Because of these approaches, the presence of psychiatrists in the army was legitimized. In addition, the presence of war neuroses acknowledged as a temporary disruption in the fighting ability of soldiers.

Peace

Soldiers coming home during or after the war faced a wall of misunderstanding. Civilians praised and honoured the veteran but at the same time feared his inability to fit in and his potential to disrupt society.[26] Veterans discovered that civilians had been fighting an entirely different war which was far more innocent, honourable, and much less violent and dramatic than the scenes they had witnessed. Many civilians thought of the war as some extended boy-scout summer adventure camp, with lots of out-door activity and excitement. During the war, the media had been tightly controlled, letters from soldiers to home were censured; even the pictures published in magazines were sanitized and brushed up. For example, in the rare occasion that they did display soldiers' dead bodies, all these bodies were relatively intact. Home-bound citizens never saw gruesome pictures of bodies ripped apart – a sight very common in war (as the platoon sergeant of the previous section could testify).[27] The war-time government public relation offices provided a fictive account of the war in which no mistakes were made, soldiers fought heroically, good and evil were clearly demarcated, and no bodies were ripped apart. The coverage of the war was characterized by a 'flight from complexity, irony, skepticism, and criticism' and an all-encompassing embrace of what Paul Fussell calls 'high-mindedness', demanding that 'analysis, criticism, evaluation, and satire yield to celebration, charm, and niceness' while accentuating the positive.[28] The war-time cinema delineated 'little but a fairy-tale world of un-complex heroism and romantic love, sustained by toupees, fake bossoms, and happy endings.'[29] The home front appeared complacent, unimaginative and innocent to the true conditions at the battle-field, either out of ignorance or denial.

The home front, high military officers, and politicians (who did not witness the conditions at the front lines) thought and spoke about the war using grand narratives of patriotic duty, masculinity, sacrifice, and service. At this point, I would like to quote a definition of grand narrative or narrative fetishism as given by Eric Santner in his work on the Holocaust:

> By narrative fetishism I mean the construction and deployment of narrative consciously or unconsciously designed to expunge the traces of the trauma or loss that called that narrative into being in the first place.... [It] is a strategy of undoing, in fantasy, the need for mourning by simulating a condition of intactness, typically by situating the site and origin of loss elsewhere. Narrative fetishism releases one from the burden of having to reconstitute one's self-identity under 'post-traumatic' conditions; in narrative fetishism, the 'post' is indefinitely postponed.[30]

Grand narratives provide harmonizing interpretations, redeeming the meaning of the war while repressing or marginalizing trauma and recuperating loss in history. One could think here of the grand narratives of Progress of Western civilization, resulting in greater welfare for more and a reduction of suffering for all, sidestepping colonialism and the Holocaust. Or the dead rhetoric of Churchill in the following speech: 'May the fathers long tell the children about this tale! May your glory ever shine! May your laurels never fade! May the memory of this glorious pilgrimage of war never die!'[31] This rhetoric seemed to be ever-present when soldiers returned home from the war. Waiting for them were parades, medals, flags, and drum-bands. The home-front had suffered its own trauma, most notably in the absence of their soldier-boys, but this trauma had now been alleviated. No wonder that veterans felt that their experiences had become inexpressible: the language that was at their disposal did not have the words for it. Veterans surely appreciated the triumph parades, laurels, medals, and honours, but, somehow, they appeared discongruent with the suffering they had been through.[32]

The immediate post-war era witnessed strong attempts to re-masculinize American society. Women were driven from their jobs while an ideology of the domestic blessings of the suburban home designed a new social role of mother and care-giver to them. Men's magazines printed an enormous amount of stories in which veterans took charge of a feminized, corrupt, and alienated home-front by showing everybody – but particularly women – their proper place in dependence and in the home. In these tales of redemption, veterans reestablished their place in society by embodying true masculine values.[33] Psychiatry immediately jumped on the band-wagon of the reconstruction of American society along the lines of an imagined bucolic past by presenting themselves as those who could provide the guidelines for raising a well-adjusted, strong, and virile post-war generation. Because of these new concerns, psychiatry did not form an exception to the wall of mis-recognition and repression of trauma that faced veterans. American psychiatrists who had stayed at home did not have much sympathy for the psychotherapeutic methods and the emphasis on environmental factors of their front-line colleagues. After the war, their concern with the predispositions for mental breakdown became dominant again. Psychotherapeutic approaches to repeat and abreact war trauma were replaced by a general concern of a threat to the masculinity of the nation. According to post-war psychiatrists, American mothers ('smothers') had raised a generation of weaklings that would inevitably break down in battle. Since the 'American Mom' attacked the masculinity in the men of tomorrow, preventive action should be directed to them. In this crusade for the restoration of masculinity, American psychiatrists joined social trends that crystallized during the Cold War.

Psychiatric problems did not stop once those suffering from war neuroses were removed from the battlefield or when the war was over. In 1943 the National Committee for Mental Hygiene organized a

Division of Rehabilitation under the directorship of Thomas A.C. Rennie, the director of a rehabilitation clinic at the Payne Whitney Clinic in New York.[34] The initial plan was to establish rehabilitation clinics all over the country to help returning veterans find their place in society again. Most veterans went to their general practitioner first; as a consequence general practitioners came to desire basic knowledge of psychotherapeutic principles. In 1948, a model training course in the basic principles of psychotherapy was organized at the University of Minnesota.[35] From about 1944 on, a great number of advice manuals were published for the 'family and friends' of the veterans.[36] With all this attention to the returning veteran, emphasis shifted from war neuroses and psychiatric problems to the general problems of adjustment that every veteran had to face. In this way, the unique trauma individual soldiers had undergone because of their battle experiences was replaced with the far more mundane and widespread problem of getting used to home conditions after an absence of several years.

When the war was over, psychiatrists offered a range of explanations for the high incidence of nervous breakdown during the war (it was believed that the American fighting forces had the highest breakdown rate of all participants in the war, despite rigid screening efforts). It was said, for example, that all soldiers had, to some extent, regressed to a child-like state as a consequence of army conditions. After all, the army made most of the daily decisions for its soldiers and thereby put a premium on dependence and obedience.[37] In this depiction, the soldier was demoted from virile fighter to a dependent and potentially maladjusted child. When all returning ex-soldiers were in a state of artificial regression, it could be expected that they would lack a fighting spirit in daily life. At the time, battle neurosis were trivialized as just one of the many problems everybody had to face on a daily basis. Combat conditions provided only an intense variation of the battles that had to be fought everyday at home. By equating the battles of war and the battles of everyday life, it became possible to state that psychoneurosis is 'in exaggerated form a type of illness whose seeds are latent in all of us.'[38] It also meant that the war had only exposed those whose maturity had lacked from the beginning – and, in this sense, war was robbed of its horrendous characteristics and given a relatively benign function.

After the war, the mental condition of soldiers before they were drafted came to be seen as the most important factor in causing breakdowns. For this reason, the 'everyday problems of normal people' as the precipitating cause of breakdowns in war and peace became a central concern for psychiatrists. Against the background of these new concerns were the unsolved and perplexing questions as to why so many Americans had to be rejected for service on psychological grounds, and why so many broke down during the war. In other words, the problem addressed by psychiatrists after the war was the seeming lack of virile and tough masculinity in American men, and, therefore, in the nation as a whole. And, not surprisingly, the feminized home-front was blamed. Psychiatry jumped on the anti-feminist post-war bandwagon that sought to shut women out of their war-time jobs and transform them into gentle and sensitive suburban home-keepers and mothers.[39] Instead of helping a few traumatized soldiers, psychiatrists set themselves the task of aiding the reconstruction of the post-war family: a far more daunting task, keeping its significance as the Cold War increased in strength.

This displacement of interest in the home-front rather than the battle-field can be witnessed in the extensive advice literature published during and after the war that would advise parents, wives, and sweethearts how to help their returning soldier-boys adjust to peace. The psychiatrist George K. Pratt gave in his *From Soldier to Civilian* the following case history to illustrate the typical hazards facing veterans. His was one of the many manuals written about the veteran problem and addressed to the 'veteran's family and friends'. Arthur Stone's face had been disfigured by a particularly vicious mortar fragment. He had received 'the most highly skilled medical attention any human being could hope for.' After he was shipped back to the U.S., he lost most of his over-sensitiveness and morbid preoccupation with his face after talking things over with a psychiatrist. He was excited and happy that he could return home and had already made dozens of plans of what he would do when he got back. His hopes, however, would soon be dashed:

> As Arthur stepped from the train Mother, Dad, and young brother Eddie waved a greeting and rushed towards him. His face broke out into what he meant for a grin of pleasure but actually it was a twisted, grotesque grimace from several muscles that would not properly behave. ... Mr. and Mrs. Stone's shock was not concealed, and Arthur's heightened sensitivity caused him to read revulsion into it. But the Stones quickly recovered. With nervous, high-pitched chatter to cover their agitation they took Arthur home.

> To the returned soldier the next few weeks were almost worse than the battle field. ... It annoyed him beyond words to have Mother tiptoe about the house, shushing everyone who talked loudly, to have

her fuss over him and to see the tears of silent pity course down her cheeks as she begged him to "rest" on the couch in the living room. He felt like screaming when he overheard snatches of muted telephone conversations behind closed doors with repeated references to "poor Arthur." He strove manfully to stifle his exasperation when his mother insisted on his reciting over and over again the intimate details of his wounding; how it happened; when it happened; did it hurt much; did he lose quantities of blood; ... how did it feel to be under enemy fire; etc., etc., until her well-meaning interrogations into these personal matters hurt worse that the surgeon's probing for embedded mortar fragments. Even Dad with all his good intentions was scarcely less irritating. He had been in World War I, and each time Arthur recounted some incident of the battlefield his father found it necessary to match it with an incident of his own, always contriving to make his experience a little more exciting.

Arthur's parents, Pratt explained, insisted on treating him like a little child who did not know yet what was best for him. His mother insisted that he would stay home and rest, rather than to go out and meet friends or find a job. This "treatment" sure proved to be effective:

> Gradually, his desire for independence weakened. Gradually, he began to take over into himself their concept of him being an invalid, and gradually he slipped back imperceptibly into his former status of 'little Arthur' until his new-found inner urgings for a normal place in the world were stifled and abandoned.[40]

At home, Arthur finally found his Waterloo. His normal and healthy urges for independence and maturity were successfully stifled by his family. This image of the defeated veteran constituted the horrors of family life to psychiatrists. To counteract the barrage fire of the home-front, most manual and articles about 'the veteran' and 'GI Joe' repeatedly emphasized that he should be given his freedom, that he needed some time to adjust but that such is nothing unusual, and that, by all means, his family should encourage him to be independent. The veteran needed to be fostered back to independence and maturity: the real man at war needed a little help in becoming a real man at home. To achieve this, everyone should learn the language of behavior, learn how to understand the *meaning* of the veteran's behavior rather than be put off by his rough talk and inept reactions.[41]

Many veterans had experienced the traumatic nature of battle, such as the horrors of facing death on a daily basis. Yet according to rehabilitation psychiatrists, it was not these conditions which led to readjustment problems after returning home. I have already mentioned the generally regressed state of the average soldier. In addition, the strong bonds between buddies, previously seen as the most important component of morale, were now seen as a liability, interfering with the conditions of family life. Rehabilitation psychiatrists viewed leading veterans out of their state of regression and the restoration of masculinity I defined as responsibility and independence – as their central task. Veterans had to be weaned from the bonds with their buddies and to be taught the emotional satisfactions of family life.

The danger mothers, wives, and sweet-hearts posed to returning veterans were generalized in the years following the war by combining them with already existing mother-blaming literature from before the war.[42] If mothers and wives could interfere with the readjustment of veterans, it could be envisaged that they had sown the seeds for maladjustment in the war before hostilities even broke out. In 1946, the Philadelphia psychiatrist Edward A. Strecker published *Their Mothers' Sons*, an indictment of the American "Mom" for raising so many sons who broke down without any exposure to battle or dangerous circumstances – the undeserving psychiatric casualties of war. Invariably, he found that behind each broken-down soldier stood an over-protective Mom who had not untied the emotional apron string which bound her children to her. By her overprotective attitude and her own emotional needs, the American 'Mom' had produced a generation of undeserving psychiatric casualties, rejectees for army service, and draft-dodgers. Everything such a Mom did was unconsciously designed 'exclusively to absorb her children emotionally and to bind them to her securely.'[43] The good mother, on the contrary, produced a proper balance of give-and-take in her children. As a consequence, they were able to attain social maturity and independence later in life. Problematizing the position of the mother became a very popular theme in American psychiatry after the second World War (although mother-blaming was certainly not new to the discipline). It fitted particularly well with the period of social reconstruction, during which women were forced to relinquish their position in the working world and urged to take up a domestic role. Psychiatrists had proven to be very successful in restoring virile masculinity in soldiers who mentally maimed by the war – could they not help preserve the masculinity of growing boys against the emotional onslaughts of their mothers?

Grinker and Spiegel translated their war experiences into a general psychosomatic approach investigating the interaction of health and environmental stress.[44] The psychiatric war experience provided a strong stimulus for research into psychosomatic medicine; war neuroses provided a compelling illustration of the influence of mental factors in health and disease. They proclaimed that the war had been a crucial experiment, a wonderful revealer of the human spirit, providing the right experimental conditions to expose those whose maturity had been lacking from the beginning. After the war, medical researchers adopted psychological research designs in order to develop generalized theories about the impact of stress on human beings. These research designs were characterized by the statistical investigations of groups, rather than of individuals. Within the army, and later within the VA hospitals, veterans were already grouped, which eased statistical research into stress. As a consequence, new forms of medical, psychiatric, and psychological knowledge were created that went beyond information gained from case histories. This generalized knowledge claimed to provide insight into the functioning of human beings in daily life; as well as under conditions of extreme stress. The statistical designs aided in the construction of an abstract individual; a statistical aggregate, suffering from rather abstract and general forms of 'stress'. In this way, the individual experiences of veterans were, in a way, over-generalized; their uniqueness and traumatic nature was erased. In this transformation, they became an illustration of the mundane stresses of daily life. Battle trauma and the experiences of American soldiers were trivialized as they were made into examples of the general effect of environmental stress on overall well-being. Research in psychosomatic medicine re-inscribed the veterans' experiences in battle in the physiology of the body.

After the conclusion of a victorious war, grand narratives about justice, democracy, liberty, and national purpose were virtually hegemonic. They made it necessary for the individual veteran to displace or actively forget his trauma. He was celebrated as a fighter for the good cause; his trauma had no place in this world. With respect to the memories that haunted him, psychology and psychiatry provided a compelling modernist discourse by erasing the traumatic pain of the individual as individual, in contrast with the larger historical process in which he participated and to which he traced his trauma. This erasure of trauma or its repression was first accomplished in discourse – that pain is the responsibility of the individual, and placed right there, detached from any historical, political or social process. Second, the redemptive practice of psychotherapy attempted to repair and remove the psychological damage by functionally erasing it.

As I mentioned, after World War II Strecker and others retroactively explained the trauma of individual soldiers as a result of the debilitating effect of American mothers. In this way, the actual trauma and pain of the soldier suffering from war neurosis was undone and remade as a replay, an almost meaningless repetition of an earlier, more fundamental trauma. This trauma figured an omnipotent and devouring mother attacking young boys who were unable to leave her sphere of influence. This strategy of replacing the working-through of actual mental wounds caused by past experiences by a mythological scheme of an eternal conflict closely resembles Freud's abandonment of the seduction hypothesis by putting the Oedipus complex in its place.[45] In the concern with the damaging influence of mothers, the historical contingencies of war are replaced by essential processes taking place on the intersection of the social and the biological: procreation, child-raising, and the family. At the end of the war, history was erased to make room for the eternal and universal structure of the family. The psychiatric discourse on the democratic family fitted particularly well with a more general Cold War ideology: The Americans did not win a particular war, but the war of democracy and liberty against totalitarianism, racism, and cruelty. Psychiatrists did not treat soldiers who were mentally maimed by particular battles, but concerned themselves with threats inherent in motherhood. Central in this displacement by psychiatrists was their desire to translate their war-time successes into peacetime gains. By uncovering a fundamental problem at the root of the American family, they assured themselves of the broadest imaginable field of application for their therapeutic interventions.

In this sense psychoanalysis in America was transformed not in the exploration or recognition of trauma but more in its displacement. Psychiatrists removed trauma from the battlefield and placed it in the haven in the heartless world – the family. With the American notion of the self-made man, any notion of motherhood becomes inherently problematic; mothers can either be reformed into a masculine model as engineers of manhood (as John Watson attempted); or depicted as dangers, sources of the subversion of the self-made man from the outset: over-protective, rejecting, or emotionally interfering (as the post-war psychoanalysts did).[46] In the psychiatric attempt at masculine rehabilitation, the pain done to men during the war is displaced – it was not inflicted by other men; nor by the social process gone mad called war. Rather than acknowledging the actual cruelty committed; it was replaced; and patients were encouraged to re-experience an imaginary Oedipal drama, where the psychiatrist became the patient's ally in combating the mother and in gaining independence. This phenomenon could, in a somewhat bold interpretation, partly be explained by the guilt of the psychiatric profession in maintaining the war machine that maimed their patients. Of course, the psychiatrist in uniform was really a co-conspirator in the trauma of the soldier; as part of the army command structure he was part of the war machine that sent soldiers to the battlefield. In redirecting their attention from the cruel nature of war to the cruel nature of mothers, the army and the army-psychiatrist were both exonerated. In addition, the psychiatrist continued an even more fundamental battle – more in the field of where the social and the biological coincide – with the family, rather than on the battlefield of history.

In this grand narrative, psychological and social categories are collapsed. The history of psychoanalysis is replete with similar examples in which society and the person were seen and analyzed as analogues. The crippled soldier became equivalent to the crippled nation; almost forced to its feet by its progenitor: the mother. In the post-war psychoanalytic view of trauma, history is denied; or, what is left of the recognition of social and political history is recognized when it is played out in the personal history of individual patients. It is the singularity of the event, the war; the senselessness and the irrevocable nature of the trauma; the loss to the soldier, that is denied. Instead, he is made a part in the progressive science of psychiatry and psychology, that triumph over superstition and cruelty in their progress in bringing the real nature of trauma to light. The number of psychoneurotic casualties was a trauma for America and for psychiatrists; it led to a widespread concern with the masculinity of the nation.

The diverse conceptualizations of war neuroses – the outcome of unbearable stress, or of overprotective mothers – had radically different implications for the organization of therapy, mental health care, and psychological advice literature. Definitions provided by psychiatrists were always contested: either by colleagues, by veterans, or by mothers who refused to follow their directives. Psychiatrists, their patients, and the friends and families of the latter collectively tried to make sense out of the horrors of war and, at the same time, define the outlines of a new society.

Conclusion

In this paper I have investigated the reaction of American society in general and the psychiatric profession in particular to the trauma of

World War II. I argued that the traumas of individual soldiers were repressed, displaced, and re-inscribed in a seemingly more fundamental battle between mothers and sons. I explored the initial open and positive reaction of the profession to traumatic experiences and the reasons for the abandonment of these insights later on. In this exploration, the interaction of social views of normality, the crisis of American masculinity, and views of individual mental health all converge and interact. It is this interaction between social views and perspectives on individual adjustment that determined this particular reaction towards trauma in American society.

As a consequence, there was no place for the experience of trauma of American ex-soldiers (in many respects, this had to wait for the Vietnam war). This convinced many veterans that the real war would never get into the books. To quote Paul Fussell again, describing the experience of veterans:

> [They had] the conviction that optimistic publicity and euphemism had rendered their experience so falsely that it would never be readily communicable. They knew that in its representation to the laity what was happening to them was systematically sanitized and Normal Rockwellized, not to mention Disneyfied... . The troops' disillusion and their ironic response, in song and satire and sullen contempt, came from knowing that the home front then (and very likely historiography later) cold be aware of none of these things. ... As experience, thus, the suffering was wasted.... America has not yet understood what the Second World War was like and has thus been unable to use such understanding to re-interpret and re-define the national reality and to arrive at something like public maturity.[47]

The comment about Disneyfying the war proved to be a fore-sight. Recently, the Walt Disney Corporation wanted to buy up one of the most important Civil War battle-fields in Virginia in order to establish an amusement park for a nice day out with the whole family. War and entertainment still appear to be closely related in today's movies. Boys receive tanks and guns as birth-day presents. This all implies that war is still seen as a rather boyish experience, a natural continuation of the games played by children. The repression of a recognition of the violence of war seems to be central in American society – the psychiatric profession only plays its part in a grander narrative more bent on denial than on working-through.

Notes

1 Previous versions of this chapter have been presented at the Richardson History of Psychiatry Research Seminar at New York Hospital-Cornell Medical Center and at a Seminar of the Centre for the History of Science, Technology, and Medicine – Wellcome Unit for the History for the History of Medicine at the University of Manchester. I thank participants at both seminars for their comments which forced me to clarify my arguments.

2 For more on Céline see: Jay Winter, "Voyage to the end of a mind: Céline, psychiatry, and war," in: Mark Micale and Paul Lerner, eds., *Traumatic Pasts: History, Psychiatry and Ttrauma in the Modern Age, 1860-1930* (New York: Cambridge University Press, forthcoming, 1998). Céline is, of course, an inherently problematic character because of his later espousal of violence, racism, and fascism.

3 Louis-Ferdinand Céline, *Journey to the End of the Night*, translated by John H. P. Marks (New York: New Directions, 1960), 6, 23, 33 (translation modified to fit closer to the French original).

4 *Ibid.*, 55, 57, 58, 90, 91, 92.

5 *Ibid.*, 95, 96, 97.

6 *Ibid.*, 87. See also the observations on the theatrical attitude as a way of denying the horrors of war in chapter 6, 'The Theater of War', in: Paul Fussell, *The Great War and Modern Memory* (New York: Oxford Univ. Press, 1975).

7 For similar comments on the necessary condition of the public and social acknowledgment of trauma in order for individuals to be able to work through their individual trauma see Judith Lewis Herman, *Trauma and Recovery: The Aftermath of Violence, from Domestic Abuse to Political Terror* (New York: Basic Books, 1992), chapter 1: A forgotten history. See also: Dominick LaCapra, 'History and Psychoanalysis', *Critical Inquiry* (1987), 13, 222-251; *Representing the Holocaust: History, Theory, Trauma* (Ithaca: Cornell Univ. Press, 1994); Cathy Caruth, ed., *Trauma: Explorations in Memory* (Baltimore: Johns Hopkins Univ. Press, 1995).

8 For the connection between individual and collective memory see: Michael S. Roth, 'Remembering forgetting: *Maladies de la Mémoire* in nineteenth-century France', *Representations* (1989), 26, 49-68; 'The Time of Nostalgia: Medicine, History, and Normality in Nineteenth-Century France', *Time and Society* (1992), 1, 271-286; Ian Hacking, 'Memoro-Politics, Trauma, and the Soul," *History of the Human Sciences* (1994), 7, 29-52; *Rewriting the Soul: Multiple Personality and the Sciences of Memory* (Princeton: Princeton Univ.

Press, 1995). For the relation of personal and collective memory in mourning over the Great War see Jay Winter's excellent study *Sites of Memory, Sites of Mourning: The Great War in European Cultural History* (Cambridge: Cambridge University Press, 1995); see also: John R. Gillis (ed.), *Commemorations: The politics of National Identity* (Princeton: Princeton Univ. Press, 1994). For another, intriguing approach see: Klaus Theweleit, *Male fantasies, Vol. 1: Women, Floods, Bodies, History* (Minneapolis, MN: Univ. of Minnesota Press, 1987). The recent interest in trauma is partly based on a re-reading of Sigmund Freud, *Beyond the Pleasure Principle*, translated by James Strachey (New York: WW Norton, 1989, or. 1920).

9   Gerald Grob states that 'World War II marked a watershed in the history of mental health policy and the evolution of American psychiatry.' In Gerald Grob, *From Asylum to Community: Mental Health Policy in Modern America* (Princeton: Princeton Univ. Press, 1991). According to Nathan Hale, 'The war accelerated vital shifts in American psychiatry from a hospital specialty relying primarily on somatic treatment to an eclectic psychodynamic model in which psychotherapy and preventive treatment in a community setting played an important role.' Nathan G. Hale Jr., *Freud and the Americans, 1917-1985: The Rise and Crisis of Psychoanalysis in the United States* (New York: Oxford Univ Press, 1995), 187.

10 For a very confident statement about the influence psychiatry could have on preventing a third World War see G. Brock Chisholm, 'The Reestablishment of Peacetime Society [the William Alanson White Memorial Lectures]', *Psychiatry* (1946) 9, 3-20. I allude to the following very influential studies: John Dollard, Neal E. Miller, Leonard W. Doob, O. H. Mowrer, and Robert R. Sears, *Frustration and Aggression* (New Haven, Ct: Yale Univ. Press for the [Yale] Institute of Human Relations, 1939); Theodore W. Adorno, *The Authoritarian Personality* (New York: Harper, 1950). For an overview of the problem of aggression within the American family see Fred Matthews, 'The Utopia of Human Relations: The Conflict-Free Family in American Social Thought, 1930-1960', *Journal for the History of the Social and Behavioral Sciences* (1983), 24, 343-362. For an interesting analysis of the application of psychiatry to international politics see Ellen Herman, *The Romance of American Psychology: Political Culture in the Age of Experts* (Berkeley: Univ. of California Press, 1995), chapter 2: 'War on the Enemy Mind'.

11 See, for example: Nancy Pottishman Weiss, 'Mother, the Invention of Necessity: Dr. Benjamin Spock's *Care for Infant and Child*, in N. Ray Hiner and Joseph M. Hawes (eds), *Growing Up in America: Children*

in Historical Perspective (Urbana: Univ. of Illinois Press, 1985).

12   See Herman, *op. cit.* (note 10), chapter 4, 'Nervous in the Service'. She mentions that a total of 1,846,000 recruits were rejected from the armed forces for neuropsychiatric (NP) reasons, a full 12 per cent of all recruits and a full 38% of all rejections. An additional 550,000 were rejected for the same reason after their initial exam. See *ibid.* 88. The psychoanalytic psychiatrist Harry Stack Sullivan occupied an important position in organizing these screening activities.

13   Roy R. Grinker and John P. Spiegel, *War Neuroses* (Philadelphia: Blakiston, 1945). Dedicated to Frank Fremont-Smith, medical director of the Josiah Macy Jr. Foundation, which continued to fund psychosomatic research extensively after the war. This book was first published as a confidential reader for army physicians as: Roy R. Grinker and John P. Spiegel, *War Neurosis in North Africa: The Tunisian Campaign, January-May 1943* (Washington D.C.: Prepared and distributed for the Air Surgeon Army Air Forces, by the Josiah Macy Foundation, 1943).

14   Martin Stone, "Shell shock and the psychologists," in: William Bynum, Roy Porter, and Michael Shepherd (eds), *The Anatomy of Madness: Essays in the History of Psychiatry*, Vol. 2: *Institutions and Society* (London: Tavistock, 1988).

15   To quote Paul Fussell: 'The war seemed so devoid of ideological content that little could be said about its positive purposes that made political or intellectual sense, especially after the Soviet Union joined the great crusade against what until then had been stigmatized as totalitarianism. ... That is, if you embraced the right attitude, you could persuade yourself that in the absence of any pressing ideological sanction, the war was about your military unit and your loyalty to it.' Fussell, *Wartime: Understanding and Behaviour in the Second World War* (New York: Oxford University Press, 1989), 136-140

16   For example, Herbert X. Spiegel. 'Preventive Psychiatry with Combat Troops', *American Journal of Psychiatry* (1944), 100, 310-315, elaborated on morale as dependent on group cohesion.

17   Grinker and Spiegel, *op. cit.* (note 13, 1945).

18   *Ibid.*, 23.

19   *Ibid.*, 93.

20   Cathy Caruth (ed.), *Trauma: Explorations in Memory* (Baltimore: Johns Hopkins Univ. Press, 1995), 10. These paragraphs rely heavily on the introductions to the other chapters in the book she provides.

21   Grinker and Spiegel, *op. cit.* (note 13, 1945), 115.

22   See the chapter on treatment, Grinker and Spiegel, *op. cit.* (note 13, 1945), 75-114; for the treatment programs developed during the war see Herman, 'Nervous in the Service', *op. cit.* (note 10).

23   Grinker and Spiegel, *op. cit.* (note 13, 1945), 87

24   *Ibid.*, 82.

25   William Menninger, 'Neuropsychiatry for the General Medical Officer', War Department Technical Bulletin, War Department, Washington, D.C., 21 Sept. 1944. TB MED 94.

26   David A. Gerber, 'Heroes and Misfits: The Troubled Social Reintegration of Disabled Veterans' in *The Best Years of Our Lives*," *American Quarterly* (1994) 46, 545-74.

27   Fussell, *op. cit.* (note 15), esp. Chapter 18: 'The real war will never get in the books.'

28   *Ibid.*, 170.

29   *Ibid.*, 189.

30   Eric L. Santner, 'History beyond the Pleasure Principle: Some Thoughts on the Representation of Trauma', in Saul Friedlander (ed.), *Probing the Limits of Representation: Nazism and the "Final Solution"* (Cambridge: Harvard Univ. Press, 1992), 144. See also the reflections of Dominick LaCapra in 'The Return of the Historically Repressed', in: *Representing the Holocaust: History, Theory, Trauma* (Ithaca, NY: Cornell University Press, 1994), 169-223.

31   Quoted in Fussell, *op. cit.* (note 15), 267.

32   The experience of returning Vietnam soldiers was much worse; rather then praise, they were blamed for atrocities committed in an unjust war. See, for example, Lt. Col. Dave Grossman. *On Killing: The Psychological Cost of Learning to Kill in War and Society* (Boston, MA: Back Bay, 1995).

33   Timothy Shuker-Haines. 'Home is the hunter: Representations of returning World War II veterans and the reconstruction of masculinity, 1944-1951', Univ. of Michigan unpublished Ph.D., 1994. Shuker-Haines analyzes the men's magazines *Bluebook* and *Argosi*, movies, and soap-operas. For veterans movies see also: Sonya Michel, 'Danger on the Home Front: Motherhood, Sexuality, and Disabled Veterans in American Postwar Films," in Miriam Cooke and Angela Woollacott (eds), *Gendering War Talk* (Princeton: Princeton Univ. Press, 1994), 260-279.

34   See Thomas A.C. Rennie, 'National Planning for Psychiatric Rehabilitation', *American Journal of Orthopsychiatry* (1944), 14, 386-395; 'A Plan for the Organization of Psychiatric Rehabilitation Clinics', *Mental Hygiene* (1944), 38; 'Psychiatric Rehabilitation Therapy', *American Journal of Psychiatry* (1945), 101, 476-485;

Thomas A.C. Rennie, and Luther E. Woodward, 'Rehabilitation of the Psychiatric Casualty', *Mental Hygiene* (1945), 29, 32-45.

35 See *Medicine and the Neuroses; Report of the Hershey Conference on Psychiatric Rehabilitation* (New York: National Committee for Mental Hygiene, 1945); Thomas A. C. Rennie, 'Psychotherapy for the General Practitioner: A Program for Training', *American Journal of Psychiatry* (1947), 103, 653-660; Helen Leland Witmer (ed.), *Teaching Psychotherapeutic Medicine, an Experimental Course for General Physicians, given by Walter Bauer and others* (New York: Commonwealth Fund, 1947).

36 For a few typical examples see 'Psychiatric toll of warfare', *Fortune Magazine* (Dec, 1943): 141-149; Herbert I. Kupper, *Back to Llife: The Emotional Adjustment of our Veterans* (New York: L.B. Fischer, 1945); Alexander G. Dumas and Grace Keen, *A Psychiatric Primer for the Veteran's Family and Friends* (Minneapolis: Univ. of Minnesota Press, 1945); Carl R. Rogers and John L. Wallen, *Counselling with Returned Servicemen* (New York: McGraw-Hill, 1946). Sociological studies include: Waller, Willard. *The Veteran comes Back* (New York: Dryden Press, 1944); Robert J. Havinghurst, *et al.*, *The American Veteran back Home: A Study of Veteran Readjustment* (New York: Longmans Green, 1951). Psychological studies include: Walter C. Alvarez, *Minds that came Back* (Philadelphia: Lippincott, 1961); Therese Benedek, *Insight and Personality Adjustment: A Study of the Psychological Effects of War* (New York: Ronald Press, 1946). For an account of the socio-political function of these advice manuals see: Susan M. Hartmann, 'Prescriptions for Penelope: Literature on Women's obligations to returning World War II Veterans', *Women's Studies* (1978), 5, 223-229.

37 Ethel Ginsburg, 'Veteran into Civilian: The Process of Readjustment', 35th Annual Meeting of the National Committee for Mental Hygiene, Nov. 8-9, 1944 [NCMH Archives, Box 11; file 2]; later published as: Ethel L. Ginsburg, 'Veteran into civilian: The process of readjustment', *Mental Hygiene* (1945) 29, 7-19.

38 Kupper, *op. cit.* (note 36), 27.

39 See also Sonya Michel, 'Danger on the Home Front: Motherhood, Sexuality, and Disabled Veterans in American Postwar Films," in Cooke and Woollacott (eds), *op. cit.* (note 33), 260-279; 'American Women and the Discourse of the Democratic Family in World War II', in Margaret Randolph Higonnet *et al* (eds), *Behind the Lines: Gender and the Two World Wars* (New Haven: Yale Univ. Press, 1987).

40 George K. Pratt, *Soldier to Civilian: Problems of Readjustment* (New York: McGraw-Hill, 1944), 7-9.

41 *Ibid.*, 9-10.

42 See, for example: Barbara Ehrenreich and Deirdre English, 'Motherhood as Pathology', in *For Her Own Good: 150 Years of the Experts' Advice to Women* (Garden City, NY: Anchor Books, 1978), 211-265; Elaine Showalter, *The Female Malady: Women, Madness, and English Culture, 1830-1980* (New York: Pantheon, 1985); John Neill, 'Whatever became of the Shizophrenogenic mother?', *American Journal of Psychotherapy* (1990), 44, 499-504.

43 Edward A. Strecker, *Their Mothers' Sons: The Psychiatrist Examines an American Problem* (Philadelphia: Lippincott, 1946), 36.

44 Roy R. Grinker and John P. Spiegel, *Man Under Stress* (Philadelphia: Blakiston, 1945).

45 See Dominick LaCapra, 'History and Psychoanalysis', *Critical Inquiry* (1987) 13, 222-251.

46 John B. Watson, *Psychological Care of Infant and Child* (New York: WW Norton, 1928); Diane E. Eyer, *Mother-Infant Bonding: A Scientific Fiction* (New Haven: Yale Univ. Press, 1992).

47 Fussell, *op. cit.* (note 15), 268.

INDEX

Printed in the United States
By Bookmasters